Essentials of Occupational Medicine

Essentials of Occupational Medicine

Edited by Kirk Anderson

AMERICAN
MEDICAL PUBLISHERS
www.americanmedicalpublishers.com

American Medical Publishers,
41 Flatbush Avenue,
1st Floor, New York,
NY 11217, USA

Visit us on the World Wide Web at:
www.americanmedicalpublishers.com

ISBN: 978-1-63927-447-5

Cataloging-in-Publication Data

Essentials of occupational medicine / edited by Kirk Anderson.
p. cm.
Includes bibliographical references and index.
ISBN 978-1-63927-447-5
1. Medicine, Industrial. 2. Medicine. 3. Occupational diseases. I. Anderson, Kirk.
RC963 .H36 2022
616.980 3--dc23

Table of Contents

Preface

Occupational medicine is a field of medicine which deals with the maintenance of health in the workplace. It focuses on the prevention of injuries and diseases in the workplace, along with their treatment. Maintenance and increase in the productivity, and social adjustment in the workplace are the main objectives of occupational medicine. The chronic ailments caused due to work or occupational activity are called occupational diseases. Some occupational lung diseases include occupational asthma, chronic obstructive pulmonary disease, bronchiolitis obliterans and lung cancer. Contact dermatitis and urticaria are two of the most common types of occupational skin diseases. Preventive methods for such diseases include personal protection of the workers, irritant replacement or removal, etc. This book unravels the recent studies in the field of occupational medicine. It is compiled in such a manner, that it will provide an in-depth knowledge about the management of occupational diseases at workplace. For all those who are interested in this field, this book can prove to be an essential guide.

This book is a comprehensive compilation of works of different researchers from varied parts of the world. It includes valuable experiences of the researchers with the sole objective of providing the readers (learners) with a proper knowledge of the concerned field. This book will be beneficial in evoking inspiration and enhancing the knowledge of the interested readers.

In the end, I would like to extend my heartiest thanks to the authors who worked with great determination on their chapters. I also appreciate the publisher's support in the course of the book. I would also like to deeply acknowledge my family who stood by me as a source of inspiration during the project.

Editor

1

Work related injury among Saudi Star Agro Industry workers in Gambella region, Ethiopia

Daniel Haile Chercos* and Demeke Berhanu

Abstract

Background: Work injury is an important cause of morbidity and mortality, much of these work injuries burden can be found in industry required heavy manual work such as, agriculture and fishers. Hence; agriculture is consistently cited as one of the most hazardous industry in the world. The objective of this study isto assess the magnitude and associated factors of work related injury among Saudi Star Agro Industry workers in Gambella region, South West Ethiopia.

Methods: An institutional based cross-sectional study design was conducted on Saudi Star Agro Industry located in Gambella region, from February - June 2014 on 449 randomly selected workers who arestratifiedby working department. Anobservation checklist, factory clinical records and a structured interview questioner were used as a data collection tools.

Result: The prevalence of work related injury was 36.7%. Marital status [AOR;1.69, 95%; CI;(1.1–2.7)], service year [AOR;1.9,95%; CI;(1.17–3.1)], working more than 48 h per week [AOR;9.87, 95%; CI;(5.95–16.28)],safety training [AOR;3.38, 95%;CI;1.14–9.98)], regular health checkup [AOR; 12.29, 95%; CI (9–51.35)] and usage of personal protective equipment [AOR; 2.36, 95%; CI; (1.06–5.25)] were significant factors for the occurrence of work related injury.

Conclusion: The prevalence of work related injury was high. Working hours, safety training and regular health checkup increases the risk of work related injury.

Keywords: Agro industry, Ethiopia, Work related injury, Working environment

Background

Occupational injuries are one of the major public health problems in the world. This is because the total consequence of occupational injury extend well beyond direct physical injury and include a wide array of social and economic burdens [1]. Work related injury is an important cause of morbidity and mortality and much of work related injury burden can be found in industries requiring heavy manual work such as agriculture and fishers [2–4]. However most of work related injuries can be prevented by using appropriate occupational safety and health service as well as by using ongoing injury surveillance [5].

* Correspondence: daniel.haile7@gmail.com
Department of Environmental and Occupational Health and Safety, Institute of Public Health, University of Gondar, P.O. Box 196, Gondar, Ethiopia

Globally, the burden of occupational injury accounts for 100 million cases per year, in which 360,000 are fatal accidents [6]. Reports showed that Developing countries have the highest injury fatality rate, in which 14 death reported per 100,000 workers due to occupational injuries [6, 7]. This results a loss of about 4% of world Gross National Product and the impact is estimated to be 10–20 times more in developing countries [8].

Agriculture is consistently cited as one of the most hazardous industry in the world. As a result, workers and their families are vulnerable to high injury and fatality rates. In 2008, the farmer and rancher occupation had a fatality rate that was 10 times more when compared with all occupations (40.3 Vs 3.7 per 100,000 workers) [5]. This indicates that workers in the agriculture sector suffer from higher rates of accidents and fatal injuries than workers found in other industries [3, 4].

Agriculture, have many organizational and environmental characteristics that can affect the health of workers including; exposure to hazardous conditions in the natural environment, use of dangerous machinery and chemicals and unconventional work arrangement [2–4]. On top of that, the introduction of new technologies and new chemical substances have led to new occupational injuries [8].

Agriculture constitutes the major economical share for most of the Sub-Saharan countries including Ethiopia. In Ethiopia, the number of industries in the agricultural sector is increasing recently and it became the backbone of the Ethiopian economy. In Ethiopia; agricultural industries accounts for almost all of the foreign exchange earnings of the country and it provides almost 50% of the country's Growth Domestic Product (GDP), with nearly 80% of the labor force working in this sector [9]. Although there are few studies done so far that had made considerable progress in protecting workers from occupational injury and illness, there are still vast unreported occupational accidents and diseases exists [10]. In addition, a geographical variation is a big factor for fatality rate of occupational injuries. Therefore it is important to study and take preventive measure related to work related injuries in agricultural sector of a country [11].

Methods

Aim of this study

The aim of this study is to assess the prevalence and associated factors of work related injury among Saudi Star Agro Industry workers, Gambella region, South West Ethiopia.

Study design

An institutional based cross-sectional study design was conducted from February - June 2014.

Study area and period

This study was conducted at Saudi Stare Agro Industry. The study area is located in South West of Ethiopia, Gambella region, Aboboworeda, which is about 813 km from the capital city, Addis Ababa. The company was established in 2007 and has a current production capacity of 12800 t of rice per year. Currently, the industry has employed 1064 workers from which 244 (22.94%) are female workers.

Source population

All workers who were working in agricultural production segment of Saudi Stare Agro Industry.

Inclusion and exclusion criteria

Inclusion criteria

All agricultural workers involved in agricultural production segment.

Exclusion criteria

Administrative staffs, workers on annual leave and workers who were absence during data collection period.

Sample size

The sample size was calculated using a single population proportion formula. It was calculated taking 95% confidence interval, marginal error 4%, and work related injury as 78.3% [12]; yielding a sample size of 449 workers.

Three departments were selected as the major area of the enterprise where workers directly involve in agricultural division. Assuming that work related injury varies with the nature of the work; the calculated sample size was distributed across the selected three departments using stratified sampling technique. Study subjects were allocated proportionally from each department and finally subjects were drawn by simple random sampling technique from each department sampling frame.

Operational definitions

- Work related injury; any physical injury condition sustained on worker in connection with the performance of his/her work but not include work related diseases that need exposure assessment and laboratory tests [13].
- Personal protective equipment (PPE); Utilization of the worker specialized clothing or equipment worn by employees for protection against health and safety hazards at the time of interview [14].
- Manual handling; the movement or support of any load effort, including; lifting put down pushing, puling, carrying and moving.
- Sleeping disorder; the presence of sleeping problems when the workers are at work in the factory [14].
- Safety guarding of machine; the machine is safe if it safe guards workers from contacts with dangerous moving parts [7].
- Agricultural injury; is defined as unintentional physical injury or poisoning which occurred during an agricultural activities and which required medical attention [5].
- Incident; any unplanned event resulting in, or having the potential for injury, illness, in health, damage or other loss [5].
- Excessive heat: heat is recorded as excessive if a worker is found sweating when naked or with light clothing; if the investigator feels a sudden heat wave when entering to the work [7].

Data collection tools and procedures

The data was collected using face to face interview administered from pre – tested structured questionnaire developed from International Labor Organization (ILO),

Occupational Safety and Health (OSH) policy 2012 standards and other studies modified for the purpose of this study. Observations were also made by principal investigator using prepared observational checklist to evaluate work environment. Moreover, record reviews from clinic and safety committee group discussion were also used as assertion to the self-reported information made by study respondents. Seven data collector, one supervisor and one principal investigator were enrolled during data collection.

Data quality control

The questionnaire was developed first in English and translated to Amharic and back to English by language experts for consistency validity. The data collectors were trained for 3 days about data collection tool, questioning technique and ethical issues. A pre-test was also conducted on similar industry to assess the validity and reliability of the questionnaire. The completeness of the questionnaires was checked before data entry.

Data processing and analysis

The data was entered in Statistical Package for Social Sciences (SPSS) 16 for analysis. All assumptions applied to binary regression including fitness of model were checked. The findings were present by using frequencies, tables, and graphs. The presence of interaction between independent factors explored. To identify factors associated with work related injury, Binary Logistic regression model was fitted and variables with a $p < 0.2$ in bivariate analysis included in the multi-variant analysis. Those predictors with p-value < 0.05, in the multi-variant analysis was considered as independent and significant predictors for work related injury and Odds ratio (OR) with 95% confidence interval was reported.

Table 1 Distribution of socio-demographic characteristics of respondents in Saudi Star Agro Industry in Gambelia region, Ethiopia, 2014 ($n = 449$)

Variable	Frequency(n)	Percent (%)
Sex		
Male	265	59%
Female	184	41%
Age		
18–29	324	72.2%
> 29	125	27.8%
Educational status		
Illiterate	10	2.2%
Read and write	132	29.4%
Primary school(1–8)	152	33.9%
Secondary school (9–12)	114	25.4%
TVT	37	8.2%
First degree and above	4	0.9%
Marital status		
Married	215	47.9%
Single	232	51.7%
Divorce	2	0.4%
Employment type		
Temporary	413	92%
Permanent	36	8%
Monthly income		
≤ 1600	382	85.1%
> 1600	67	14 .9%
Working experience		
≤ 3	269	59.9%
> 3	180	40.1%

Results

Socio-demographic factors

Majority of a study participants, 265 (59%) were male. The minimum and maximum age was 18 and 41 respectively and 232 (51.6%) of respondent were single.

From a total of 449 respondent 152 (33.9%) were primary school (1–8 grade) and 269 (59.9%) respondents had 3 years and below service year experience. Regarding employment pattern, 413 (92%) were temporarily employed and 382 (85.1%) of the respondent were earned less than 1600 ETB (Table 1).

Work related injury characteristics

Prevalence of work related injuries

Among the study participants, 165 (36.7%) had work related injury in the last 12 months with the overall prevalence rate of 367 per 1000 exposed worker per year. Moreover, 18 (4%) respondent were also injured at job in the last 2 weeks. With respect to the frequency of injury occurrence in the last 12 months, 110 (24.5%) respondents were injured once, and 55 (12.2%) injured more than once (Fig. 1).

Cause, type and affected body part

From Injured respondents, predominantly affected parts of the body were; hand 46 (27.9%), leg 34 (20.6%), eye 25 (15.15%) and toe 23 (13.93%) (Table 2). With respect to type of injuries, 61 (37.0%) laceration, 25 (15.15%) eye injury, 24 (14.54%) cut and 23 (13.94%) puncture were the most type of injury reported by respondents (Table 3). Hand tool 63 (38.20%), machine 32 (20%), splinting objects 26 (15.75%) and lifting objects 17 (10.3%) were the top sources of work related injures (Table 4).

With regard to the specific days of injuries, 80 (48.48%) were on Monday, 52 (31.51%) were on Tuesday and most respondent injured in the morning at the time of 6A.M – 6P.M (Fig. 2). When we see Absenteeism due

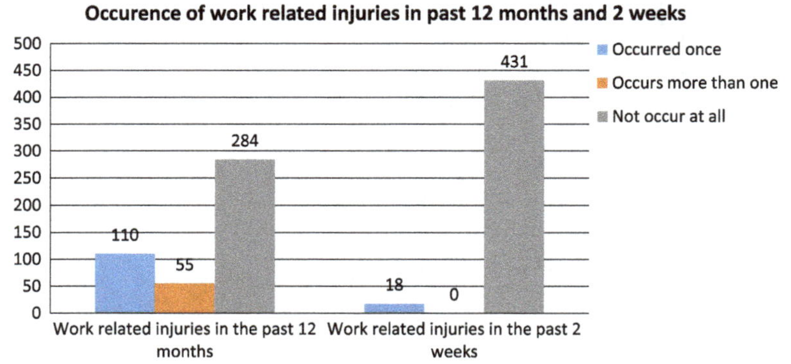

Fig. 1 The prevalence and frequency of work related injuries in the past 12 months and 2 weeks among Saudi Star Agro Industry workers in Gambella region, Ethiopia, 2014

to work related injuries in the industry in the last 12 months, 75 (16.7%) absenteeism occurred for 1 day, 10 (2.2%) for 2 days and 3 (0.2%) for 3 days.

Of those injured respondents 101 (61.2%) workers injured while in production department (cultivating, irrigation, and loading unloading) and 36 (21.8%) were injured in agro mechanization department (mechanic, tractor operator, loader operator and welder). The most frequent reason given by the respondents for the occurrence of injury were working behavior 79 (47.87%).

Severity of work related injury

Out of 165 injured respondents six (1.3%) were hospitalized and 87 working days were lost as the result of work related injury.

Description of work environment

Concerning with working hour, 338 (75.27%) respondents were working for 48 h per week and 111 (24.8%) were working for more than 48 h. From all respondents, 94.2% realized that they have no safety training and 96.88% of the respondents responded lack of supervision at work place (Fig. 3).

Behavioral characteristics

Among 449 respondents, 59 (13%) were drinking alcohol, 20 (4.5%) were chewing chat, 18 (4%) were smoking cigarette and 42 (4.5%) had sleep disorder. From all respondents 376 (83.75) were not using PPE. Reasons given by respondents for not using PPE are 307 (81.64%) were no PPE, 26 (6.91%) were lack of awareness, 10 (2.65%) don't know how to use the PPE, 15 (3.98%) not comfortable and 18 (4.8%) were due to decrease performance of PPE.

Observation of work environment

During the observation, we have seen that most working section were with excessive heat and dust. In addition, there were no safety division and personnel in the enterprise that help in promoting health and safety condition at work place. Warning sign and health and safety instructions or procedure did not exist in all working section; similarly all working section lacks first aid equipment except they had clinic at central level (Table 5).

Associated factors of work related injury

From the socio-demographic variables, marital status and service years of workers showed significant association

Table 2 Parts of the body injured and types of injury among workers in Saudi Star Agro Industry in Gambelia region, Ethiopia, 2014($n = 165$)

Part of the body affected	Frequency	Percent (%)
Hand	46	27.9%
Toe	23	13.9%
Back	17	10.3%
Eye	25	15.2%
Finger	2	1.2%
Leg	34	20.6%
Ear	2	1.2%
Chest	8	4.8%
Upper arm	1	0.6%
Other	7	4.3%

Table 3 Type OF INJURES among injured worker in Saudi Star Agro Industry in Gambelia region, Ethiopia, 2014 ($n = 165$)

Types of injury	Frequency	Percent (%)
Abrasion/Laceration	61	37.0%
Cut	24	14.5%
Puncture	23	13.9%
Back pain	14	8.5%
Eye injury	25	15.2%
Ear injury	2	1.2%
Others	16	9.7%

Table 4 Source of injury among injured workers in Saudi Star Agro Industry in Gambelia region, Ethiopia, 2014 ($n = 165$)

Source of injury	Frequency	Percent (%)
Machine	33	20%
Falling object	15	9.1%
Splinting object	26	15.8%
Collision	2	1.2%
Acid and acidic substance	8	4.8%
Hand tool	63	38.2%
Lifting object	17	10.3%
Other	1	0.6%

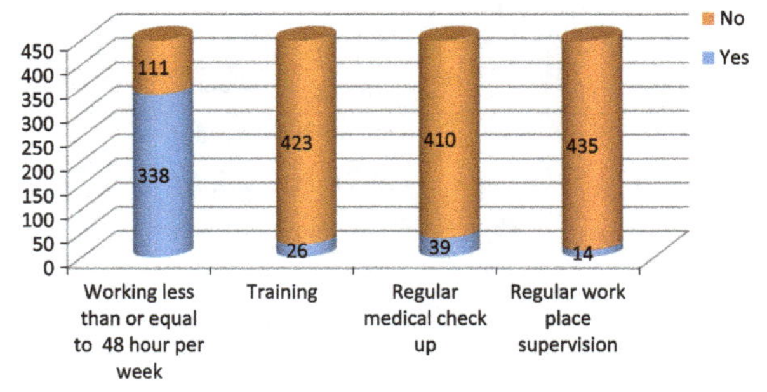

Fig. 3 Work environment related factors among workers in Saudi Star Agro Industry in Gambella region, Ethiopia, 2014

with work related injury. Workers who are single were 1.73 times more likely to report work related injury than workers who are in marriage [AOR; 1.73; 95%; CI (1.09–2.75) and workers whose service year less than or equal to 3 were 1.89 times more likely to report work related injury than whose service year above 3 years [AOR; 1.89; 95%; CI; (1.16–3.08). However sex, age, educational status, income and type of employment have no significance association with work related injury in this study.

Among work environment variables, hours worked per week, safety training and regular health checkup showed significant association with work related injury. Workers who worked more than 48 h per week were 8.33 times more likely to be injured than workers who spend their time in the work place for 48 h and less [AOR; 8.33; 95%; CI (4.87–14.41)]. Similarly, workers without safety and health training were 4.56 times more likely to be injured than who had training [AOR; 4.56; 95%; CI;(1.299–16.1)].In addition, workers who had no regular health checkup were 5.84 times more likely to be injured than who had regular health checkup [AOR; 5.56; 95%; CI (2.04–16.73)]. However, supervision of work place had no significant association with work related injury.

Among behavioral factors, usage of personal protective equipment was significantly associated with work related injury. Workers who did not used personal protective equipment's were 2.58 times more likely to reported work related injury than workers who did use PPE in the work place [AOR; 2.58, 95%; CI (1.17–5.68]. However, smoking cigarettes, drinking alcohol, sleep disorder and chewing chat were not significantly associated with work related injury (Table 6).

Discussion

Magnitude and severity of work related injury

Determining the prevalence of work related injuries and identifying associated factors are essential in the development of injury prevention strategy at the work place. The overall prevalence of work related injury in this study was 36.7% or 367 per 1000 workers per year. This finding is similar with studies done in agricultural workers stating that workers suffer markedly high rate of injuries than any other workers [5, 15]. In addition, most workers in this study are temporary workers (92%) and temporary workers and daily laborers are among the most vulnerable groups in agricultural workplaces [16].

This study indicates high rate of injury compared to a study made on other industries [2, 17, 18]. This could be due to poor promotion and preventive work related to safety and health such as, lack of safety training, lack of regular health checkup, lack of poor usage of personal protective equipment's, and being temporary worker

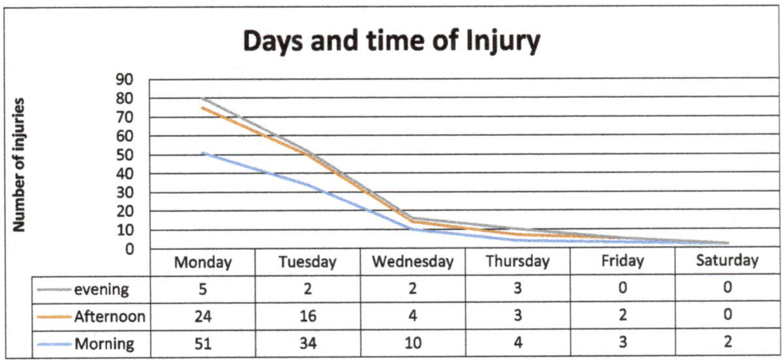

	Monday	Tuesday	Wednesday	Thursday	Friday	Saturday
evening	5	2	2	3	0	0
Afternoon	24	16	4	3	2	0
Morning	51	34	10	4	3	2

Fig. 2 Days and time of work related injuries among Saudi Star Agro Industry workers in Gambella region, Ethiopia, 2014

Table 5 Occupational health and safety hazards identified in working section, Saudi Star Agro Industry in Gambelia region, Ethiopia, 2014

Type of workplace	Work department	Hazard Identified
Agro mechanization	Farm mechanization	Excessive heat, dust, sharps, gasoline and Sulfuric acid
	Work shop/Garage	Excessive heat, sharps, gasoline and Sulfuric acid
Workshop/Garage	Pest control department	Pesticide and chemicals, and PPE are not Standardized
Others	Seed preparation and rice packing	Noise, Poor ventilation, sharps, dust, and have loaded materials
	Unit farm Irrigation	Excessive heat and dust, Snack bits Dust, and sharps

Table 6 Summery of logistic regression analysis of the relative effect of work related injuries among SAUDI STAR AGRO INDUSTRY IN GAMBELLA REGION, ETHIOPIA, 2014

Characteristics	WRI		COR 95% CI	AOR 95% CI
	Yes	No		
Sex				
Male	86	176	0.719(0.49–1.06)^{x}	0.63(0.4–1.01)^{0}
Female	76	108	1.00	
Age				
≤ 29	126	198	1.04(0.9–2.18)^{0}	1.28(0.76–2.17)^{0}
> 29	39	86	1.00	
Marital status				
Single	107	127	2.28(1.54–3.39)^{xxx}	1.6 (1.01–2.57)^{x}
Married	58	157	1.00	1.00
Service				
≤ 3	123	146	2.77(1.8–4.22)^{xxx}	2.05(1.22–3.29)^{xx}
> 3	42	138	1.00	1.00
Safety				
No	161	262	3.38(1.14–9.98)^{x}	4.89(1.37–17.4)^{x}
Yes	4	22	1.00	1.00
PPE				
No	155	221	4.42(2.19_8.89)^{xxx}	2.54(1.15–5.64)^{x}
Yes	10	63	1.00	1.00
Health checkup				
No	161	248	5.84(2.04–16.73)^{xx}	4.06(1.1–14.99)^{x}
Yes	4	36	1.00	1.00
Chewing chat				
No	5	15	0.55(0.2–1.57)^{0}	0.66(0.14–3.04)^{0}
Yes	160	269	1.00	
Working hour				
≤ 48	81	257	1.00	1.00
> 48	84	27	9.87(5.98–16.28)^{xxx}	8.53(4.9–14.73)^{xxx}

^{0}NB variable whose P-value < 0.3 in bivariate; ^{x}significant at $P < 0.05$; ^{xx}significant at $P < 0.01$; ^{xxx}significant at $P < 0.001$

(temporary workers does not get equal benefits with permanent workers in most industries) may contribute to high rate of injury in this study.

Major work related injury types, part of the body affected, and source of injury

The finding of this study indicates that, abrasion/laceration, eye injury, cut and punctures as the most frequent types of injuries. These findings are consistent with studies conducted in Ethiopia; study conducted in Tendaho agricultural industry and a study done in Gondar on small and medium scale industries [8, 18]. These findings are also consistent with a study done on risk of agricultural injury among African-American farm works from Alabama and Mississippi and a study conducted on eye health and safety among Latino farm workers [19, 20]. In addition literature revealed that the stated findings are common in work related injury [3, 21].

This study also revealed that hand tools, machine and splinting objects are the common source of injury. This finding is consistence with a study done in agricultural injury in rural California [21]. The reason for this may be due to the fact that most of the workers were temporary and daily laborer. These workers are characterized by manual handling and working on environment which is full of pieces of stone and dry soil. The risk of temporary workers and manual worker as the most exposed group in agricultural activities is well documented in study done in Easter U.S [22]. These findings are also in agreement with other studies done in Ethiopia such as Tendho agricultural industry, large scale metal manufacturing industry in Addis Ababa, and on small and medium scale industry in Gondar [7, 8, 18].

In this study we have found that hand, leg, eye and toe were the most common parts of the body injured. This finding is in agreement with the study done in Tendaho agricultural industry in Afar, Ethiopiaand a study done on farm related injury on older Kentucky farmers in U.S. [8, 23].

Determinant of work related injury

The finding of the studies revealed several factors that related to the occurrence, severity and types of injury.

Among the assessed socio-demographic determinant of work related injury marital status and service year were significantly associated with work related injury. This finding is consistent with the study done in Tendho agricultural industry, study done on large scale manufacture industries in Addis Ababa and study done on small and medium scale enterprise in Gondar [7, 8, 17]. In addition, this finding is also consistent with studies done on Kentucky farmers [18].

The finding of this study showed that from all work environmental factors, working hour per week, safety training and regular health checkup were significantly associated with work related injury. These are in agreement with studies done in Tendho manufacturing industry, large manufacturing industries in Addis Ababa, a study done in small and medium enterprise in Gondar, Ethiopia and a study done on occupational injuries in Kombolcha textile factory, Ethiopia [7, 8, 13, 18]. Similarly, the finding of the study is consistent with the studies done on fatal occupational injury among non-governmental employee in Malaysia and injuries and fatalities on older farmers in U.S. [3, 22].

Among the assessed behavioral determinant of work related injury, using of personal protective equipment was significantly associated with injury. This finding is in agreement with studies done in large manufacturing industry in Addis Ababa, study done in Tendho agricultural industry in Afar, study done on small and medium enterprise in Gondar, and study done on occupational injuries among Addis Ababa city municipal solid waste collectors [7, 8, 18, 24]. Similar finding is also observed on studies done on injuries and fatalities in U.S farmers and agricultural injuries on older farmers in Kentucky [22, 23].

Conclusion

The prevalence of work related injury in Saudi Star Agro Industry was high. Marital status, service year, usage of personal protective equipment, safety training regular health checkup and working hours per week were significantly associated with work related injuries.

Abbreviations

AOR: Adjusted odds ratio; CI: Confidence interval; GDP: Growth domestic product; ILO: International Labor Organization; IRB: Institutional Review Board; OR: Odds ratio; OSH: Occupational safety and health; PPE: Personal protective equipment; SPSS: Statistical package for social sciences

Acknowledgements

We would further like to thank University of Gondar, College of Medicine and Health Sciences for providing ethical clearance for his study. We also like to express our gratitude to Saudi Star Agro Industry office, State Farm management staffs and study participants.

Funding

This research is funded by University of Gondar, Research and Community Service directorate as an award of winning research projects among academician within the University.

Authors' contributions

DHC participated in proposal research design process, data analysis, and presentation and interpretation process of result, preparation of scientific paper or the manuscript, and corresponding author of the manuscript. DB was responsible for generating the concept of this research paper, literature review and organization, preparation of draft research proposal document, organizing data collection process, and preparation of draft data analysis and interpretation. All authors read and approved the final manuscript.

Competing interests

The authors declare that they have no competing interests.

References

1. Smith TD, DeJoy DM. Occupational injury in America: an analysis of risk factors using data from the General Social Survey (GSS). J Safety Res. 2012;43(1):67–74.
2. Lee SJ, et al. Work-related injuries and fatalities among farmers in South Korea. Am J Ind Med. 2012;55(1):76–83.
3. Abas AB, et al. Fatal occupational injuries among non-governmental employees in Malaysia. Am J Ind Med. 2013;56(1):65–76.
4. Fransen M, et al. Shift work and work injury in the New Zealand Blood Donors' Health Study. Occup Environ Med. 2006;63(5):352–8.
5. Earle-Richardson GB, et al. Improving agricultural injury surveillance: a comparison of incidence and type of injury event among three data sources. Am J Ind Med. 2011;54(8):586–96.
6. Uehli K, et al. Sleep problems and work injuries: a systematic review and meta-analysis. Sleep Med Rev. 2014;18(1):61–73.
7. Habtu Y, Kumie A, Tefera W. Magnitude and factors of occupational injury among workers in large scale metal manufacturing industries in Ethiopia. Open Access Library Journal. 2014;1(08):1.
8. Yiha O, Kumie A. Assessment of occupational injuries in Tendaho Agricultural Development SC, Afar Regional State. Ethiop J Health Dev. 2010;24(3):167–74.
9. Andrews D, et al., The Federal Democratic Republic of Ethiopia: Selected Issues and Statistical Appendix. International Monetary Fund Country Report. 2006(06/122)
10. Kolben K. Labor rights as human rights. Va J Int'l L. 2009;50:449.
11. Karttunen JP, Rautiainen RH. Occupational injury and disease incidence and risk factors in Finnish agriculture based on 5-year insurance records. J Agromedicine. 2013;18(1):50–64.
12. Aderaw Z, Engdaw D, Tadesse T. Determinants of occupational injury: a case control study among textile factory workers in Amhara Regional State, Ethiopia. J Trop Med. 2011;2011:657275.
13. Yessuf Serkalem S, Moges Haimanot G, Ahmed Ansha N. Determinants of occupational injury in Kombolcha textile factory, North-East Ethiopia. Int J Occup Environ Med. 2014;5(2):84–93.
14. Lovelock K, et al. Occupational injury and disease in agriculture in North America, Europe and Australasia: a review of the literature. Dunedin: University of Otago; 2008.
15. ILO. Safety and Health in Agriculture, in SafeWork, h.a.t.e. Programme on safety, Editor. Geneva: International Labour Office; 2000. p. 22.
16. Ezenwa AO. A study of fatal injuries in Nigerian factories. Occup Med (Lond). 2001;51(8):485–9.
17. Tadesse T, Kumie A. Prevalence and factors affecting work-related injury among workers engaged in Small and Medium-scale industries in Gondar wereda, North Gondor zone, Amhara Regional State, Ethiopia. Ethiop J Health Dev. 2007;21(1):25–34.
18. McGwin Jr G, Enochs R, Roseman JM. Increased risk of agricultural injury among African-American farm workers from Alabama and Mississippi. Am J Epidemiol. 2000;152(7):640–50.
19. Verma A, et al. Eye health and safety among Latino farmworkers. J Agromedicine. 2011;16(2):143–52.
20. McCurdy SA, Kwan JA. Agricultural injury risk among rural California public high school students: prospective results. Am J Ind Med. 2012;55(7):631–42.
21. Myers JR, Layne LA, Marsh SM. Injuries and fatalities to U.S. farmers and farm workers 55 years and older. Am J Ind Med. 2009;52(3):185–94.

Work participation of patients with musculoskeletal disorders: is this addressed in physical therapy practice?

Wiebke Oswald[1,2], Nathan Hutting[1*], Josephine A. Engels[1], J. Bart Staal[3,4], Maria W. G. Nijhuis-van der Sanden[4] and Yvonne F. Heerkens[1]

Abstract

Background: Musculoskeletal disorders are the main complaints for visiting a physical therapist (PT) in primary health care; they have a negative effect on an individual's quality of life and result in a major cost to society. Qualitative research has shown that physical therapists (PTs) treating patients with these disorders experience barriers in the integration of occupational factors within their practice, and also revealed a lack of cooperation between PTs and (other) occupational healthcare providers. The aim of this study is to quantitatively investigate how generalist PTs in the Netherlands, who treat patients with musculoskeletal disorders, currently integrate occupational factors within their practice, and to identify their opinions and needs with regard to enhancing the integration of the patient's work within physical therapy practice.

Methods: A cross-sectional survey was conducted among generalist PTs who treat working-age (18–67 years) patients with musculoskeletal disorders. Generalist PTs were contacted for participation via digital news-mails and asked to fill out an online survey which was developed based on the results of a recent qualitative study. The survey consisted of: i) demographics of the participants, ii) questions on how generalist PTs currently integrate occupational factors within their practice, and iii) asked their opinion about the integration of occupational factors within physical therapy. The PTs were also asked about their needs with regard to the integration of occupational factors and with regard to cooperation with other (occupational) health professionals. All answers (using Likert scales) are presented as the *number* and *percentage* of the respondents reporting those specific answers, whereas all other answers are presented as means and standard deviations.

Results: Of the 142 respondents, 64% indicated that occupational factors should be addressed to a greater extent within physical therapy. To have the possibility to bill for a workplace assessment (60.6%) and more knowledge about laws and regulations (50%) were identified as needs of the respondents. Only 14.8% of the respondents indicated that they communicate with or consult a PT specialized in occupational health. Only 12.7% of the participants who do not have a specialized PT within their practice sometimes/regularly refer patients to a specialized PT.

Conclusions: Although generalist PTs address occupational factors within their practice, there is room for improvement. This study also identified a lack of cooperation between generalist PTs and PTs specialized in occupational health.

Keywords: Musculoskeletal disorders, Physical therapy, Occupational health, Work participation

* Correspondence: Nathan.Hutting@han.nl
[1]Faculty of Health and Social Studies, Research Group Occupation & Health, HAN University of Applied Sciences, P.O. Box 6960, 6503 GL Nijmegen, Netherlands
Full list of author information is available at the end of the article

Background

The main complaints for visiting a physical therapist (PT) in primary healthcare worldwide are musculoskeletal disorders (MSDs) [1]. MSDs have a negative effect on an individual's quality of life and are a major cost to society [2, 3]. The most common MSDs (e.g. back and neck/shoulder problems) are the main cause of disability among the working-age (18–67 years) population [2]. In Great Britain in 2013–2014, the prevalence of work-related MSDs was 1680 per 100,000 employees, and the incidence of new cases was 550 per 100,000 employees [4].

Work-related MSDs are disorders whereby work activities and conditions significantly contribute to the onset or progression of the disorder, but are not necessarily the sole cause of the disorder [5]. In the development of MSDs, in addition to other risk factors, the work environment and its characteristics can play an important role. For example, adverse working conditions, psychosocial problems, lack of proper attention to ergonomics, postural problems during work, and mental overload/underload [5]. Even though it remains unclear whether work exposure is responsible for the onset or progression of MSDs, work-related MSDs play a considerable role in the financial burden on society, which continues to increase [6–8].

Although work exposure can cause health problems, work also has a beneficial influence on the individual's wellbeing [9]. Moreover, work participation is an important factor of perceived quality of life [10, 11]. Long periods of absenteeism lead to a smaller chance of return to work and an increased risk of problems related to physical, mental and social wellbeing [11, 12]. Research has shown that return to work can be an important component of rehabilitation [13]. For example, if interventions are provided within a few weeks after the complaints started, or in the early stage of absenteeism, they can contribute to the prevention of long-lasting absenteeism [13–16].

In the Netherlands, primary healthcare and occupational healthcare are two separate systems. Dutch patients with work-related MSDs often consult health professionals in primary healthcare rather than in occupational healthcare. Although participating in work is an important factor of wellbeing [10], most caregivers in primary healthcare -including physical therapists (PTs)- pay insufficient attention to the relation between MSDs and occupational factors among their working patients [17]. Absenteeism can be reduced by improving primary healthcare and by improving the communication between health professionals, occupational health professionals, the workplace, the patient and the insurer [18, 19]. Therefore, the Social and Economic Council of the Netherlands (SER) recommended to improve the quality of primary, secondary and tertiary healthcare, by increasing knowledge about and by focusing on prevention of absenteeism, return to work, and accessibility to occupational healthcare for all employees [17]. More attention, knowledge and collaboration in occupational-related healthcare could lead to a cost reduction of more than 1 billion euro a year [17, 20].

In 2016, almost 25% of the Dutch working-age population visited a PT in primary healthcare due to MSDs in the past year [21]. With their expertise on MSDs, complemented by knowledge and skills in managing occupational factors, PTs can play an important role in facilitating rehabilitation, return to work (RTW) and prevention of absenteeism [19, 22]. There is strong evidence in both the occupational health and physiotherapy literature to support the role of PTs as primary care providers for injured workers with MSDs [22]. Provision of treatments to address specific MSD pathology is integral to recovery, which can facilitate earlier RTW. The interventions that consistently demonstrate greater efficacy for positive work outcomes tend to be multi-modal and multi-disciplinary, including PTs [22]. Common modalities used by PTs include advice and education, manual therapy, and exercise [22]. One review found that i) patient education had some effect on RTW for workers with low back pain, ii) physical exercise was effective in subacute and chronic low back pain workers, and iii) graded activity had positive effects on RTW, pain and functional status [23]. However, studies in the UK show that primary healthcare providers, including PTs, do not provide guidance and support to workers with regard to their work problems [24, 25].

In a recent qualitative study performed by our group in the Netherlands [26], PTs stated that they experience barriers in the integration of occupational factors in their practice. The Netherlands has an educational program in which generalist PTs can specialize in occupational physical therapy or work-related physical therapy; nevertheless, less than 1% of the PTs is registered as an occupational physical therapist (OPT) or work-related physical therapist (WPT). The OPT is specialized in creating a healthy work environment and reducing sick leave within an organization, whereas the WPT is specialized in enhancing the capacity for recovery of employees with occupational health complaints. Work-related PTs are geared towards the reintegration of employees through individual and work-orientated exercises and treatment; they treat employees in a private practice setting or (if necessary and/or relevant) within the organization itself [27]. Although generalist PTs treat working-age patients with MSDs, they may hesitate to include occupational factors in their treatment, irrespective of whether or not they found work an important factor. Furthermore, PTs do not always cooperate with occupational physical therapists (OPTs) in order to provide sufficient care to their working-age patients [26].

Based on the results of the qualitative study [26] it was concluded that a quantitative study is needed to investigate (on a broader scale) how generalist PTs in the Netherlands integrate their patients' occupational factors within the physical therapy, and which barriers and facilitators influence the integration.

Therefore, this study aims to i) quantitatively investigate how PTs is the Netherlands, who treat patients with MSDs, currently integrate occupational factors within their practice, and ii) identify their opinions and needs with regard to enhancing the integration of the patient's work within physical therapy.

Methods

Procedures and participants

A cross-sectional survey was conducted among PTs who treat working-age patients with MSDs. PTs in the Netherlands were contacted (during November–December 2016) for participation via calls in digital news-mails of the Royal Dutch Society for Physical Therapy (KNGF), the Dutch Institute of Allied Health Professions (NPi), and social media networks of the researchers (LinkedIn). Included for this survey were generalist PTs who treat working-age patients with MSDs, whereas OPTs and work-related physical therapists (WPTs) were excluded in order to get a clear view of the opinions of generalist PTs who have not specialized in occupational healthcare. The call in the news-mails explained the purpose of the study and the voluntary nature of participation. The PTs were asked to fill out an online survey, provided via Parantion Easion Survey version 3.63. A link to log on to the website anonymously was included in the digital newsletter. To encourage participation, all PTs who filled in the survey had the option to fill in their e-mail address (voluntary) in order to win a gift card of 60 euro.

Survey

Based on the results of our recent qualitative study [26], a survey was developed for the present investigation. The qualitative study investigated how PTs integrate occupational factors within their practice, what they need for a better cooperation with other occupational health professionals, and which factors can facilitate a better integration of occupational factors within physical therapy [26]. An overview of the main categories and underlying themes identified in the earlier qualitative study are presented in Additional file 1: Appendix 1. The survey was pretested by two generalist PTs and reviewed by the members of the research group. No major modifications of the survey were found to be necessary.

The first part of the survey assessed demographics of the participating PTs in terms of gender, age, years of experience as PT, and PTs' specialization. With regard to specialization and referral to occupational health professionals, it was possible to choose more than one specialization. The survey consisted of questions on how PTs currently integrate occupational factors within their practice, and on their opinion on the integration of occupational factors within physical therapy. The PTs were also asked about their needs with regard to the integration of occupational factors (need of knowledge, skills and tools) and with regard to cooperation with WPTs, OPTs, and other occupational health professionals.

Part of the survey was based on the concepts awareness, attitude, social influences, and self-efficacy of the I-Change model [28]. Awareness of the importance of involving occupational factors in their practice was investigated (Table 2, question 1a–d). Attitude was assessed by asking the PTs whether they had a positive (Table 2, question 2a-e, 2k) or a negative attitude (Table 2, question 2f-g, 2i-j) towards involving occupational factors in their practice. Social influences were assessed in terms of norms, modeling, support, and pressure (Table 2, question 3a–e). Furthermore, self-efficacy was assessed (Table 2, question 4a–f). For all questions, unless stated otherwise, a 5-point Likert scale was used for response, ranging from strongly disagree to strongly agree, or ranging from never to always.

Data analysis

Demographics are presented as means and standard deviations (SDs), while gender and specialization are presented as number and percentage. All answers using Likert scales are presented as the *number* and the *percentage* of the respondents reporting that specific answer, whereas all other answers are presented as means and standard deviations (SDs).

The Statistical Package for the Social Science (SPSS, version 22) was used to analyze the data.

Results

In this study, a total of 142 PTs completed the survey. The mean age of the PTs was 42.4 (SD 13.3) years, 49.3% were male and 50.7% were female. The average years of work experience was 18.4 (SD 13.0) years. The most common postgraduate specializations were manual therapy (38.7%) and sports physical therapy (14.1%). Psychosomatic physical therapy was reported as a specialization by 8.5% of the PTs, and edema physical therapy was reported by 5.6%. A minority of the PTs were specialized in orofacial physical therapy (2.1%), haptonomy (1.4%), and pelvic physical therapy (0.7%). The category 'other' was chosen by 40.8% of the PTs. The participating PTs estimated that 67.6% (SD 18.2)

Table 1 Number and percentage of generalist physical therapists (n = 142) addressing several occupational factors within physical therapy practice

	Never, n (%)	Rarely, n (%)	Sometimes, n (%)	Regularly, n (%)	Always, n (%)
1. To what extent do you address the following items within the patient interview in patients with paid work?					
a) Load and capacity in relation to work activities	0	1 (0.7)	7 (4.9)	36 (25.4)	98 (69.0)
b) Work tasks/work operations of the patient	0	1 (0.7)	14 (9.9)	56 (39.4)	71 (50.0)
c) Work method/work technique of the patient	0	10 (7.0)	35 (24.6)	49 (34.5)	48 (33.8)
d) Workplace of the patient	1 (0.7)	8 (5.6)	36 (24.5)	54 (38.0)	43 (30.3)
e) Working hours of the patient	2 (1.4)	20 (14.1)	37 (26.1)	49 (34.5)	34 (23.9)
f) Work pressure of the patient	0	7 (4.9)	24 (16.9)	60 (42.3)	51 (35.9)
g) Workplace absenteeism	1 (0.7)	20 (14.1)	32 (22.5)	42 (29.6)	47 (33.1)
h) Working together with supervisor/colleagues	8 (5.6)	38 (26.8)	51 (35.9)	25 (17.6)	20 (14.1)
i) Return to work (in case of absenteeism)	1 (0.7)	5 (3.5)	21 (14.8)	67 (47.2)	48 (33.8)
j) Importance of work participation for the patient	1 (0.7)	3 (2.1)	32 (22.5)	61 (43.0)	45 (31.7)
k) Degree to which the patient thinks that there is a relationship between the complaints and the patient's work	2 (1.4)	5 (3.5)	23 (16.2)	65 (45.8)	47 (33.1)
l) Recovery options within the work situation	1 (0.7)	3 (2.1)	32 (22.5)	61 (43.0)	45 (31.7)
m) Recovery options outside the work situation	2 (1.4)	5 (3.5)	23 (16.2)	65 (45.8)	47 (33.1)
2. To what extent do you address the patient's work/work activities during the following phases of practice?					
a) Physical examination	3 (2.1)	13 (9.2)	38 (26.8)	45 (31.7)	43 (30.3)
b) Treatment goals/treatment plan	1 (0.7)	4 (2.8)	12 (8.5)	60 (42.3)	65 (45.8)
c) Treatment	2 (1.4)	2 (1.4)	15 (10.6)	79 (55.6)	44 (31.0)
d) Evaluation	1 (0.7)	2 (1.4)	16 (11.3)	61 (43.0)	62 (43.7)
3. To what extent do you advise/give information (to) the patient during treatment about the following items?					
a) Load and capacity in relation to work activities	1 (0.7)	0	9 (6.3)	54 (38.0)	78 (54.9)
b) Work tasks/work operations of the patient	1 (0.7)	2 (1.4)	28 (19.7)	67 (47.2)	44 (31.0)
c) Work method/work technique of the patient	1 (0.7)	6 (4.2)	32 (22.5)	56 (39.4)	47 (33.1)
d) Workplace of the patient	3 (2.1)	7 (4.9)	33 (23.2)	70 (49.3)	29 (20.4)
e) Working hours of the patient	7 (4.9)	32 (22.5)	52 (36.6)	35 (24.6)	16 (11.3)
f) Work pressure of the patient	2 (1.4)	10 (7.0)	37 (26.1)	63 (44.4)	30 (21.1)
g) Workplace absenteeism	3 (2.1)	24 (16.9)	44 (31.7)	45 (31.7)	26 (18.3)
h) Working together with supervisor/colleagues	9 (6.3)	40 (28.2)	46 (32.4)	32 (22.5)	15 (10.6)
i) Return to work (in case of absenteeism)	1 (0.7)	3 (2.1)	29 (20.4)	69 (48.6)	40 (28.2)
j) Importance of work participation for the patient	1 (0.7)	5 (3.5)	31 (21.8)	71 (50.0)	34 (23.9)
k) Degree to which the patient thinks that there is a relationship between the complaints and the patient's work	1 (0.7)	5 (3.5)	31 (21.8)	66 (46.5)	39 (27.5)
4. To what extent do you perform the following actions during treatment?					
a) Let the patient imitate work activities	4 (2.8)	14 (9.9)	44 (31.0)	67 (47.2)	13 (9.2)
b) Let the patient make photos/videos of the workplace	62 (43.7)	38 (26.8)	26 (18.3)	14 (9.9)	2 (1.4)
c) Visit the patient's workplace	80 (56.3)	40 (28.2)	16 (11.3)	6 (4.2)	0
d) Use questionnaires or screening lists about work or aspects of work	50 (35.2)	46 (32.4)	23 (16.2)	20 (14.1)	3 (2.1)
5. When I refer patients to a professional in the field of occupational health it is:					
a) Directly after the history taking	45 (31.7)	51 (35.9)	36 (25.4)	9 (6.3)	1 (0.7)
b) In case of disappointing recovery	19 (13.4)	18 (12.7)	64 (45.1)	32 (22.5)	9 (6.3)
c) In case of failure of recovery	18 (12.7)	16 (11.3)	49 (34.5)	37 (26.1)	22 (15.5)
d) In case of recurrent complaints	16 (11.3)	28 (19.7)	71 (50.0)	23 (16.2)	2 (2.8)

of their patients were of working age and that 66.9% (SD 20.5) of their patients had paid work.

Table 1 describes to what extent PTs address occupational factors of patients with paid work within the patient interview, pay attention to their patients work/ work activities during the phases of physical therapy, give advice about occupational factors during treatment, and perform actions to investigate the workplace of their patients. Table 1 also describes in what situations PTs refer their patients to an occupational health professional.

The participating PTs stated that, if they communicate with or consult other occupational health professionals, then they mainly have contact with occupational health/ insurance physicians (72.5%; in the Netherlands, insurance physicians assess the disability claims of injured workers) and occupational therapists (31.7%). A minority of the PTs has contact with employers (17.6%), WPTs (14.8%), Human Resource managers (12%), OPTs (11.3%) and labor experts (10.6%).

The majority of the PTs (76.8%) had no direct OPT or WPT colleague. Of this 76.8%, the majority (60%) never refer to a WPT outside their practice/company, 27.3% rarely refer to a WPT, 10% sometimes refer to a WPT, and 2.7% regularly refer their patients to a WPT outside their practice. Of the generalist PTs who have a WPT as colleague, 6.1% never and 18.2% rarely work together. About 64% of the generalist PTs do not want to have more intensive cooperation with a WPT, whereas 53.5% would like to have more contact with OPTs within the patient's company. Also, 54.9% of the PTs would like to have more intensive cooperation with occupational health and insurance physicians.

Table 2 describes the proportion of the opinions of PTs with regard to addressing occupational factors within physical therapy in terms of awareness, attitude, social influences, and self-efficacy. Table 3 presents the needs of PTs with regard to the involvement of occupational factors within physical therapy.

Discussion

This study investigated to what extent generalist PTs in the Netherlands currently integrate occupational factors in their treatment of patients with MSDs within primary care and evaluated their opinions/needs with regard to enhancing integration of the patient's work within physical therapy.

Importance of addressing occupational factors

Most respondents were aware of the importance of involving occupational factors within their care. Most of the respondents had a positive attitude towards paying (more) attention to occupational factors. They found it important to address the patient's work because it has a positive effect on the patient's performance. This is consistent with findings from our recent qualitative research [26]. In general, the respondents had high self-efficacy (i.e. beliefs about their capabilities to produce designated levels of performance) with regard to integrating occupational factors within their practice. With regard to social support, the perceived support of colleagues and supervisors of the respondents was not clearly shown in this study. However, with regard to the social support of patients, most respondents received appreciation with regard to involving occupational factors within their care.

Addressing occupational factors in practice

In this study, most respondents stated that they integrate occupational factors of patients in their care. Generally, respondents indicated that they regularly or always address occupational factors within their patient interview. However, almost a quarter of the respondents indicated that they only sometimes pay attention to work methods, the workplace, and absenteeism of their patients. Respondents had a positive attitude and experienced awareness, social support, and high self-efficacy with regard to integrating occupational factors within their practice. However, although these positive findings and the fact that most respondents stated that they involve the occupational factors of their patients within their practice, 64.1% indicated that occupational factors should be addressed to a greater extent. It seems that fulfilling the items mentioned in the I-Change model [28], does not necessarily lead to adequate behavior with regard to addressing occupational factors within generalist physical therapy. Thus, although respondents do address occupational factors, most respondents think that the patient's work should be more extensively addressed.

With regard to working together with supervisor/ colleagues, most respondents indicated that they rarely or only sometimes address this topic. Relationships at work is one important psychosocial factor and bad relationships at work are an important barrier for recovery for, e.g., chronic low back pain [29]. This is line with previous qualitative research in which participants emphasized that patients need to be questioned about their work, including all work features and psychosocial factors [26]. Another study showed that psychosocial factors are a major barrier for return to work [30]. Also, musculoskeletal PTs are aware of the potential benefits of incorporating psychological interventions within their practice, but feel insufficiently trained to use such interventions and do not sufficiently integrate these psychosocial factors within their practice [31, 32]. However, in the present study, work pressure (also a psychosocial factor) was addressed regularly or always by most respondents.

Table 2 Number and percentage of the opinions of generalist physical therapists (n = 142) with regard to addressing occupational factors within physical therapy practice in terms of awareness, attitude, social influences and self-efficacy

	Totally disagree, n (%)	Disagree, n (%)	Neutral, n (%)	Agree, n (%)	Totally agree, n (%)
1. Awareness *Instruction: Please indicate to what extent you agree or disagree with the following statements:*					
a) The border where general physical therapy ends and occupational health physical therapy starts is clear to me.	10 (7.0)	64 (45.1)	38 (26.8)	27 (19.0)	3 (2.1)
b) I am aware of the fact that, on average, the majority of my patients have paid work.	5 (3.5)	8 (5.6)	15 (10.6)	61 (43.0)	53 (37.3)
c) I see the way my patients work (performance) as a possible treatment option.	3 (2.1)	4 (2.8)	21 (14.8)	78 (54.9)	36 (25.4)
d) I see the extent of work participation of my patient as a possible treatment option.	4 (2.8)	4 (2.8)	24 (16.9)	81 (57.0)	29 (20.4)
2. Attitude *Instruction: The following statements are about your opinion regarding physical therapy in general, not just about your own actions.*					
a) The patient's work should have a larger place within the physical therapy than it currently does	2 (1.4)	12 (8.5)	37 (26.1)	66 (46.5)	25 (17.6)
b) I consider the patient's work as a major barrier or facilitator for recovery.	3 (2.1)	5 (3.5)	14 (9.9)	81 (57.0)	39 (27.5)
c) I consider the patient's work as a major cause of complaints.	4 (2.8)	13 (9.2)	(46 (32.4)	58 (40.8)	21 (14.8)
d) Addressing the patient's work in practice has positive effects on the patient's performance.	1 (0.7)	0	14 (9.9)	82 (57.7)	45 (31.7)
e) Addressing the patient's work in physical therapy practice has a positive effect on the patient's work absenteeism.	2 (1.4)	4 (2.8)	31 (21.8)	73 (51.4)	32 (22.5)
f) It is not important to address the patient's work/work activities within physical therapy practice because the patients visit the physical therapist for treating his/her physical complaints.	87 (61.3)	39 (27.5)	5 (3.5)	8 (5.6)	3 (2.1)
g) There is insufficient opportunity to address the patient's work/work activities within the regular physical therapy treatment.	51 (35.9)	59 (41.5)	5 (10.6)	16 (11.3)	1 (0.7)
h) Cooperation with the business community about occupational health offers a possibility to put more focus on physical therapy and create a different business model.	4 (2.8)	4 (2.8)	31 (21.8)	68 (47.9)	35 (24.6)
i) The domain 'work' belongs to the company/occupational health physical therapist, whereas generalist physical therapists have little to do with it.	47 (33.1)	63 (44.4)	21 (14.8)	8 (5.6)	3 (2.1)
j) The specific knowledge that is required in the field of occupational health is not sufficiently accessible to the generalist physical therapist.	17 (12.0)	31 (21.8)	55 (38.7)	34 (23.9)	5 (3.5)
k) The patient's demand of care is rarely related to his/her work.	44 (31.0)	58 (40.8)	23 (16.2)	14 (9.9)	3 (2.1)
3. Social influences *Instruction: The following statements relate to your personal situation and about your personal opinion. Please indicate to what extent you agree or disagree with the following statements:*					
a) My colleagues think that I should not address the patient's work in my practice.	69 (48.6)	49 (34.5)	20 (4.1)	4 (2.8)	0
b) The majority of my colleagues pay sufficient attention to their patient's work in their practice.	5 (3.5)	30 (21.1)	47 (33.1)	53 (37.3)	7 (4.9)
c) I notice that patients like it when I discuss their work situation with them.	3 (2.1)	6 (4.2)	21 (14.8)	88 (62.0)	24 (16.9)
d) My colleagues support me to pay attention to the work of my patient.	6 (4.2)	15 (10.6)	62 (43.7)	50 (35.2)	9 (6.3)
e) My supervisor supports me to pay attention to the work situation of my patient.	6 (4.2)	12 (8.5)	69 (48.6)	40 (28.2)	15 (10.6)

Table 2 Number and percentage of the opinions of generalist physical therapists (n = 142) with regard to addressing occupational factors within physical therapy practice in terms of awareness, attitude, social influences and self-efficacy *(Continued)*

4. Self-efficacy *Instruction: Please indicate to what extent you agree or disagree with the following statements:*					
a) I am able to address the work of my patient within my practice, despite the ever-changing laws and regulations in this area.	3 (2.1)	12 (8.5)	38 (26.8)	75 (52.8)	14 (9.9)
b) I am able to ask my patient about his/her working situation and to adapt my treatment accordingly.	1 (0.7)	3 (2.1)	16 (11.3)	96 (67.6)	26 (18.3)
c) Based on my current knowledge, I am optimally able to treat patients who work and to advise them with regard to work tasks/work technique, workplace working hours, workload, and work absenteeism.	6 (4.2)	34 (23.0)	43 (30.3)	44 (31.0)	15 (10.6)
d) I find it difficult to assess to what extent the patient's complaint is work related.	14 (9.9)	61 (43.0)	29 (20.4)	36 (25.4)	2 (1.4)
e) I am able to hold a substantive discussion about the patient with an occupational health physician or occupational health physical therapist.	2 (1.4)	14 (9.9)	28 (19.7)	71 (50.0)	27 (19.0)
f) Based on my knowledge of the field of occupational therapy, I am able to refer patients to the occupational health physical therapist if indicated.	9 (6.3)	29 (20.4)	38 (26.8)	45 (31.7)	21 (14.8)

Addressing the patient's work/work activities is done by the majority of respondents in all phases of care. However, during physical examination, 38.1% of the respondents stated that they never, rarely, or only sometimes pay attention to the work of their patients. Respondents indicated that they give advice to their patients about their workplace, and most respondents let the patient imitate/show their work activities. However, the majority of respondents do not use pictures/videos, nor do they visit the workplace, and 67.4% never or only rarely uses a work-related questionnaire. This indicates that the advice given by generalist PTs is mainly general advice and not based on the specific workplace/work situation of the patient.

Lack of knowledge and needs of respondents

In previous qualitative research in the Netherlands [26], lack of knowledge of generalist PTs was seen as a barrier for addressing work within PT practice. Participants felt particularly uncertain about what kind of advice they are 'allowed' to give patients, and about their knowledge related to workplace laws and regulations. Other topics requiring attention were: knowledge about work-related factors, how to address work-related factors, the workplace, workplace investigations, and knowledge about occupational healthcare providers [26]. In the present study, only 41.6% of the respondents agree or totally agree that, based on their current knowledge, they are optimally able to treat patients who work and to advise them about occupational factors. Of all respondents, 36.6% mentioned that they need more knowledge about work tasks/work activities, work methods/technique, workplace, working hours, and workload. Although most respondents indicated that they were able to address the patient's work despite the ever-changing laws and regulations, half of the respondents indicated 'more knowledge about occupational health-related laws and regulations' as one of their needs.

About 36% of the respondents stated that they need more work-specific knowledge and skills to carry out a basic workplace assessment. Since 60.6% of the respondents indicated that they have a need for the possibility to bill for a workplace assessment, financial considerations might be an additional reason for the low percentage of workplace visits. However, in the Netherlands, from 2017 onwards several insurance companies provide billing opportunities for workplace visits, which meets the need of the respondents. Therefore, upgrading the knowledge and skills of generalist PTs who will carry out these workplace assessments seems necessary.

Other needs of over 50% of the respondents were: questionnaires about work participation and screening lists to assess to what extent the patient's complaint is work related (this was also an outcome of the previous qualitative research) [26]. Almost 40% of the respondents stated that attention to occupational factors should play a greater role in the basic physical therapy educational programs and in physical therapy guidelines.

Cooperation with occupational healthcare providers

Our earlier qualitative study revealed that a major issue to be addressed is the lack of cooperation between the PT and (other) occupational healthcare providers, especially between the generalist PT and the WPT/OPT and the occupational health physician [26]. Moreover, the difference between generalist physical therapy and work-related physical therapy/occupational physical therapy was unclear. It was emphasized by the participating PTs and WPTs/OPTs that WPTs/OPTs have specific knowledge and that WPT/OPT is a valuable specialization.

Table 3 Overview of the needs of physical therapists with regard to the involvement of occupational factors within physical therapy practice

	n (%)
To have the possibility to bill for a workplace assessment.	86 (60.6)
Questionnaires about the work participation of the patient.	75 (52.8)
Screening lists to assess to what extent the patient's complaint is work related.	74 (52.1)
More knowledge about occupational health-related laws and regulations.	71 (50.0)
More knowledge about the domain and the position of the occupational health physical therapist.	61 (43.0)
More knowledge about the domain and position of occupational health professionals such as the occupational health nurse, occupational health physician, insurance physician, medical consultant and human resources consultant.	58 (40.8)
More attention to the factor work in the basic physical therapy educational programs.	56 (39.4)
More attention to work within the physical therapy guidelines.	55 (38.7)
More knowledge about work tasks/work activities, work methods/technique, workplace, working hours, workload.	52 (36.6)
More time in the treatment session to discuss work-related factors.	52 (36.6)
More practical tools to integrate work within my practice.	51 (35.9)
More practical skills to carry out a basic workplace assessment.	51 (35.9)
More opportunities to give 'work' a proper place within the electronic patient's file.	40 (28.2)
More attention to the factor work in the Master educational programs for physical therapy specializations (if applicable).	25 (17.6)

However, some respondents mentioned that they were able to address most of the work-related factors themselves [26]. In the present survey, for most of the respondents the difference in competences and responsibilities between generalist PT and OPT was unclear but 77.5% of the respondents do see a role for themselves within the domain of 'work'. However, for at least part of the respondents, the specific knowledge that is required in the field occupational health is not sufficiently accessible to the generalist PT. Also, more than 40% of the respondents also stated that they need more knowledge about the domain and position of WPTs and other occupational health professionals.

Generalist PTs do refer patients to an occupational health professional. However, this referral process could be improved, especially after the patient interview and in case of a disappointing recovery. Another question is: to which occupational health professional should patients be referred to. It seems that generalist PTs mostly communicate about the patient with the occupational health physician/insurance physician and the occupational therapist. Only 14.8% of the respondents indicated that they communicate with or consult a WPT. If generalist PTs have a colleague WPT within their practice they often do work together. However, if no WPT is present within their practice, only 12.7% of the PTs sometimes/regularly refer patients to a WPT. Only 35.9% of the respondents answered that they had a need for more intensive cooperation with the WPT, whereas 46.5% had a need for a more intensive cooperation with the OPT. Based on the results of qualitative research it was concluded that the cooperation/networking between PTs and WPTs, and knowledge about the WPT, should be enhanced [26]. However, based on the present survey, it seems that although there is little cooperation between generalist PTs and OPTs/WPTs, generalist PTs do not feel the need to work more closely together. Moreover, since almost 50% of the respondents indicated that they have sufficient knowledge of the domain of the WPT to refer patients, they do not see a need for cooperation or have insufficient insight into the additional value of the WPT. In the earlier qualitative study [26], the interaction between participants (WPTs, OPTs and PTs) during the focus group meetings might have contributed to a better perspective with regard to cooperation with the generalist PT and the OPT/WPT.

Strengths and limitations

Although some studies have evaluated the experiences/perspectives of PTs with regard to RTW [19, 30] or managing a condition in the context of work [33], to our knowledge this is the first study to use a survey to investigate how generalist PTs currently integrate work participation within their practice, and to evaluate their opinions/needs with regard to enhancing the integration of the patient's work within physical therapy. The developed survey was based on our earlier qualitative research [26], which ensured that a variety of clinically important topics was included in the survey. Moreover, this survey provides a triangulation of the results of the previous qualitative study and evaluated the results of the qualitative study on a broader scale in a group of generalist PTs. Thus, the present study contributes to the body of knowledge with regard to addressing occupational factors within physical therapy practice.

This study also has some limitations. Although the use of digital news-mails and social media increased the chance of reaching almost all PTs in the Netherlands, it was still difficult to find respondents for this study. This was also the case in previous qualitative research, probably indicating that the relevance of this topic was judged as low by PTs [26]. Since potential respondents were recruited by news-mails and announcements, this implies that mainly PTs already interested in work/occupation filled in the survey, which could have led to selection bias and influenced our results. Also, in this study, 23.2% of the respondents had a WPT within their practice. From a total of 19,557 PTs in the Netherlands who are a member of the Royal Dutch Society for Physical Therapy, only 169 are registered with the professional Dutch OPT/WPT association. Therefore, in this study, a relatively large number of respondents had a WPT in their practice, which may have led to more knowledge about occupational factors and a more pronounced positive attitude with regard to the WPT.

It is also possible that some respondents gave wished-for answers on some of the questions in the survey. This could be possible in most of the questions, because we assume that the ideal answers are known by the respondents. In addition, respondents can also have insufficient insight in their own knowledge and skills and overestimate their actual knowledge and skills, which could lead to too positive results of the survey.

Due to the varying background, age, gender and specializations of the respondents, it is a representative sample of generalist PTs. However, the 142 respondents represent only a small proportion of the Dutch PTs, which limits the generalizability of the results. Therefore, the results of this study should be interpreted with caution. Nevertheless, we think that this study is a valuable addition to our previous qualitative research, in which 21 generalist PTs and 9 WPTs/OPTs participated in the focus groups [26].

Recommendations

Although most respondents were aware of the importance of integrating occupational factors and perceived that they addressed occupational factors within their practice, it seems that the patient interview and clinical reasoning process were based on subjective procedures and impressions. It seems that a more systematic approach to obtain insight into occupational factors by means of questionnaires, observations, and workplace visits could increase effectiveness. This was also supported by the respondents, as the majority indicated that occupational factors should be more extensively addressed within physical therapy. Therefore, it seems valuable to support and facilitate generalist PTs in addressing these factors, i.e. by providing more information about work-related factors, laws and regulations, questionnaires and screening lists, and by incorporating work-related factors in guidelines. This can be done by developing (online) courses and integration of these factors within physical therapy educational programs. Moreover, an easy-to-use guideline to address occupational factors could be developed and it seems valuable to provide an overview of all these topics (e.g. via an online toolbox) [26]. Also, facilitating a systematic approach for addressing work participation within PT practice seems valuable. There is also a lack of knowledge about the domain and added value of the WPT and OPT, and a lack of cooperation. Although enhancing the cooperation with the WPT was not a specific need of most of the respondents (only 35.9% mentioned they want more intensive cooperation with a WPT), cooperation between generalist PTs and WPT should be enhanced [17, 26]. To achieve this, an overview or decision tree could be useful. To facilitate cooperation, a role might be played by the professional associations and the individual therapists [26].

It is also recommended to investigate the actual situation in practice by observations or investigation of the medical files. This would allow to explore areas in which generalist PTs might be unaware of missing competences and knowledge. In addition, it would be interesting to examine how generalist PTs in other countries integrate occupational factors within their practice.

Conclusions

This study provides insight into how generalist PTs in the Netherlands currently integrate occupational factors within their practice and also identified their opinions/needs with regard to enhancing the integration of the patient's work within physical therapy practice. Most generalist PTs address occupational factors within their care. However, it seems that occupational factors should me more extensively addressed within physical therapy practice. Many respondents reported that they need more information about work-related factors, laws and regulations, questionnaires, and screening lists. Another need was to have the possibility to bill for a workplace assessment, as well as more knowledge on the domain/position of WPTs and other occupational health professionals. This study also identified a lack of cooperation between generalist PTs and WPTs. The results of this survey can be used to facilitate the integration of occupational factors within physical therapy practice and to enhance cooperation between generalist PTs and WPTs.

Abbreviations

MSDs: Musculoskeletal disorders; OPT: Occupational physical therapist; OPTs: Occupational physical therapists; PT: Physical therapist; PTs: Physical therapists; RTW: Return to work; SD: Standard deviations; WPT: Work-related physical therapist; WPTs: Work-related physical therapists

Acknowledgements

The authors thank all physical therapists who participated in this study.

Funding

This study was funded by the Scientific College Physical Therapy (WCF) of the Royal Dutch Society for Physical Therapy (KNGF).

Authors' contributions

NH, WO, JBS, JE, MN and YH developed the initial study proposal and acquired funding for the study. All authors helped to develop the survey, which was first drafted by WO and NH. WO and NH developed the online survey. All data were analysed by WO and NH. All authors provided valuable input to the design of this paper, which was drafted by WO and NH. All authors commented on the draft versions. All authors have read and approved the final manuscript.

Consent for publication

All participants gave informed consent that their data were used for publication.

Competing interests

The authors declare that they have no competing interests.

Author details

[1]Faculty of Health and Social Studies, Research Group Occupation & Health, HAN University of Applied Sciences, P.O. Box 6960, 6503 GL Nijmegen, Netherlands. [2]Faculty of Health and Social Studies, Physical Therapy, HAN University of Applied Sciences, Nijmegen, Netherlands. [3]Faculty of Health and Social Studies, Research Group Musculoskeletal Rehabilitation, HAN University of Applied Sciences, Nijmegen, Netherlands. [4]Radboud Institute for Health Sciences, IQ Healthcare, Radboud University Medical Center, Nijmegen, Netherlands.

References

1. Shaw WS, Main CJ, Johnston V. Addressing occupational factors in the management of low back pain: implications for physical therapist practice. Phys Ther. 2011;91(5):777–89. https://doi.org/10.2522/ptj.20100263.
2. Vos TB, Barber RM, Bell B, Bertozzi-Villa A, Biryukov S, Bolliger I, et al. Global, regional, and national incidence, prevalence, and years lived with disability for 301 acute and chronic diseases and injuries in 188 countries, 1990-2013: a systematic analysis for the global burden of disease study 2013. Lancet. 2015;386(9995):743–800. doi:10.1016/S0140-6736(15)60692-4.
3. Du S, Yuan C, Xiao X, Chu J, Qiu Y, Qian H. Self-management programs for chronic musculoskeletal pain conditions: a systematic review and meta-analysis. Patient Educ Couns. 2011;85(3):e299–310. doi:10.1016/j.pec.2011.02.021.
4. Health and Safety Executive. Musculoskeletal Disorders in Great Britain 2014. Health and Safety Executive; 2014.
5. World Health Organization. Identification and control of work-related diseases: report of a WHO expert committee [meeting held in Geneva from 28 November to 2 December 1983]. Geneva: World Health Organization; 1985.
6. Public Health Agency of Canada. Economic burden of illness in Canada, 2005–2008. Public Health Agency of Canada; 2014. http://www.phac-aspc.gc.ca/publicat/ebic-femc/2005-2008/assets/pdf/ebic-femc-2005-2008-eng.pdf.
7. Trimbos-instituut. Factsheet ziekteverzuim in Nederland [Factsheet absenteeism in the Netherlands]. Psychische en somatische aandoeningen bij werkenden. Trimbos-instituut; 2013.
8. Australian Institute of Health and Welfare. Australia's health 2016. Australian Institute of Health and Welfare; 2016. http://www.aihw.gov.au/WorkArea/DownloadAsset.aspx?id=60129555788.
9. Huber M, van Vliet M, Giezenberg M, Winkens B, Heerkens Y, Dagnelie PC, et al. Towards a 'patient-centred' operationalisation of the new dynamic concept of health: a mixed methods study. BMJ Open. 2016;6(1):e010091. doi:10.1136/bmjopen-2015-010091.
10. Chorus AM, Miedema HS, Boonen A, Van Der Linden S. Quality of life and work in patients with rheumatoid arthritis and ankylosing spondylitis of working age. Ann Rheum Dis. 2003;62(12):1178–84.
11. Waddell G, Burton AK. Is work good for your well-being? London: The Stationary Office; 2006.
12. van Tulder M, Becker A, Bekkering T, Breen A, del Real MT, Hutchinson A, et al. Chapter 3. European guidelines for the management of acute nonspecific low back pain in primary care. Eur Spine J. 2006;15(Suppl 2):S169–91. doi:10.1007/s00586-006-1071-2.
13. Institute for Safety, Compensation and Recovery Research. New online education program will help physiotherapists promote Return to Work. Institute for Safety, Compensation and Recovery Research; 2016. http://www.iscrr.com.au/about-iscrr/news-and-events/news/2016/online-education-program-physios-rtw.
14. Bishop A, Wynne-Jones G, Lawton SA, van der Windt D, Main C, Sowden G, et al. Rationale, design and methods of the study of work and pain (SWAP): a cluster randomised controlled trial testing the addition of a vocational advice service to best current primary care for patients with musculoskeletal pain (ISRCTN 52269669). BMC Musculoskelet Disord. 2014;15:232. doi:10.1186/1471-2474-15-232.
15. Schaafsma FG, Whelan K, van der Beek AJ, van der Es-Lambeek LC, Ojajarvi A, Verbeek JH. Physical conditioning as part of a return to work strategy to reduce sickness absence for workers with back pain. Cochrane Database Syst Rev. 2013;8:CD001822. doi:10.1002/14651858.CD001822.pub3.
16. Cancelliere C, Donovan J, Stochkendahl MJ, Biscardi M, Ammendolia C, Myburgh C, et al. Factors affecting return to work after injury or illness: best evidence synthesis of systematic reviews. Chiropractic & manual therapies. 2016;24(1):32. doi:10.1186/s12998-016-0113-z.
17. Sociaal Economische Raad. Betere zorg voor werkenden [Better care for workers]. Den Haag: Social and Economic Council of the Netherlands; 2014.
18. Wevers CW, van Genabeek J. Meer oog voor arbeid in de gezondheidszorg [More focus on work in health care]. Hoofddorp TNO; 2010.
19. Johnston V, Nielsen M, Corbiere M, Franche RL. Experiences and perspectives of physical therapists managing patients covered by workers' compensation in Queensland, Australia. Phys Ther. 2012;92(10):1306–15. doi:10.2522/ptj.20110194.
20. Kremer AM, Steenbeek R. Avoidable sickness absence in a Dutch working population. J Occup Rehabil. 2010;20(1):81–9. doi:10.1007/s10926-009-9200-5.
21. Statline. Gezondheid en zorggebruik [Health and use of healthcare]. CBS, Den Haag/Heerlen. 2016. http://statline.cbs.nl/Statweb/publication/?DM=SLNL&PA=83005ned&D1=17-19. Accessed 17 Feb 2017.
22. Peters S, Johnston V. Literature review about physiotherapy in the management of musculoskeletal conditions prepared for the Australian physiotherapy association. St. Lucia: School of Health and Rehabilitation Sciences, The University of Queensland; 2014.
23. Staal JB, De Rijk A, Houkes I, Heymans MW. Clinical interventions to reduce work disability in workers with musculoskeletal disorders or mental health problems. In: JR LPA, editor. Handbook of work disability. New York: Springer; 2013.
24. Coole C, Watson PJ, Drummond A. Staying at work with back pain: patients' experiences of work-related help received from GPs and other clinicians. A qualitative study. BMC Musculoskelet Disord. 2010;11:190. doi:10.1186/1471-2474-11-190.
25. Pincus T, Greenwood L, McHarg E. Advising people with back pain to take time off work: a survey examining the role of private musculoskeletal practitioners in the UK. Pain. 2011;152(12):2813–8. doi:10.1016/j.pain.2011.09.010.
26. Hutting N, Oswald W, Staal JB, Engels JA, Nouwens E, Nijhuis-van der Sanden MWG, et al. Physical therapists and importance of work participation in patients with musculoskeletal disorders: a focus group study. BMC Musculoskelet Disord. 2017;16;18(1):196.
27. NVBF. Occupational and work-related physical therapy. 2011.
28. de Vries H, Mesters I, Riet JV, Willems K, Reubsaet A. Motives of Belgian adolescents for using sunscreen: the role of action plans. Cancer Epidemiol Biomark Prev. 2006;15(7):1360–6. doi:10.1158/1055-9965.EPI-05-0877.
29. Staal JB, Hendriks EJM, Heijmans M, Kiers H, Lutgers-Boomsma AM, Rutten G, et al. KNGF-richtlijn Lage rugpijn [physical therapy guideline low back pain]. Amersfoort: Koninklijk Nederlands Genootschap voor Fysiotherapie; 2013.
30. Gosling C, Keating J, Iles R, Morgan P, Hopmans R. Strategies to enable physiotherapists to promote timely return to work following injury. Frankston Victoria Department of Physiotherapy, Monash University, Australia; 2015.
31. Alexanders J, Anderson A, Henderson S. Musculoskeletal physiotherapists' use of psychological interventions: a systematic review of therapists' perceptions and practice. Physiotherapy. 2015;101(2):95–102. doi:10.1016/j.physio.2014.03.008.
32. Oostendorp RA, Elvers H, Mikolajewska E, Laekeman M, van Trijffel E, Samwel H, et al. Manual physical therapists' use of biopsychosocial history taking in the management of patients with back or neck pain in clinical practice. Sci World J. 2015;2015:170463. doi:10.1155/2015/170463.
33. Wynne-Jones G, van der Windt D, Ong BN, Bishop A, Cowen J, Artus M, et al. Perceptions of health professionals towards the management of back pain in the context of work: a qualitative study. BMC Musculoskelet Disord. 2014;15:210. doi:10.1186/1471-2474-15-210.

3

Comparison between the musician-specific seating position of high string bow players and their habitual seating position – a video raster stereographic study of the dorsal upper body posture

Daniela Ohlendorf[1*], Jennifer Marx[1], Kathrin Clasen[2], Eileen M. Wanke[1], Stefan Kopp[2], David A. Groneberg[1] and Stefanie Uibel[1]

Abstract

Background: Effects of playing high stringed bow instruments on the upper body posture have not been analysed so far. The instrument-specific seating position when playing in an orchestra is compared to the habitual seating position.

Methods: Three dimensional back scans were performed in 13 professional violinists and viola players of a radio orchestra (8 f / 5 m). Trunk position in their habitual seating position and in the instrument- specific seating position imitating playing was compared. Statistical differences were calculated using Wilcoxon Matched Pairs Test with Bonferroni Holm correction.

Results: Significant differences were found between the seated position with instrument and without ($p < 0.001$, 0.03, 0.02 or 0.01) in the spine (trunk length, sagittal trunk decline, lumbar bending angle, maximal rotation, standard deviation rotation, lumbar lordosis), the shoulder (scapula distance, scapula rotation, scapula angle right) and pelvis distance.

Conclusions: Playing an instrument changes the static seating position by increased rotation of the spine and specific shoulder adaptations holding the instrument (left arm) and the bow (right arm), with minor effects on the pelvis. This forced position may result in chronic health effects. The method used in this study is an approach to better understand the involved muscular structures and possible resulting health damages.

Keywords: Stringed bow player, Upper body posture, Three-dimensional back scan, Musician-specific seating position

Background

Professional musicians frequently suffer from ailments due to forced postures demanded by a specific instrument. This has been shown as early as 1985 [1] and 1986 [2] in questionnaire-based surveys and is confirmed in a recent review [3]. Most importantly, the physical demands of playing a specific instrument facilitate musculoskeletal disorders, e.g. by asymmetrical and/or repetitive motions and forced postures [4]. Approximately 50% of professional musicians report these injuries [5, 6], with the highest incidence in high string bow players (viola and violin players) [7]. Künzel [8] reports that 70% of the movement apparatus problems are induced by the typical forced unfavourable playing posture combined with the restricted compensation possibilities.

These problems are especially pronounced in the cervical and lumbar spinal column and the upper extremities [5, 9] as shown in interview- and questionnaire-based studies. In string bow instrumentalists, during their training period, similar physical problems and intensive health impairments have been found in questionnaire studies, partly

* Correspondence: ohlendorf@med.uni-frankfurt.de
[1]Institute of Occupational Medicine, Social Medicine and Environmental Medicine, Goethe-University Frankfurt/Main, Theodor-Stern-Kai 7, Building 9A, 60590 Frankfurt/Main, Germany

necessitating medical treatment [5, 10–15]. If not balanced by muscular activities the resulting posture deviations from the perpendicular line of the body may lead to malpostures and impaired playing ability [5]. These findings emphasize the importance of early preventive measures.

Early in the nineteenth century educational, physiotherapeutic, sports and musician interventions have been developed and implemented [5, 16, 17]. So far, their effectiveness in preventing or treating musician specific ailments has not been proven [5, 10]; modern techniques may be able to show effects of specific interventions for treatment and prevention.

For high string bow musicians, several publications deal with the effects of performing on the movement apparatus [18–23]. Video recordings or motion capture systems were used most often; they document instrument related movements [18–20, 24]. Kruta de Araújo et al. [21] used video detection of angular changes in body sections to record arm and head motions of playing violinists. Subsequent computer based evaluation was able to document posture differences. Due the camera position the video analysis is hampered by their two-dimensional recording planes (horizontal and vertical) [25]. Wasmer & Eickhoff [22] compared violinists in standing and seated playing position. In the playing motion while seated the upper trunk was more and the shoulder section less involved in the playing movements. Even the position of a violinist at the musical stand was important and resulted in different curvatures of the spinal column. Philipson et al. [26] used EMG to show higher activity in the *M. deltoideus*, M. biceps brachii and in the upper section of the M. trapezius in high bow instrumentalists reporting pain than those without pain. Levy et al. [27] compared violinists playing with or without shoulder support and found a reduced EMG activity in M. trapezius, M. sternocleidomastoideus and in the frontal part of *M. deltoideus* but without changes in M. biceps brachii. This is supported in an EMG-study of Berque & Gray [28] with an increased activity in the M. trapezius in pain free musicians, and by Wilkinson & Grimmer [29] quantifying tendon size by ultrasound.

No three-dimensional posture analysis of high string bow players has yet been published which included the differential analysis of all spinal sections as well as the shoulder and pelvis region. However, video raster stereography would allow this analysis. These data will allow the quantification of the strains on the musculoskeletal system and lead the therapy selection. In the present study the upper trunk position of high bow players is measured in their natural position, i.e. seated without an instrument, and compared to their typical playing seated position with their instrument. Using this approach, we will show and quantify the differences in posture within the shoulder, spine, and pelvis parameters.

Material and methods

Subjects

All 13 (8 w / 5 m) professional musicians playing bow instruments (violin / viola) of the "HR 3" radio orchestra in Frankfurt/Main (Germany) participated in this study. The mean age was 43.6 ± 9.9 years (range 32 to 59 years) and they have been playing their instrument for 36.9 ± 9.1 years, 6.12 days per week up to 4.19 h per day. All musicians were right–handed.

Exclusion criteria were acute trauma lesions, e.g. fractures, herniated discs and torn ligaments, surgery within the last six months, analgesics or muscle relaxant medication, genetic muscular or neurological diseases. All participants gave written informed consent to participate in this study, which was approved by the ethics committee of the Medical Faculty of the Goethe-University (Nr. 305/12), in accordance with the 1964 Helsinki Declaration and its later amendments. Furthermore, the individual of Figs. 1 and 2 in this manuscript has given written informed consent to publish these pictures.

Measurement system

The back scanner "ABW-BodyMapper" (ABW GmbH; Frickenhausen / Germany) scanned the upper body posture by video raster stereography (Fig. 1) with 30 frames per second in the standard mode and a maximum of 50 frames per second. The camera resolution was 640–480 pixel over an area of 640 × 400 mm; depth resolution of the resulting image was 1 / 100 mm, lateral resolution < 1 mm as specified by the manufacturer. In repeated measurements using skin markers for reference positions the localization of a given point was accurate by an error margin of < 0.5 mm.

A sensitivity of 98%, a specificity of 84% and 13.9% false-positive values were published for the video raster stereographic survey [30]. Furthermore, raster stereography and radiological angle values presented excellent correlation according to Drerup (correlation coefficient 0.8 to 0.93; Drerup [31, 32]). Six self-adhesive markers were used to indicate anatomical landmarks as shown in Fig. 1. Drerup et al. [33] found this technique to be reliable with an intraindividual variation of 1 mm for the lumbar spine dimple.

This measurement system has been used in several studies [34–38]. It is a fast non-contact method to quantify body posture and it is suitable for measuring pathological postures like scoliosis, kyphosis or leg length discrepancies.

Evaluation parameter

All parameters derived from the marker positions are listed in Table 1.

Investigation protocol

All participants were seated on a regular musician chair and the upper body posture was measured with and

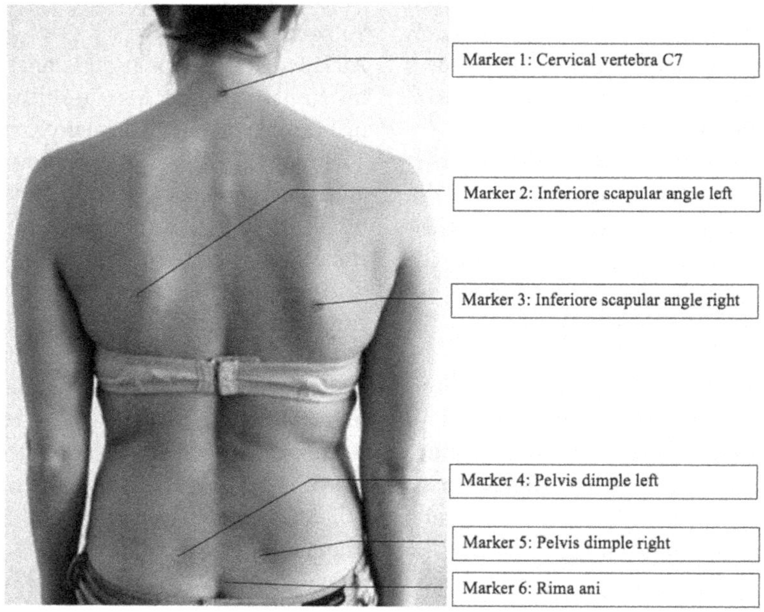

Fig. 1 Location of the 6 marker

without instrument in a randomized order. For measurements in the position without instrument, the markers were fixed on the bare back, and the participants took their preferred position (height, habitus, looking forward and hanging arms) with bared trunk. For measurements with their instrument the participants sat on their chair and played a medium pitch tone in the anticipated loudness "forte" with the middle of the bow. The left hand is placed on the 1st position of the fingerboard. They looked directly at the music stand, which is marked on the wall in front of them (Fig. 2). The posture was scanned for each position for 2 s, 3 scans were taken within 2 min and the parameters were calculated from the average of these data sets. In between the measurements the participants were allowed to relax for at least 2 min, all measurements including preparations lasted no longer than 15 min.

Statistical evaluation

Statistical calculations were performed using the software BiAS 10.03 (Epsilon-Verlag, Darmstadt, Germany). Normal data distribution was tested by Kolmogoroff Smirnoff Lilliefors test. As the data sets were not normally distributed the Wilcoxon-Matched Pairs Test including a Bonferroni-Holm correction was used to test for significance. Significance is assumed at a difference level of 5%; significant differences are gives as: * $= p < 0.05$; ** $= p < 0.01$; *** $= p < 0.001$.

Results

Posture differences in the upper body were quantified by comparing the parameters (Table 1), the results are presented in Table 2. The trunk length D is reduced from position 1 to position 2 with a mean of 497.65 ± 27.85 mm to 490.30 ± 25.22 mm ($p < 0.001$) in the sagittal plane.

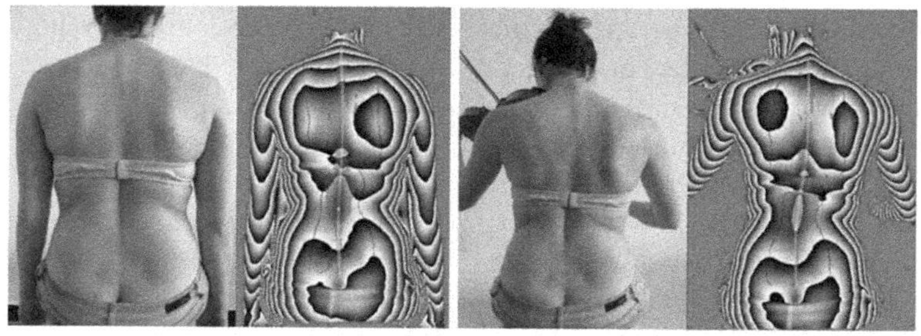

Fig. 2 Group 1: Showing comparative positions 1 / 2

Table 1 List and description of back scan parameters

Parameter	Description
Spine parameter	
Trunk length D (TLD) (mm)	Spatial distance between the markers VP and DM
Trunk length S (TLS) (mm)	Spatial distance between the markers VP and SP
Sagittal trunk decline (STD) (°)	Inclination of the trunk length D marked line from the perpendicular to the sagittal plane. Tilt ventrally (negative values) = flexion Tilt dorsally (positive values) = extension
Frontal trunk decline (FTD) (°)	Inclination of the trunk length D marked line from the perpendicular to the frontal plane. Tilt anteriorly (negative values) = possible lordosis Tilt dorsally (positive values) = possible kyphosis
Axis decline (AD) (°)	Deviation of the line of the area marked by the trunk length D line of the 90° rotated distance DL-DR ➔decline between upper body and pelvis
Thoracic bending angle (TBA) (°)	Deviation of the distance VP - KA from the perpendicular
Lumbar bending angle (LBA) (°)	Deviation of the distance KA - LA from the perpendicular
Standard deviation lateral deviation (SDLD) (mm)	Root mean squared deviation of the median line of the distance VP - DM
Maximal lateral deviation (MLD) (mm)	Maximum deviation of the median line of the distance VP - DM Negative values = deviation to the left Positive values = deviation to the right
Standard deviation rotation (SDR) (°)	Root mean square deviation of surface rotation of the median line (torsion of the spinous processes of the spine)
Maximal rotation (MR) (°)	Maximum positive or negative surface rotation on the median line
Kyphosis angle (KA) (°)	In the sagittal plane measured angle between the upper inflection point of the spine at the thoracolumbar and VP inflection point IP; point of greatest negative surface decline
Lordosis angle (LA) (°)	Angle between the inflection point at DM and the thoracolumbar inflection point IP
Pelvis parameter	
Pelvis distance (PD) (mm)	Spatial distance between SIPS L and SIPS R.
Pelvis height (PH) (°)	Decline of the connecting line between SIPS L and SIPS R to the horizontal in the frontal plane in degrees
Pelvis height (mm)	Decline of the connecting line between SIPS L and SIPS R to the horizontal in the frontal plane in millimeter
Pelvis torsion (°)	Angle between the surface normal on the two dimples SIPS L and SIPS R Negative differential angle = Normal at point SIPS L is stronger upward as at point SIPS R Positive difference angle = Normal at point SIPS L is stronger downward as at point SIPS R.
Pelvis rotation (°)	Rotation of the distance SIPS L – SIPS R in the transversal plane
Shoulder parameter	
Scapular distance (SDI) (mm)	Distance between the left (AISL) and the lower right scapular angle (AISR).
Scapular height (SH) (°)	Height difference between the points AISL and AISR Positive value = AISR higher than AISL Negative value = AISR deeper than AISL
Scapular rotation (SR) (°)	Rotation of the distance DL-DR in the transversal plane
Scapular angle left (SAL) (°) / Scapula angle right (SAR) (°)	Best fit straight line on the shoulders to the horizontal. The center point of the regression line is set vertically above AISL / AISR. The greater the angle, the more caudally located the shoulder.

Concurrently, the trunk length S decreases (position 1: 551.29 ± 30.64 mm; position 2: 542.80 ± 28.24 mm; $p \le 0.001$). Sagittal trunk decline is characterized by a reduction from position 1 (– 7.67 ± 2.16°) to position 2 (– 3.73 ± 2.51°, $p < 0.001$), indicating a lower degree of leaning ventrally of the trunk. The lumbar lordosis increases as seen by the increasing lumbar bending angle from position 1 (6.29 ± 3.83°) to position 2 (8.53° ± 3.83°, $p < 0.03$). Holding the instrument results in an increased spinal rotation to the right; this is seen in the standard deviation rotation and maximal rotation from position 1 (SDR 4.25 ± 2.25°, MR 3.10 ± 7.47°) to position 2 (SDR 7.17 ± 4.84°, MR 12.42 ± 14.16°), with $p < 0.001$ for SDR and $p < 0.01$ for MR.

For the pelvis position a significant change has been found for the pelvis distance, which decreases from 92.46 ± 7.14 mm (position 1) to 91.32 ± 7.48 mm (position 2, $p < 0.02$) indicating an "inflare" motion of the os ilium.

As consequence, shoulder parameters were also effected by holding an instrument. The scapula distance increases from 165.81 mm ± 22.48 mm to 176.98 mm ± 20.62 mm ($p < 0.001$) due to abduced scapulae. The scapula rotation increased as well in position 2 from 2.87 ± 3.18° to 5.76 ± 5.82°, positioning the right angulus inferior scapulae further dorsally than the left one ($p < 0.02$) as caused by a left backward shoulder inclination and rotation). The right scapula angle decreased from 34.04 ± 9.99° to 27.07 ± 5.51° ($p < 0.001$), the positive values indicates a lower right shoulder while playing the instrument. In conclusion, differences in shoulder, spine and pelvis posture are detectable after adjusting to the instrument. All significances are shown graphically in Fig. 3.

Table 2 Mean values (MV) and standard deviations (SD) of the all parameters with respect to position 1 and 2 as well as the calculated *p*-values of the Wilcoxon-Matched-Pairs-Test

Spinal parameters	Position 1		Position 2		*p*-value
Spinal parameters	MV	SD	MV	SD	*p*-value
Trunk length D (mm)	497.65	27.85	490.30	25.22	0.001***
Trunk length S (mm)	551.29	30.64	542.80	28.24	0.001***
Sagittal trunk decline (°)	−7.67	2.16	−3.73	2.51	0.001***
Frontal trunk decline (°)	0.53	1.03	1.34	1.99	0.13
Axis decline (°)	1.21	2.47	2.16	2.59	0.09
Thoracic bending angle (°)	13.53	4.42	14.14	3.33	0.45
Lumbar bending angle (°)	6.29	3.83	8.53	3.83	0.03*
Standard lateral deviation (mm)	3.45	2.37	4.06	3.31	0.64
Maximal lateral deviation (mm)	−3.24	6.31	−0.81	9.27	0.20
Standard deviation rotation (°)	4.25	2.25	7.17	4.84	0.001***
Maximal rotation (°)	3.10	7.47	12.42	14.16	0.01**
Kyphosis angle (°)	48.28	12.84	44.58	13.73	0.76
Lordosis angle (°)	32.89	24.58	24.79	11.10	1.00
Pelvis parameters					
Pelvis distance (mm)	92.46	7.14	91.32	7.48	0.02*
Pelvis height (°)	0.90	2.73	0.91	2.11	0.62
Pelvis height_2 (mm)	1.36	4.38	1.46	3.43	0.97
Pelvis torsion (°)	−0.08	2.23	0.81	3.77	0.42
Pelvis rotation (°)	0.87	3.51	2.41	5.63	0.31
Shoulder parameters					
Scapula distance (mm)	165.81	22.48	176.98	20.62	0.001***
Scapula height (mm)	0.26	8.35	−3.98	11.05	0.09
Scapula rotation (°)	2.87	3.18	5.76	5.82	0.02*
Scapula angle left (°)	29.05	5.55	40.55	19.16	0.13
Scapula angle right (°)	34,04	9,99	27,07	5,51	0.001***

Legend: * = $p < 0.05$; ** = $p < 0.01$; *** = $p < 0.001$

Discussion

The results show that playing a violin or viola induces major changes in the upper body posture. In order to quantify these changes, we compared the upper posture while playing with the participant's habitual upper body posture, which has been chosen as the baseline position.

Playing the instrument increases spinal extension (TLD, TLS, STL), reduces the truncal inclination by spinal flexion (STL), increases lumbar lordosis (LBA) and rotated the upper body to the right (SR).

Habitual seating occurs spontaneously and results in an extension of the pelvis in the iliosacral joints with a corresponding decrease in lumbar lordosis [39]. This position centers the pelvis between the most anterior and the most posterior possible pelvis positions. Although it ideally distributes the static load it is difficult to sustain. However, this position is similar to the seated body position when playing a violin [39, 40].

Holding the instrument with the chin and positioning the left arm under the instrument causes a right sided dorsal upper body rotation. This rotation is increased by the requirement of looking at the centrally placed music stand in our setup, with the head rotated to the left to gaze at the imaginary music stand. This posture also changes the shoulder area as characterized by an abduced scapula (SD), a dorsal right shoulder (SR) and a lowered right shoulder with a cranially positioned scapula (SAR). This necessitates unfamiliar tonicity, especially for the right side and affects the M. levator scapulae and M. trapezius.

The changes in the shoulder area are caused by holding the instrument itself and the bow while playing. The shoulder of the instrument arm (left side) is held with the shoulder flexed, abduced, and externally rotated (Fig. 2).

In the pelvis area only the distance of the upper posterior iliacal crest markers is decreased and causes an "inflare" motion of the os ilium. If this also affects the tonicity it would impair the *M. quadratus* lumborum.

This study shows specific changes in the posture of violinists and viola players. They affect various sections of the upper body including the shoulder, pelvis and spine. Major alterations were observed in the spinal rotation and shoulder position and rotation with smaller effects in the spine length and pelvic distance verifying the working hypothesis. These changes can be explained by the specific demands of violin and viola playing. Corresponding findings were reported by Fishbein [2] and Kok [3]. Since the instrument-specific posture has to be held for many hours every day over many years they may result in chronic health effects.

In further studies, musicians of different playing levels could be differentiated with regard to playing related musculoskeletal disorder [41]. Here, however, the difficulty must be taken into account that professional musicians in particular are scheduled for rehearsals and concerts in such a way that participation in a scientific investigation is not top priority.

Since the physical constitution of the musicians cannot be changed and the postural demands cannot be altered it is advisable to optimize health prevention like as has already been done with exposure factors of farmers or fishermen [42–44]. One possibility would be to use the Cornell Musculoskeletal Discomfort Questionnaire to get a better insight of MSD [45].

Conclusion

Professional musicians often complain about musculoskeletal problems from playing their instrument already early in their professional training [5, 10–15]. The method presented in this study illustrates the magnitude

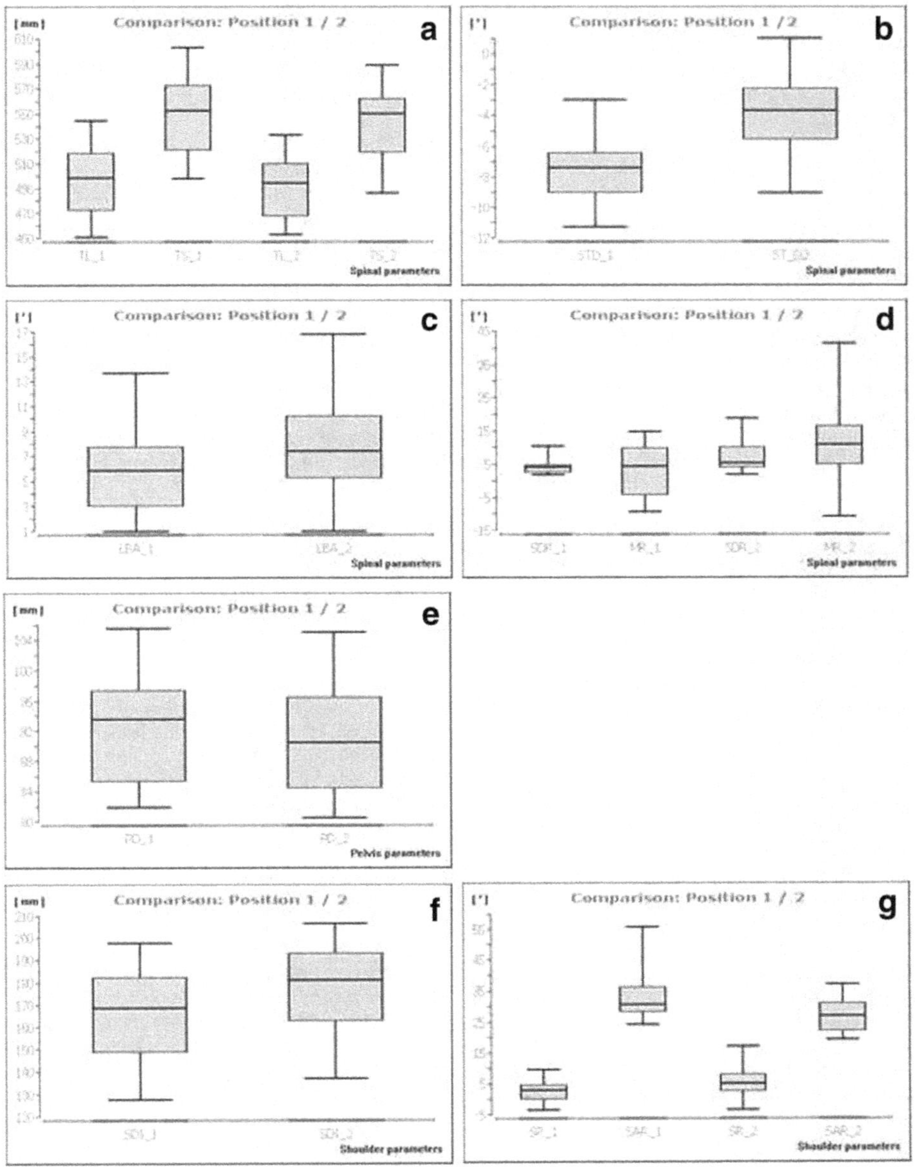

Fig. 3 Upper body posture in high string bow instrument players. Legend: **a** trunk length S/D; **b** sagittal trunk decline; **c** lumbal bending angle; **d** standard deviation of the rotation/maximal rotation; **e** pelvis distance; **f** scapula distance; **g** scapula rotation; scapula angle right; for definition of the parameters see Table 1. Summarizes the significant differences induced when playing the instrument

of the muscular changed in string bow players while playing their instrument. While playing the instrument spinal extension (TLD, TLS, STL) increases, the truncal inclination is reduced by spinal flexion (STL), lumbar lordosis (LBA) is increased and the upper body is rotated to the right (SR). Therefore, this information can be used to support physiotherapeutic treatment and to adjust prevention and/or rehabilitation. Due to the muscular changes that can be detected with this method, it should be discussed in the future whether a physical therapy should be a MUST HAVE for a professional orchestra in the future.

Abbreviation

EMG: Elektromyography

Acknowledgements

Not applicable

Funding

There is no funding.

Authors' contributions

DO, JM, KC, EMW, SK, DAG and SU made substantial contributions to the conception and design of the manuscript, DO, JM and SU made substantial contributions to the construction of the measurement protocol and DO and JM has been involved in the statistical data analysis. All authors have read and approved the final manuscript.

Competing interests

The authors declare that they have no competing interests.

Author details

[1]Institute of Occupational Medicine, Social Medicine and Environmental Medicine, Goethe-University Frankfurt/Main, Theodor-Stern-Kai 7, Building 9A, 60590 Frankfurt/Main, Germany. [2]School of Dentistry, Department of Orthodontics, Goethe University Frankfurt/Main, Theodor-Stern-Kai 7, Building 9A, 60590 Frankfurt am Main, Germany.

References

1. Schmale H, Schmidtke H. Der Orchestermusiker: seine Arbeit u. seine Belastung: eine empirische Untersuchung. Mainz [u.a.]: Schott; 1985.
2. Fishbein M, Middlestadt SE, Ottati V, Straus S, Ellis A. Medical problems among ICSOM musicians: overview of a national survey. Med Probl Perform Art. 1988;3(1):1–8.
3. Kok LM, Huisstede BM, Voorn VM, Schoones JW, Nelissen RG. The occurrence of musculoskeletal complaints among professional musicians: a systematic review. Int Arch Occup Environ Health. 2015;89(3):373–96. https://doi.org/10.1007/s00420-015-1090-6.
4. Lee HS, Park HY, Yoon JO, Kim JS, Chun JM, Aminata IW, Cho WJ, Jeon IH. Musicians' medicine: musculoskeletal problems in string players. Clinics in orthopedic surgery. 2013;5(3):155–60.
5. Spahn C, Blum J. MusikerMedizin: Diagnostik, Therapie und Prävention von musikerspezifischen Erkrankungen. Stuttgart: Schattauer Verlag; 2011.
6. Zaza C. Playing-related musculoskeletal disorders in musicians: a systematic review of incidence and prevalence. CMAJ. 1998;158(8):1019–25.
7. Davies J, Mangion S. Predictors of pain and other musculoskeletal symptoms among professional instrumental musicians: elucidating specific effects. Med Probl Perform Art. 2002;17(4):155–68.
8. Künzel E. Die Anatomie des Geigenspiels: Der Weg zur Überwindung der Geigerschäden. Schneider Verlag: Tutzing; 2002.
9. Blum J. Das Orchester als Ort körperlicher und seelischer Harmonie? Eine Erhebung unter bundesdeutschen Streichern. Das Orchester. 1995;4:23–9.
10. Zander MF. Musiker zwischen Gesundheit und Krankheit: Evaluation des Freiburger Präventionsmodells. In: Freiburger Beiträge zur Musikermedizin. edn. Bochum [u.a.]: Projektverlag; 2006. p. 1–235.
11. Pratt RR, Jessop SG, Niemann BK. Performance related disorders among music majors at Brigham Young university. Int J Arts Med. 1992;1:7–20.
12. Roach KE, Martinez MA, Anderson N. Musculoskeletal pain in student instrumentalists: a comparison with the general student population. Med Probl Perform Art. 1994;9(4):125–30.
13. Spahn C, Richter B, Zschoke I. Health attitudes, preventive behavior, and playing-related health problems among music students. Med Probl Perform Art. 2002;17(1):22–8.
14. Cayea D, Manchester RA. Instrument-specific rates of upper-extremity injuries in music students. Med Probl Perform Art. 1998;13(1):19–25.
15. Larsson LG, Baum J, Mudholkar GS. Nature and impact of musculoskeletal problems in a population of musicians. Med Probl Perform Art. 1993;8(3):73–6.
16. Zaza C. Research-based prevention for musicians. Med Probl Perform Art. 1994;9(1):3–6.
17. van de Klashorst GO. The disposition of the musician. Amsterdam: Broekmans & van Poppel; 2002.
18. Tulchinsky E, Riolo L. A biomechanical motion analysis of the violinist's bow arm. Med Probl Perform Art. 1994;9(4):125–30.
19. Shan G, Visentin P. A quantitative three-dimensional analysis of arm kinematics in violin performance. Med Probl Perform Art. 2003;18(1):3–10.
20. Yagisan N, Karabork H, Goktepe A, Karalezli N. Evalution of three-dimensional motion analysis of the upper right limb movements in the bowing arm of violinists through a digital photogrammetric method. Med Probl Perform Art. 2009;24(4):181–4.
21. Kruta de Araújo NC, Gatto Gárdia MC, Soares Másculo F, Gomes Lucena NM. Analysis of the frequency of postural flaws during violin performance. Med Probl Perform Art. 2009;24(3):108–12.
22. Wasmer C, Eickhoff F. Vergleichende Untersuchungen zur Spielbewegung bei Geigern. In: Freiburger Beiträge zur Musikermedizin edn. Bochum: Projekt Verlag; 2011. p. 1–123.
23. Turner-Stokes L, Reid K. Three-dimensional motion analysis of upper limb movement in the bowing arm of string-playing musicians. Clinical biomechanics (Bristol, Avon). 1999;14(6):426–33.
24. Verrel J, Woollacott M, Lindenberger U. Articulated coordination of the right arm underlies control of bow parameters and quick bow reversals in skilled cello bowing. Front Psychol. 2014;5:885.
25. Buckley T, Manchester R. Overuse injuries in non-classical recreational instrumentalists. Med Probl Perform Art. 2006;21(2):80–7.
26. Philipson L, Sorbye R, Larsson P, Kaladjev S. Muscular load levels in performing musicians as monitored by quantitative electromyography. Med Probl Perform Art. 1990;5(2):79–82.
27. Levy CE, Lee WA, Brandfonbrener AG, Press J, Levy AE. Electromyographic analysis of muscular activity in the upper extremity generated by supporting a violin with and without a shoulder rest. Med Probl Perform Art. 1992;7(4):103–9.
28. Berque P, Gray H. The influence of neck-shoulder pain on trapezius muscle activity among professional violin and viola players. Med Probl Perform Art. 2002;17(2):68–75.
29. Wilkinson M, Grimmer K. Ultrasound of the left shoulder girdle in professional violists and violinists. Med Probl Perform Art. 2001;2(16):58–65.
30. Asamoah V, Mellerowicz H, Venus J, Klockner C. Measuring the surface of the back. Value in diagnosis of spinal diseases. Der Orthopade. 2000;29(6):480–9.
31. Drerup B. Improvements in measuring vertebral rotation from the projections of the pedicles. J Biomech. 1985;18(5):369–78.
32. Drerup B, Hierholzer E. Objective determination of anatomical landmarks on the body surface: measurement of the vertebra prominens from surface curvature. J Biomech. 1985;18(6):467–74.
33. Drerup B, Hierholzer E. Automatic localization of anatomical landmarks on the back surface and construction of a body-fixed coordinate system. J Biomech. 1987;20(10):961–70.
34. Marini I, Alessandri Bonetti G, Bortolotti F, Bartolucci ML, Gatto MR, Michelotti A. Effects of experimental insoles on body posture, mandibular kinematics and masticatory muscles activity. A pilot study in healthy volunteers. J Electromyogr Kinesiol : official journal of the International Society of Electrophysiological Kinesiology. 2015;25(3):531–9.
35. Marini I, Gatto MR, Bartolucci ML, Bortolotti F, Alessandri Bonetti G, Michelotti A. Effects of experimental occlusal interference on body posture: an optoelectronic stereophotogrammetric analysis. J Oral Rehabil. 2013;40(7):509–18.
36. Ohlendorf D, Himmelreich M, Mickel C, Groneberg DA, Kopp S. Does a temporary leg length discrepancy have an influence on upper body posture and lower jaw position in competitive athletes? Sportverletz Sportschaden : Organ der Gesellschaft fur Orthopadisch-Traumatologische Sportmedizin. 2015;29(3):157–63.
37. Ohlendorf D, Turbanski S, Kopp S, Piwowarczyk A. Effects of a temporary asymmetrical occlusion block on upper body posture. J Craniomand Func. 2011;3(4):293–308.
38. Ohlendorf D, Lehmann C, Heil D, Horzer S, Kopp S. The impact of a total hip replacement on jaw position, upper body posture and body sway. Cranio : the journal of craniomandibular practice. 2015;33(2):107–14.
39. Suppé B. FBL Klein-Vogelbach Functional Kinetics: Die Grundlagen: Bewegungsanalyse, Untersuchung, Behandlung, vol. 6. Auflage. Heidelberg: Springer Verlag; 2007.
40. Szende O. Handbuch des Geigenunterrichts. Düsseldorf: Sandvoß, F.K.; 1990.
41. Ohlendorf D, Wanke EM, Filmann N, Groneberg DA, Gerber A. Fit to play: posture and seating position analysis with professional musicians - a study protocol. J Occup Med Toxicol (London, England). 2017;12:5.
42. Berg-Beckhoff G, Ostergaard H, Jepsen JR. Prevalence and predictors of musculoskeletal pain among Danish fishermen - results from a cross-sectional survey. J Occup Med Toxicol (London, England). 2016;11:51.
43. Bhattarai D, Singh SB, Baral D, Sah RB, Budhathoki SS, Pokharel PK. Work-related injuries among farmers: a cross-sectional study from rural Nepal. J Occup Med Toxicol (London, England). 2016;11:48.
44. Girbig M, Freiberg A, Deckert S, Druschke D, Kopkow C, Nienhaus A, Seidler A. Work-related exposures and disorders among physical therapists: experiences and beliefs of professional representatives assessed using a qualitative approach. J Occup Med and Toxicol (London, England). 2017;12:2.

4

Association between mental demands at work and cognitive functioning in the general population – results of the health study of the Leipzig research center for civilization diseases (LIFE)

Francisca S Then[1,2*], Tobias Luck[1,2], Melanie Luppa[1], Katrin Arélin[2,3], Matthias L Schroeter[2,3], Christoph Engel[2,4], Markus Löffler[2,4], Joachim Thiery[5], Arno Villringer[3] and Steffi G Riedel-Heller[1]

Abstract

Background: The level of mental demands in the workplace is rising. The present study investigated whether and how mental demands at work are associated with cognitive functioning in the general population.

Methods: The analysis is based on data of the Health Study of the Leipzig Research Centre for Civilization Disease (LIFE). 2,725 participants aged 40–80 years underwent cognitive testing (Trail-Making Test, Verbal Fluency Test) and provided information on their occupational situation. Participants over the age of 65 years additionally completed the Mini-Mental State Examination. Mental demands at work were rated by a standardized classification system (O*NET). The association between mental demands and cognitive functioning was analyzed using Generalized Linear Modeling (GENLIN) adjusted for age, gender, self-regulation, working hour status, education, and health-related factors.

Results: Univariate as well as multivariate analyses demonstrated significant and highly consistent effects of higher mental demands on better performance in cognitive testing. The results also indicated that the effects are independent of education and intelligence. Moreover, analyses of retired individuals implied a significant association between high mental demands at work of the job they once held and a better cognitive functioning in old age.

Conclusions: In sum, our findings suggest a significant association between high mental demands at work and better cognitive functioning. In this sense, higher levels of mental demands – as brought about by technological changes in the working environment – may also have beneficial effects for the society as they could increase cognitive capacity levels and might even delay cognitive decline in old age.

Keywords: Cognition, Cognitive abilities, Occupation, Work, Demands, Self-regulation, Population-based study

Introduction

There is a continuous trend of rising mental demands in the general working environment, particularly in economically advanced countries [1]. The shift away from physical jobs to occupations with higher mental demands apparently encompasses all educational groups [2]. The motor of this shift seems to be skill-based technological changes which bring about a greater contingent of professional, technical, and associate jobs [1]. The ongoing accelerated technological advances push companies to compete at increased quality standards which then involve higher mental demands for the worker [3]. The trend of increasing levels of mental demands in the working environment raises the question of how mental work demands may affect the individual.

High mental demands encountered on a daily level, as in the workplace, might exert a harmful or beneficial effect on cognitive functioning. Experimental studies, for example, have shown that very demanding tasks lead to decrements of performance in cognitive testing (e.g.,

* Correspondence: francisca.then@medizin.uni-leipzig.de
[1]Institute of Social Medicine, Occupational Health and Public Health (ISAP), Medical Faculty, University of Leipzig, Philipp-Rosenthal-Str. 55, 04103 Leipzig, Germany
[2]LIFE – Leipzig Research Center for Civilization Diseases, University of Leipzig, Leipzig, Germany

[4-6]). Moreover, high mental demands might embody a stressor that, if chronic, could impair cognitive functioning [7]. However, studies have shown that whether high mental demands really impair cognitive performance depends on task difficulty and neuroendocrinological effects [8]. Hence, it is possible that – under particular conditions – high mental demands can affect cognitive functioning in a harmful manner. On the other hand, there is evidence that high mental demands may have a beneficial effect on cognitive functioning. Findings of epidemiologic studies in the elderly (aged 70 years or older) imply that individuals with mentally demanding jobs may have a lower risk of cognitive impairment in old age [9,10] and a reduced risk of dementia [11,12]. Similarly, studies examining manual work [13,14] or complexity of work tasks [15,16] suggest that lower mental demands at work may be associated with a higher dementia risk. Essentially, mental activity throughout the life-course is thought to build up a cognitive reserve that enhances the capacity of the cerebral neural network to efficiently compensate for pathogenic damages and, thus, delays the symptomatic onset of severe neuropsychiatric diseases such as dementia [17]. The motivational reserve model adds another component to the cognitive reserve: It argues that innate motivation determines the amount of highly demanding conditions confronted with during life [18]. Hence, a high motivational reserve seems to reduce the risk of cognitive impairment in old age [19]. In light of the available research results, we are faced with two sets of studies predicting either a harmful or a beneficial effect of mental demands at work on cognitive functioning.

Considering evidence on a beneficial effect of high mental demands on cognitive functioning, we need to be aware that these studies have all been conducted in the elderly population. Evidence for younger individuals is extremely sparse – nonetheless, it is extremely important because, if mental demands impact cognitive functioning, then they do that already when the individuals are still an active part of the workforce. Moreover, evidence on a beneficial effect of high mental demands on cognitive functioning in population-based studies commonly involves threshold level examinations (either by a clinical diagnosis or by using cutoffs). These types of analyses may be difficult to interpret in particular for individuals with initially poorer performance skills (e.g., low education). Analyzing effects on cognitive functioning in a dimensional space (using metric variables; as experimental studies do) could add valuable insights. Hence, the present study aimed at examining cognitive functioning via dimensional measures in a population-based sample of individuals aged 40–80 years old.

In addition, we considered it as relevant that the present study applied a comprehensive and objective definition of mental demands at work. Previous studies investigated either very specific types of mental demands at work (i.e., complexity with people, time pressure, etc.) or a crude indicator of mental demands (i.e., manual vs. non-manual labor, Dictionary of Occupational Titles, etc.). Then again other studies used subjective assessment methods for job demands by asking the participants, for example, how intellectually stimulating they perceive their job to be. Subjective assessment of job demands, however, could be biased. In the present study, we therefore focused on a comprehensive as well as objective indication of mental demands at work.

As the currently available evidence on high mental demands predicts two different outcomes, either a detrimental or a beneficial effect on cognitive functioning, the present study investigated the association between mental demands at work and cognitive functioning in a representative sample of the general population aged 40–80 years old.

Methods

Study design

The health study of the Leipzig Research Centre for Civilization Diseases (LIFE) is a large population-based study of a representative sample of the inhabitants of the city of Leipzig in Germany. An age- and gender-stratified random selection of inhabitants aged 40 to 80 years old was obtained from the population registry office. The target sample of the LIFE study is 10,000 participants with 1,250 participants per 5-year age group of which 50% are male and 50% are female. The only exclusion criterion is not being pregnant. Letters of invitation to participate in the study were sent out by mail. By February 2013, 11,825 letters of invitation were sent out. Of the invited individuals, 3,101 already participated in the study and about 30% refused participation. The recruitment process is still ongoing and response of the remaining invited individuals is pending. At the study center, the participants filled out an informed consent form. They then underwent a set of assessment batteries, including structured interviews (socio-demographic information, medical history, medications, and lifestyle factors like tobacco, alcohol, physical activity, sleep, eating behavior) and medical examinations (anthropometry, blood samples, cognitive functioning, heart anatomy & functioning, allergy, eye assessment, and others). The participants received a financial compensation of 20€.

The study was approved by the ethics committee of the University of Leipzig.

Assessment of cognitive functioning

The assessment of cognitive functioning was always performed in the morning in an interview setting in a separate enclosed room. The instructions for the examiners were computerized and the examiners documented the participants' results in an electronic data mask. All participants at the LIFE study center were asked to take part in the interview assessing cognitive performance level via the Trail Making Test (TMT) and the Verbal Fluency Test (VFT) - both subtests of the neuropsychological test battery of the Consortium to Establish a Registry for Alzheimer's disease (CERADplus) [20-22]. All participants aged 65 years or older were asked to take part in an additional cognitive assessment at another day, which included the Mini-Mental State Examination (MMSE). The TMT is a test measuring the cognitive abilities working memory, task-switching ability [23,24] and executive control [25,26]. Furthermore, the TMT is an extensively used neuropsychological assessment for individuals of all age groups [24,27]. In the TMT, the participants have to connect numbers in an ascending order as fast as they can. The version B of the TMT has an increased task difficulty: The participants have to connect numbers and letters alternatingly. The participant's score is the number of seconds needed to complete the test. A smaller score signifies a better cognitive functioning and a high score a poor cognitive functioning. The VFT measures verbal abilities, semantic fluency, and semantic memory [28,29]. In clinical practice, the VFT is used to assess cerebral lesions and progressive degenerating disorders for patients of all ages [30,31]. In the VFT, the participants have to name as many animals as possible in one minute. The score equals the number of correct animals named. A higher score represents a better cognitive functioning and a low score indicates a poor cognitive functioning. The MMSE is a screening tool for dementia and was completed only by participants over the age of 65 years. It contains 30 items that assess the level of global cognitive functioning. The highest possible score is 30, which indicates better cognitive functioning.

Participants who had difficulties completing the test (visual impairments, tremor, exhausted from a nightshift, etc.) or who had difficulties understanding the instructions due to language problems or with interruptions during the testing session were excluded from the analysis (n = 91). We also excluded individuals with chronic neuropsychiatric diseases/disorders, i.e., dementia, Parkinson's disease, epilepsy, polyneuropathy, muscle atrophy, multiple sclerosis, schizophrenia, narcolepsy, or others (n = 83).

Occupational information

Information on the participants' occupation was obtained in personal standardized interview. The participants were asked "Are you temporarily working?", "If yes, how many hours a week are you working?", and "What occupational title has the job that you are/were mainly working in?".

For the analysis, we first matched the participants' occupations to O*NET 17.0 standard occupational classification categories (www.onetonline.org). The O*NET database was developed by the US Department of Labor/Employment and Training Administration (USDOL/ETA) and provides a comprehensive set of occupational descriptors indicating worker characteristics, worker requirements, experience requirements, occupational requirements, workforce characteristics, and occupation-specific information for every type of occupation. The process of matching the participants' occupations to O*NET codes was subject to stringent criteria such as corresponding task descriptions, comparable levels of responsibilities, and equivalent technical equipment used. Some participants could not be matched to an O*NET code since they did not provide their occupational title (n = 32) or there was no corresponding occupational group in the O*NET database (n = 10). These occupational groups included "master", "helping my husband", "service provider", "demonstration worker", and "expert". Furthermore, some O*NET codes (e.g., 11–9199.00 "Managers, All Other", 21–2011.00 "Clergy", 15–1143.01 "Telecommunications Engineering Specialists") had an incomplete set of O*NET descriptors and hence could not be used for analysis. All together n = 202 participants had to be excluded from analysis due to incomplete occupational data.

In a second step, we created an index of mental demands by using all O*NET descriptor variables of "Cognitive Abilities" at work (O*NET variables 1.A.1.a - 1.A.1.g.2, see Appendix). In order to obtain the index of mental demands, the average of these variables was calculated. The cronbach's alpha of the index of mental demands was 0.97, respectively. We then categorized the mental demands in three categories: high, medium, and low demands.

In a last step, we additionally created an index of self-regulation at work by calculating the averages of the O*NET descriptor variables that describe job requirements with a high degree of self-regulation (O*NET

Table 1 Correlations between the dependent variables

	Mental demands	Age	Self-regulation	Intelligence	Working hours status	Education
Mental demands§	1	0.169***	0.183***	0.280***	0.056**	0.461***
Age§	0.169***	1	−0.071***	0.178***	0.719***	0.092***
Self-regulation§	0.183***	−0.071***	1	0.084***	−0.086***	0.226***
Intelligence§	0.280***	0.178***	0.084***	1	0.035	0.452***
Working hour status#	0.056***	0.719***	−0.086***	0.035	1	−0.032
Education#	0.461***	0.092***	0.226***	0.452***	−0.032	1

Notes: § - Pearson's correlation, # - Spearman-Rho correlation, level of significance: **p < 0.01, ***p < 0.001.

Table 2 Prevalence of health-related events by the level of mental demands at work

	Diabetes	High blood pressure	Stroke	Liver disease	Elevated blood lipids	Stroke
Mental demands (low)	*14.9%***	48.0%	4.3%	8.6%	40.6%	3.4%
Mental demands (middle)	*10.8%*	48.9%	2.7%	11.8%	36.2%	2.1%
Mental demands (high)	*15.3%*	52.1%	3.4%	12.3%	40.0%	2.4%
Demands & education (low & low)	*14.9%**	*48.5%**	5.1%	9.0%	44.0%	3.8%
Demands & education (middle & low)	*13.0%*	*49.2%*	2.5%	9.6%	37.8%	2.7%
Demands & education (middle & middle OR high & low)	*11.2%*	*49.9%*	3.3%	12.6%	35.6%	1.5%
Demands & education (high & middle)	*9.0%*	*47.3%*	2.3%	12.4%	34.3%	2.2%
Demands & education (high & high)	*16.1%*	*54.4%*	4.0%	14.0%	42.4%	2.0%

Notes: level of significance by Pearson's x^2-test: *p < 0.05, **p < 0.01, ***p < 0.001.

Table 3 Cognitive functioning of the study sample according to socio-demographic and work-related characteristics

	n (%)	Trail making test - B mean (SD)	Verbal fluency mean (SD)
Female§	1500 (51.2)	*87.98 (45.64)****	*23.85 (6.12)***
Male	1427 (48.8)	*97.97 (52.70)*	*23.20 (6.32)*
Age (70–79 years)#	680 (23.2)	*116.79 (57.00)****	*22.19 (5.86)****
Age (60–69 years)	867 (29.6)	*99.81 (49.00)*	*22.92 (5.95)*
Age (50–59 years)	776 (26.5)	*82.96 (40.40)*	*23.74 (6.30)*
Age (40–49 years)	604 (20.6)	*68.58 (35.09)*	*25.64 (6.31)*
Education (high)#	957 (32.9)	*82.33 (38.06)****	*25.24 (6.25)****
Education (middle)	836 (28.7)	*93.40 (46.71)*	*23.61 (5.92)*
Education (low)	1119 (38.2)	*101.66 (57.87)*	*22.04 (6.06)*
Not working#	1487 (51.1)	*109.22 (55.20)****	*22.41 (5.95)****
Working <15h/week	54 (1.8)	*95.20 (53.67)*	*23.84 (6.00)*
Working 15-34h/week	275 (9.4)	*78.67 (36.64)*	*25.44 (6.83)*
Working 35 + h/week	1096 (37.6)	*74.30 (34.00)*	*24.61 (6.17)*
Demands (high)#	379 (13.9)	*87.58 (38.85)****	*24.31 (6.34)****
Demands (medium)	1997 (84.3)	*91.59 (48.85)*	*23.70 (6.13)*
Demands (low)	344 (12.6)	*105.52 (59.78)*	*21.69 (6.06)*
Self-regulation (high)#	199 (7.3)	*82.09 (41.54)****	*26.04 (6.09)****
Self-regulation (medium)	2295 (84.3)	*92.18 (48.63)*	*23.48 (6.17)*
Self-regulation (low)	230 (8.4)	*108.08 (58.75)*	*21.91 (5.99)*
Stroke (no)§	2819 (97.7)	*92.10 (48.18)****	*23.61 (6.19)****
Stroke (yes)	66 (2.3)	*130.27 (81.01)*	*21.14 (7.10)*
Blood lipids (normal)§	1665 (63.0)	*89.88 (48.23)****	*23.98 (6.23)****
Blood lipids (elevated)	976 (37.0)	*99.26 (51.52)*	*22.99 (6.17)*
Liver disease (no)§	2368 (88.7)	*93.09 (50.15)***	*23.64 (6.26)*
Liver disease (yes)	301 (11.3)	*98.32 (49.61)*	*23.09 (5.96)*
Heart attack (no)§	2792 (69.9)	*92.36 (49.48)****	*23.62 (6.20)**
Heart attack (yes)	88 (3.1)	*109.82 (45.44)*	*21.89 (6.39)*
Blood pressure (normal)§	1391 (50.9)	*85.61 (45.16)****	*24.16 (6.29)****
Blood pressure (high)	1340 (49.1)	*100.98 (52.55)*	*22.96 (6.09)*
Diabetes (no)§	2534 (88.0)	*90.87 (48.37)****	*23.75 (6.23)****
Diabetes (yes)	346 (12.0)	*108.01 (54.74)*	*22.13 (5.91)*

Notes: SD standard deviation, § - Mann–Whitney-U-Test, # - Kruskal-Wallis-Test, level of significance: *p < 0.05, **p < 0.01, ***p < 0.001.

variables 1.C.4.a Self-Control, 1.C.4.b Stress-Tolerance, 1. C.4.c Adaptability/Flexibility). The cronbach's alpha of the self-regulation index was 0.88. We also categorized the self-regulation index in three categories: high, medium, and low.

Statistical analyses

All statistical analyses were conducted using SPSS (Version 20).

To test for group differences, Mann–Whitney-U-Tests, Kruskal-Wallis-Tests, and Pearson's x^2-tests were performed as appropriate. The intercorrelation of the dependent variables was significant but the coefficients were low (see Table 1). Yet in order to avoid problems of multicollinearity, we (i) categorized the dependent variables, (ii) used a very large sample size, and additionally (iii) combined the variables demands and education in one variable.

Associations between mental demands and cognitive functioning were analyzed using Generalized Linear Modeling (GENLIN). An advantage of GENLIN is that it can be performed even when the distribution deviates from normal. In Model 1, the main effect of mental demands (low/medium/high) on cognitive functioning (score in TMT-B and VFT) was investigated. In Model 2, main effects of mental demands (low/medium/high) were adjusted for age (40-49/50-59/60-69/70-79), gender (female/male), self-regulation (low/medium/high), working hours status (not working/<15 h per week/15-34 h per week/35 + h per week), the level of education completed (primary/secondary/tertiary), having had a stroke (yes/no), having had a heart attack (yes/no), having had a liver disease (yes/no), and having high blood pressure (yes/no), elevated blood lipids (yes/no), and diabetes (yes/no). Information on the individuals' health was obtained in a personal interview by the questions "Have you even been diagnosed with stroke/ heart attack/ liver disease/ high blood pressure/ elevated blood lipids/ diabetes?" In Model 3, we additionally analyzed additive effects of the level of education and mental demands. An additive score of education and demands was created by 1) scoring education and mental demands and 2) adding the scores. Scores were the following: primary education = 1, secondary education = 2, tertiary education = 3, low demands = 1, medium demands = 2, high demands = 3. The scores were added, so that each individual received one additive score for education and demands. For example, an individual with only primary education (=1) and a job with low mental demands (=1) received an additive score of 2. A person with completed tertiary education (=3) and a job with high mental demands (=3) received an additive score of 6. Possible additive scores comprised: 2 – primary education and low demands, 3 – primary education and medium demands, or secondary education and low demands, 4 – primary education and high demands, or secondary education and medium demands, or tertiary education and low demands, 5 – secondary education and high demands, or tertiary education and medium demands, 6 – tertiary education and high demands.

We conducted two further analyses: First, we addressed the potential impact of intelligence on the association

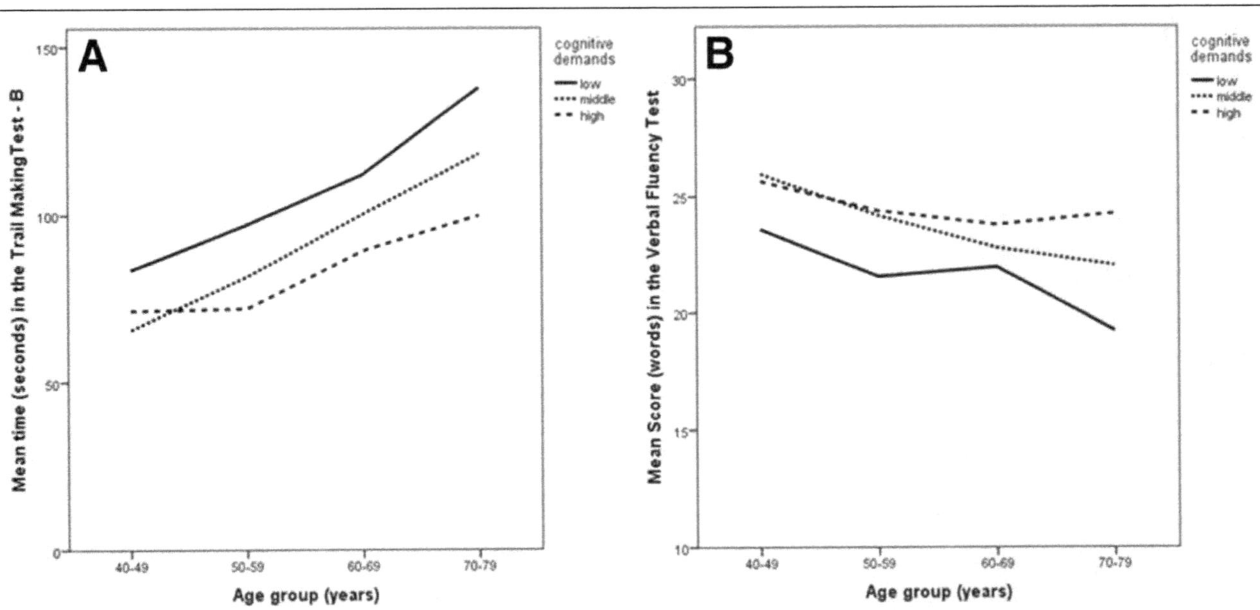

Figure 1 Means in cognitive testing (Trail Making Test - B and Verbal Fluency Test) by the level of demands over the age groups. **A.** Mean seconds needed to complete the Trial Making Test - B with lower scores indicating a better performance. **B.** Mean number of words named in the Verbal Fluency Test with higher scores indicating a better performance.

Table 4 Generalized linear model analysis on the effect of mental demands at work on cognitive functioning

	Model 1				Model 2					Model 3			
	Trail making test - B		Verbal fluency		Trail making test - B		Verbal fluency			Trail making test - B		Verbal fluency	
	β	p	β	P	β	p	β	p		β	p	β	P
Constant	4.659	0.000	3.077	0.000	4.437	0.000	3.126	0.000	Constant	4.422	0.000	3.130	0.000
Demands (high)	−0.186	0.000	0.114	0.000	−0.161	0.000	0.068	0.002	Demands & education (high & high)	−0.346	0.000	0.192	0.000
Demands (medium)	−0.141	0.000	0.089	0.000	−0.096	0.000	0.047	0.005	Demands & education (high & middle)	−0.257	0.000	0.158	0.000
Demands (low)	REF		REF		REF		REF		Demands & education (middle & middle OR high & low)	−0.160	0.000	0.094	0.000
Age (70–79 years)					0.406	0.000	−0.120	0.000	Demands & education (middle & low)	−0.067	0.036	0.048	0.020
Age (60–69 years)					0.292	0.000	−0.098	0.000	Demands & education (low & low)	REF		REF	
Age (50–59 years)					0.189	0.000	−0.076	0.000	Age (70–79)	0.406	0.000	−0.121	0.000
Age (40–49 years)					REF		REF		Age (60–69)	0.291	0.000	−0.098	0.000
Female					−0.103	0.000	0.019	0.078	Age (50–59)	0.188	0.000	−0.076	0.000
Male					REF		REF		Age (40–49)	REF		REF	
Self-regulation (high)					−0.071	0.089	0.080	0.003	Female	−0.101	0.000	0.019	0.078
Self-regulation (medium)					−0.029	0.338	0.016	0.410	Male	REF		REF	
Self-regulation (low)					REF		REF		Self-regulation (high)	−0.079	0.058	0.081	0.003
Not working					0.167	0.000	−0.028	0.090	Self-regulation (medium)	−0.033	0.269	0.014	0.478
Working <15h/week					0.145	0.023	−0.020	0.624	Self-regulation (low)	REF		REF	
Working 15-34h/week					0.048	0.107	0.042	0.026	Not working	0.169	0.000	−0.029	0.085
Working 35 + h/week					REF		REF		Working <15h/week	0.144	0.024	−0.020	0.610
Education (high)					−0.194	0.000	0.120	0.000	Working 15-34h/week	0.050	0.093	0.042	0.027
Education (medium)					−0.070	0.001	0.052	0.000	Working 35 + h/week	REF		REF	
Education (low)					REF		REF		Stroke (yes)	0.115	0.038	−0.028	0.414
Stroke (yes)					0.112	0.042	−0.028	0.428	Stroke (no)	REF		REF	
Stroke (no)					REF		REF		Blood lipids (elevated)	−0.015	0.393	−0.006	0.568
Blood lipids (elevated)					−0.015	0.397	−0.006	0.580	Blood lipids (normal)	REF		REF	
Blood lipids (normal)					REF		REF		Liver disease (yes)	0.022	0.379	−0.004	0.817
Liver disease (yes)					0.022	0.380	−0.004	0.787	Liver disease (no)	REF		REF	
Liver disease (no)					REF		REF		Heart attack (yes)	0.009	0.842	−0.026	0.380
Heart attack (yes)					0.006	0.890	−0.027	0.370	Heart attack (no)	REF		REF	
Heart attack (no)					REF		REF		Blood pressure (high)	0.009	0.617	0.000	0.970
Blood pressure (high)					0.009	0.597	0.000	0.984	Blood pressure (normal)	REF		REF	

Table 4 Generalized linear model analysis on the effect of mental demands at work on cognitive functioning *(Continued)*

Blood pressure (normal)	REF		REF		Diabetes (yes)	0.019	0.474	−0.027	0.101
Diabetes (yes)	0.018	0.500	−0.026	0.117	Diabetes (no)	REF		REF	
Diabetes (no)	REF		REF						

Notes: β - regression coefficient, p - level of significance, *REF* reference category.

between mental demands and cognitive functioning. Thus, we additionally adjusted Model 3 for estimated intelligence as measured by the German Version of the Mill Hill Vocabulary Scale [32]. Secondly, we were interested in possible long-term effects of mental demands at work on cognitive functioning. In order to evaluate whether there might be a long-term effect, we included only participants that were over the age of 65 and examined the association between the level of mental demands of the job that they had before retirement and current cognitive functioning as measured by the MMSE. The association was analyzed in the same types of models (Models 2 &-3) as described above.

Results

Within the final sample (n = 2,725), 13.9% of the participants had jobs with high mental demands, 84.3% jobs with medium mental demands, and 12.6% jobs with low mental demands. Examples of jobs with high mental demands included chief executives, physicists, civil engineers, manufacturing engineering technologists, mathematicians, and others. Medium levels of mental demands at work are faced by participants in jobs such as administrative service managers, archivists, graphic designers, dispatchers, preschool teachers, or electrical power-line installers, etc. Jobs with low mental demands were, for example, stock clerks, packers, slaughterers, janitors, bartenders, or maids.

Within the group of participants in jobs with high mental demands, 9.6% had completed primary education, 24.6% secondary education, and 65.8% tertiary education. Of participants in jobs with medium levels of mental demands, 36.2% had completed primary education, 30.9% secondary education, and 32.8% tertiary education. Regarding, however, the participants in jobs with low mental demands, 66.9% had completed primary education, 27.9% secondary education, and 5.2% tertiary education.

The prevalence of having had a stroke, a heart attack, liver disease, high blood pressure or elevated blood lipids did not differ significantly by the level of mental demands at work (see Table 2). However, individuals in jobs with medium levels of mental demands had significantly lower rates of diabetes (10.8%) than individuals in jobs with low (14.9%) or high metal demands (15.3%).

Findings on cognitive functioning of the study population are shown in Table 3. Participants who worked in jobs with high mental demands had significantly better scores in the cognitive tests TMT-B and VFT than participants who worked in jobs with low mental demands ($p < 0.001$). Moreover, participants who were younger, female, who worked fulltime, had a better health status, a higher education, and worked in a job with a higher self-regulation level performed also significantly better in the cognitive tests ($p < 0.01$) (Figure 1).

Findings of univariate analyses using GENLIN modeling supported such a significant association between higher mental demands and better cognitive functioning ($p < 0.001$ for scores in the TMT-B and VFT; see Table 4, Model 1). The associations remained significant after adjustment for age, gender, self-regulation, working status, level of education, having had a stroke, heart attack, liver disease, high blood pressure, elevated blood lipids, and diabetes (see Table 4, Model 2). In the multivariate model (Model 2), also a high level of education and a younger age was also significantly associated with better scores in cognitive testing. Moreover, we found significantly lower scores in the TMT-B in individuals with male gender and who have had a stroke or were not working (see Table 4).

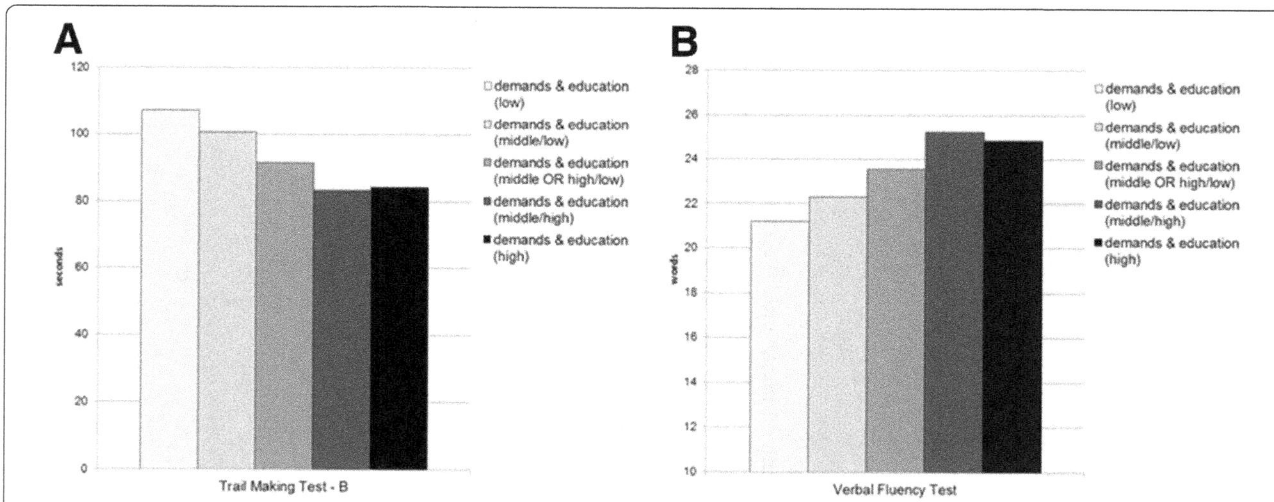

Figure 2 Means in cognitive testing (Trail Making Test - B and Verbal Fluency Test) by the level of demands and education. A. Mean seconds needed to complete the Trial Making Test - B with lower scores indicating a better performance. **B**. Mean number of words named in the Verbal Fluency Test with higher scores indicating a better performance.

In a third GENLIN model, we inspected a potential additive effect of mental demands and education on cognitive functioning (Model 3). We observed a highly significant additive effect of mental demands and education on better performance in the TMT-B and VFT ($p < 0.001$; see Table 4). The effect sizes of the factors in Model 3 were comparable to those in Model 2. The means in cognitive testing (TMT-B, VFT) by the level of demands and education are shown in Figure 2.

In order to dismiss a potential influence of intelligence on the association between mental demands and cognitive functioning, we included intelligence as independent variable in the GENLIN Model 3. The association between mental demands as well as education and cognitive functioning remained significant after including IQ in the model (see Table 5).

In a last step, we were interested in possible long-term effects of mental demands at work on cognitive functioning. Thus, in a subset of participants that were over the age of 65 years (mean age = 71; n = 422), we examined the association between the level of mental demands of the job that they had before retirement and current cognitive functioning as measured by the MMSE. Results are shown in Table 6 (Model 4 and 5). Model 4 shows significant associations between higher MMSE scores and high mental demands at work ($p = 0.010$), a high educational level ($p = 0.003$), NOT having had a stroke ($p = 0.025$), and NOT having elevated blood lipids ($p = 0.049$). Model 5 shows the same associations with a strong additive effect of mental demands and education ($p < 0.001$) – indicating that having had a job with high mental demands and having a high educational level is associated with a better cognitive functioning in old age.

Table 5 Generalized linear model analysis on the effect of mental demands at work on cognitive functioning, including intelligence as covariate

	Model 3			
	Trail making Test - B		Verbal fluency	
	β	p	β	P
Constant	4.473	0.000	3.070	0.000
Demands & education (high & high)	*−0.189*	*0.000*	*0.135*	*0.000*
Demands & education (high & middle)	*−0.124*	*0.001*	*0.092*	*0.000*
Demands & education (middle & middle OR high & low)	*−0.072*	*0.052*	*0.062*	*0.018*
Demands & education (middle & low)	*−0.046*	*0.202*	*0.035*	*0.167*
Demands & education (low & low)	REF		REF	
Age (70–79)	*0.312*	*0.000*	*−0.113*	*0.000*
Age (60–69)	*0.286*	*0.000*	*−0.101*	*0.000*
Age (50–59)	*0.170*	*0.000*	*−0.063*	*0.000*
Age (40–49)	REF		REF	
Female	*−0.104*	*0.000*	0.030	0.015
Male	REF		REF	
Self-regulation (high)	−0.053	0.235	0.057	0.071
Self-regulation (medium)	−0.004	0.916	−0.005	0.833
Self-regulation (low)	REF		REF	
Not working	*0.076*	*0.003*	0.002	0.928
Working <15h/week	−0.086	0.235	−0.045	0.365
Working 15-34h/week	−0.031	0.277	*0.044*	*0.031*
Working 35+h/week	REF		REF	
Intelligence (high)	*−0.296*	*0.000*	*0.220*	*0.000*
Intelligence (middle)	*−0.187*	*0.000*	*0.119*	*0.000*
Intelligence (low)	REF		REF	
Stroke (yes)	−0.038	0.572	0.020	0.662
Stroke (no)	REF		REF	
Blood lipids (elevated)	0.008	0.671	−0.021	0.106
Blood lipids (normal)	REF		REF	
Liver disease (yes)	0.037	0.180	−0.001	0.974
Liver disease (no)	REF		REF	
Heart attack (yes)	−0.048	0.420	0.029	0.493
Heart attack (no)	REF		REF	
Blood pressure (high)	0.012	0.541	−0.003	0.850
Blood pressure (normal)	REF		REF	
Diabetes (yes)	0.033	0.272	−0.038	0.076
Diabetes (no)	REF		REF	

Notes: β - regression coefficient, p - level of significance, REF - reference category.

Discussion

Our study aimed at examining the association between mental demands at work and cognitive functioning in the general population. Univariate as well as multivariate findings consistently demonstrated significant associations between higher mental demands and a better performance in cognitive tests. The results also indicate that the effects are independent of education. The data revealed no interaction effects but additive effects, meaning that high mental demands at work seem to be associated with cognitive functioning *additionally* to the level of education. Moreover, analyses of retired individuals confirmed a significant association between high mental demands at work and a better cognitive functioning in old age. Hence, it may be possible that jobs with high mental demands may constitute a beneficial factor for cognitive functioning in old age.

A possible explanation for the observed findings is that high mental demands at work might function like a training of cognitive abilities. A great number of studies indicated that cognitive abilities generally can be trained (e.g., [33,34]). Training effects, however, strongly depend on the level of demands: it has been demonstrated experimentally that only in high demand conditions participants can actually improve their performance [35].

Table 6 Generalized linear model analysis of mental demands at work before retirement on cognitive functioning in old age (65+ years)

	Model 4			Model 5	
	MMSE			MMSE	
	β	p		β	p
Constant	3.284	0.000	Constant	3.261	0.000
Demands (high)	*0.036*	*0.010*	Demands & education (high & high)	*0.082*	*0.000*
Demands (medium)	*0.027*	*0.031*	Demands & education (high & middle)	*0.072*	*0.000*
Demands (low)	REF		Demands & education (middle & middle OR high & low)	*0.046*	*0.005*
			Demands & education (middle & low)	*0.052*	*0.002*
Age (70–79 years)	0.002	0.734	Demands & education (low & low)	REF	
Age (60–69 years)	REF				
Female	0.010	0.111	Age (70–79)	0.002	0.727
Male	REF		Age (60–69)	REF	
Self-regulation (high)	0.026	0.100	Female	0.011	0.075
Self-regulation (medium)	0.014	0.229	Male	REF	
Self-regulation (low)	REF		Self-regulation (high)	0.027	0.082
Education (high)	*0.023*	*0.003*	Self-regulation (medium)	0.013	0.248
Education (medium)	−0.002	0.767	Self-regulation (low)	REF	
Education (low)	REF		Stroke (yes)	*−0.041*	*0.021*
Stroke (yes)	*−0.040*	*0.025*	Stroke (no)	*REF*	
Stroke (no)	REF		Blood lipids (elevated)	0.011	0.060
Blood lipids (elevated)	*0.012*	*0.049*	Blood lipids (normal)	REF	
Blood lipids (normal)	REF		Liver disease (yes)	0.003	0.726
Liver disease (yes)	0.003	0.724	Liver disease (no)	REF	
Liver disease (no)	REF		Heart attack (yes)	−0.009	0.631
Heart attack (yes)	−0.014	0.478	Heart attack (no)	REF	
Heart attack (no)	REF		Blood pressure (high)	−0.002	0.769
Blood pressure (high)	−0.002	0.745	Blood pressure (normal)	REF	
Blood pressure (normal)	REF		Diabetes (yes)	0.000	0.962
Diabetes (yes)	−0.001	0.881	Diabetes (no)	REF	
Diabetes (no)	REF				

Notes: β - regression coefficient, *MMSE* mini-mental status examination, p - level of significance; *REF* reference category.

Such experimental findings are also supported by findings of imaging studies showing that the training of highly demanding tasks obviously increases the activity of the fronto-parietal network in the brain and strengthens fronto-parietal as well as parietal-striatal connections [36,37]. As previous findings suggest a connection between the training of tasks with high mental demands and improved neural network efficiency, longitudinal studies are necessary in order to evaluate whether the association between high mental demands at work and a better cognitive functioning is subject to this particular effect as well.

Having a job with high mental demands might additionally contribute to a good cognitive reserve which protects cognitive functioning in old age. A good cognitive reserve is built up by the confrontation with mentally demanding conditions throughout the life-course, for example, obtaining a higher level of education [38]. Being confronted with high mental demands in the workplace for quite a long period of time may also constitute a life-course condition that builds up a cognitive reserve. Neuroimaging studies generally observed that with older age, the connectivity of the neural network in frontal brain regions gets disrupted [39]. Having a good cognitive reserve, however, seems to guard the brain against these age-related changes as neural imaging studies showed that older individuals with a higher cognitive reserve have a larger cortical thickness [40], a larger gray matter volume [41], and more efficiently functioning neural networks [42,43] than individuals of the same age but with a smaller cognitive reserve. A cognitive training that ameliorates the efficiency of the neural network – maybe in the form of high mental demands at work – might help building up a cognitive reserve and, hence, prolong the lifetime period during which we function well and stay symptom-free (compression of morbidity [44]). Further studies will have to validate this hypothesis.

Cognitive functioning, especially in old age, is also influenced by other factors. One important factor influencing old-age cognitive functioning is cardiovascular health. In our analysis, we have adjusted for cardiovascular factors. The association between high mental demands at work and a better cognitive functioning, however, was not modified by cardiovascular risk factors like heart attack, high blood pressure, or stroke. The prevalence of cardiovascular risk factors was similar across the different levels of mental demands at work, suggesting that the association between mental demands at work and cognitive functioning is independent of cardiovascular risk factors. Notwithstanding, further studies should investigate potentially mediating effects in more detail.

Our study is not without limitations. First, the study provides only cross-sectional findings. Longitudinal data are necessary to confirm the assumed causal association between high mental demands at work and better cognitive functioning. Secondly, it is unclear in how far a reversed causality might influence the results. Individuals may self-select or be recruited for particular occupations based on their capacities which then could reflect their performance. Only a longitudinal study design can reveal more details. In the present study, we adjusted the analysis for intelligence as measured by the German Version of the Mill Hill Vocabulary Scale. However, the vocabulary scale is only a crude proxy for intelligence. Consideration should also be given to the fact that occupational mental demands were exclusively operationalized by objective classification measures (O*NET descriptor variables). These measures, however, might differ from subjectively perceived levels of demands, as the latter strongly depend on factors like personality [45] and individual stress coping capacities [46]. Including subjective measures as well might thus help differentiating the general beneficial effects of high mental demands from those situations when high mental demands lead to decrements in cognitive performance. More research is needed to clearly understand the synergistic effect of mental demands with other influencing factors on an individual's cognitive functioning.

A general methodological challenge arising in population-based studies is the problem of multicollinearity. In the present study we attempted to avoid problems of multicollinearity by (i) categorizing dependent variables, (ii) using a very large sample size, and (iii) combining dependent variables into one variable. However, we cannot be sure that we have completely ruled out any confounding.

In sum, our findings suggest a significant association between high mental demands at work and better cognitive functioning. In this sense, higher levels of mental demands – as brought about by technological changes in the working environment – may also have beneficial effects for the society as they could increase cognitive capacity levels and might even delay cognitive decline in old age. With this in mind, the debate about changes and challenges in the world of work should give a strong consideration to such potentially beneficial effects as well.

Appendix

O*NET descriptor variables included in the index "mental demands"

1.A.1 Cognitive Abilities

1.A.1.a Verbal Abilities

1.A.1.a.1 Oral Comprehension: The ability to listen to and understand information and ideas presented through spoken words and sentences.

1.A.1.a.2 Written Comprehension: The ability to read and understand information and ideas presented in writing.

1.A.1.a.3 Oral Expression: The ability to communicate information and ideas in speaking so others will understand.

1.A.1.a.4 Written Expression: The ability to communicate information and ideas in writing so others will understand.

1.A.1.b Idea Generation and Reasoning Abilities

1.A.1.b.1 Fluency of Ideas: The ability to come up with a number of ideas about a topic (the number of ideas is important, not their quality, correctness, or creativity).

1.A.1.b.2 Originality: The ability to come up with unusual or clever ideas about a given topic or situation, or to develop creative ways to solve a problem.

1.A.1.b.3 Problem Sensitivity: The ability to tell when something is wrong or is likely to go wrong. It does not involve solving the problem, only recognizing there is a problem.

1.A.1.b.4 Deductive Reasoning: The ability to apply general rules to specific problems to produce answers that make sense.

1.A.1.b.5 Inductive Reasoning: The ability to combine pieces of information to form general rules or conclusions (includes finding a relationship among seemingly unrelated events).

1.A.1.b.6 Information Ordering: The ability to arrange things or actions in a certain order or pattern according to a specific rule or set of rules (e.g., patterns of numbers, letters, words, pictures, mathematical operations).

1.A.1.b.7 Category Flexibility: The ability to generate or use different sets of rules for combining or grouping things in different ways.

1.A.1.c Quantitative Abilities

1.A.1.c.1 Mathematical Reasoning: The ability to choose the right mathematical methods or formulas to solve a problem.

1.A.1.c.2 Number Facility: The ability to add, subtract, multiply, or divide quickly and correctly.

1.A.1.d Memory

1.A.1.d.1 Memorization: The ability to remember information such as words, numbers, pictures, and procedures.

1.A.1.e Perceptual Abilities

1.A.1.e.1 Speed of Closure: The ability to quickly make sense of, combine, and organize information into meaningful patterns.

1.A.1.e.2 Flexibility of Closure: The ability to identify or detect a known pattern (a figure, object, word, or sound) that is hidden in other distracting material.

1.A.1.e.3 Perceptual Speed: The ability to quickly and accurately compare similarities and differences among sets of letters, numbers, objects, pictures, or patterns. The things to be compared may be presented at the same time or one after the other. This ability also includes comparing a presented object with a remembered object.

1.A.1.f Spatial Abilities

1.A.1.f.1 Spatial Orientation: The ability to know your location in relation to the environment or to know where other objects are in relation to you.

1.A.1.f.2 Visualization: The ability to imagine how something will look after it is moved around or when its parts are moved or rearranged.

1.A.1.g Attentiveness

1.A.1.g.1 Selective Attention: The ability to concentrate on a task over a period of time without being distracted.

1.A.1.g.2 Time Sharing: The ability to shift back and forth between two or more activities or sources of information (such as speech, sounds, touch, or other sources).

Competing interests

The authors declare that they have no competing interests.

Authors' contributions

FST has been involved in the acquisition of data, analyzed and interpreted the data, and wrote the first draft. TL has been involved in the acquisition of data, supervised the study, analyzed and interpreted the data, and critically commented and revised the manuscript. MLu supervised the study, analyzed and interpreted the data, and critically commented and revised the manuscript. KA has been involved in the acquisition of data and critically commented and revised the manuscript. MLS has been involved in the acquisition of data and critically commented and revised the manuscript.
CE has been involved in the acquisition of data and critically commented and revised the manuscript. MLö conceived and designed the study, and critically commented and revised the manuscript. JT conceived and designed the study, and critically commented and revised the manuscript. AV conceived and designed the study, and critically commented and revised the manuscript. SGRH conceived and designed the study, supervised the study, analyzed and interpreted the data, and critically commented and revised the manuscript. All authors read and approved the final version of the manuscript.

Acknowledgements

We would like to thank all participants and the whole team at the LIFE study center who made this study possible.

This publication is supported by LIFE – Leipzig Research Center for Civilization Diseases, Universität Leipzig. LIFE is funded by means of the European Union, by the European Regional Development Fund (ERDF) and by means of the Free State of Saxony within the framework of the excellence initiative. This project was funded by means of the European Social Fund and the Free State of Saxony.

Author details

[1]Institute of Social Medicine, Occupational Health and Public Health (ISAP), Medical Faculty, University of Leipzig, Philipp-Rosenthal-Str. 55, 04103 Leipzig, Germany. [2]LIFE – Leipzig Research Center for Civilization Diseases, University of Leipzig, Leipzig, Germany. [3]Max-Planck-Institute for Human Cognitive and Brain Sciences, Leipzig, and Clinic for Cognitive Neurology, University Hospital Leipzig, Leipzig, Germany. [4]Institute for Medical Informatics, Statistics and Epidemiology (IMISE), University of Leipzig, Leipzig, Germany. [5]Institute of Laboratory Medicine, Clinical Chemistry and Molecular Diagnostics (ILM), University of Leipzig, Leipzig, Germany.

References

1. Handel MJ: **Trends in job skill demands in OECD countries.** In *OECD Social, Employment and Migration Working Papers*. Edited by Organisation for Economic Co-operation and Development; 2012:143. 1–119.
2. Johnson RW: **Trends in job demands among older workers, 1992–2002.** *Mon Labor Rev* 2004, **127**:48–56.
3. Bundesverband BKK: *Kein Stress mit dem Stress: Eine Handlungshilfe für Betriebs- und Personalräte*. Dortmund: Bundesanstalt für Arbeitsschutz und Arbeitsmedizin; 2013.
4. Galy E, Cariou M, Melan C: **What is the relationship between mental workload factors and cognitive load types?** *Int J Psychophysiol* 2012, **83**:269–275.
5. Gonzalez C: **Task workload and cognitive abilities in dynamic decision making.** *Hum Factors* 2005, **47**:92–101.
6. Hancock PA, Williams G, Manning CM, Miyake S: **Influence of task demand characteristics on workload and performance.** *Int J Aviat Psychol* 1995, **5**:63–86.
7. Conrad CD: **A critical review of chronic stress effects on spatial learning and memory.** *Prog Neuropsychopharmacol Biol Psychiatry* 2010, **34**:742–755.
8. Lupien SJ, Maheu F, Tu M, Fiocco A, Schramek TE: **The effects of stress and stress hormones on human cognition: Implications for the field of brain and cognition.** *Brain Cogn* 2007, **65**:209–237.
9. Bosma H, van Boxtel MPJ, Ponds RWHM, Houx PJ, Burdorf A, Jolles J: **Mental work demands protect against cognitive impairment: MAAS prospective cohort study.** *Exp Aging Res* 2002, **29**:33–45.
10. Potter GG, Plassman BL, Helms MJ, Foster SM, Edwards NW: **Occupational characteristics and cognitive performance among elderly male twins.** *Neurology* 2006, **67**:1377–1382.
11. Seidler A, Nienhaus A, Bernhardt T, Kauppinen T, Elo AL, Frolich L: **Psychosocial work factors and dementia.** *Occup Environ Med* 2004, **61**:962–971.
12. Smyth KA, Fritsch T, Cook TB, McClendon MJ, Santillan CE, Friedland RP: **Worker functions and traits associated with occupations and the development of AD.** *Neurology* 2004, **63**:498–503.
13. Bonaiuto S, Rocca WA, Lippi A, Giannandrea E, Mele M, Cavarzeran F, Amaducci L: **Education and occupation as risk-factors for dementia - a population-based case-control study.** *Neuroepidemiology* 1995, **14**:101–109.
14. Fratiglioni L, Winblad B, von Strauss E: **Prevention of Alzheimer's disease and dementia. Major findings from the Kungsholmen project.** *Physiol Behav* 2007, **92**:98–104.
15. Karp A, Andel R, Parker MG, Wang HX, Winblad B, Fratiglioni L: **Mentally stimulating activities at work during midlife and dementia risk after age 75: follow-up study from the Kungsholmen project.** *Am J Geriatr Psychiatr* 2009, **17**:227–236.
16. Kröger E, Andel R, Lindsay J, Benounissa Z, Verreault R, Laurin D: **Is complexity of work associated with risk of dementia? The Canadian Study of Health And Aging.** *Am J Epidemiol* 2008, **167**:820–830.
17. Stern Y: **What is cognitive reserve? Theory and research application of the reserve concept.** *J Int Neuropsychol Soc* 2002, **8**:448–460.

18. Forstmeier S, Maercker A: **Motivational reserve: lifetime motivational abilities contribute to cognitive and emotional health in old age.** *Psychol Aging* 2008, **23**:886–899.
19. Forstmeier S, Maercker A, Maier W, van den Bussche H, Riedel-Heller S, Kaduszkiewicz H, Pentzek M, Weyerer S, Bickel H, Tebarth F, Luppa M, Wollny A, Wiese B, Wagner M: **Motivational reserve: motivation-related occupational abilities and risk of mild cognitive impairment and alzheimer disease.** *Psychol Aging* 2012, **27**:353–363.
20. Aebi C, Monsch AU, Berres M, Brubacher D, Staehelin HB: **Validation of the German CERAD-neuropsychological assessment battery.** *Neurobiol Aging* 2002, **23**:S27–S28.
21. Chandler MJ, Lacritz LH, Hynan LS, Barnard HD, Allen G, Deschner M, Weiner MF, Cullum CM: **A total score for the CERAD neuropsychological battery.** *Neurology* 2005, **65**:102–106.
22. Satzger W, Hampel H, Padberg F, Burger K, Nolde T, Ingrassia G, Engel RR: **Practical application of the CERAD test battery in screening for neuropsychological dementia.** *Nervenarzt* 2001, **72**:196–203.
23. Sanchez-Cubillo I, Perianez JA, Adrover-Roig D, Rodriguez-Sanchez JM, Rios-Lago M, Tirapu J, Bercelo F: **Construct validity of the Trail Making Test: role of task-switching, working memory, inhibition/interference control, and visuomotor abilities.** *J Int Neuropsychol Soc* 2009, **15**:438–450.
24. Salthouse TA: **What cognitive abilities are involved in trail-making performance?** *Intelligence* 2011, **39**:222–232.
25. Etnier JL, Chang YK: **The effect of physical activity on executive function: a brief commentary on definitions, measurement issues, and the current state of the literature.** *J Sport Exerc Psychol* 2009, **31**:469–483.
26. Arbuthnott K, Frank J: **Trail making test, part B as a measure of executive control: validation using a set-switching paradigm.** *J Clin Exp Neuropsychol* 2000, **22**:518–528.
27. Drane DL, Yuspeh RL, Huthwaite JS, Klingler LK: **Demographic characteristics and normative observations for derived-trail making test indices.** *Neuropsychiatry Neuropsychol Behav Neurol* 2002, **15**:39–43.
28. Kraan C, Stolwyk RJ, Testa R: **The abilities associated with verbal fluency performance in a young, healthy population are multifactorial and differ across fluency variants.** *Appl Neuropsychol: Adult* 2013, **20**:159–168.
29. Henry JD, Crawford JR, Phillips LH: **Verbal fluency performance in dementia of the AlzheimerGÇÖs type: a meta-analysis.** *Neuropsychologia* 2004, **42**:1212–1222.
30. Tombaugh TN, Kozak J, Rees L: **Normative data stratified by age and education for two measures of verbal fluency: FAS and animal naming.** *Arch Clin Neuropsychol* 1999, **14**:167–177.
31. Parks RW, Loewenstein DA, Dodrill KL, Barker WW, Yoshii F, Chang JY, Emran A, Apicella A, Sheramata WA, Duara R: **Cerebral metabolic effects of a verbal fluency test - a pet scan study.** *J Clin Exp Neuropsychol* 1988, **10**:565–575.
32. Schmidt KH, Metzler P: *Wortschatztest (WST)*. Göttingen: Hogrefe-Verlag; 1992.
33. Tranter LJ, Koutstaal W: **Age and flexible thinking: An experimental demonstration of the beneficial effects of increased cognitively stimulating activity on fluid intelligence in healthy older adults.** *Aging Neuropsychol Cognit* 2008, **15**:184–207.
34. Jaeggi SM, Buschkuehl M, Jonides J, Perrig WJ: **Improving fluid intelligence with training on working memory.** *Proc Natl Acad Sci U S A* 2008, **105**:6829–6833.
35. Fairclough SH, Venables L, Tattersall A: **The influence of task demand and learning on the psychophysiological response.** *Int J Psychophysiol* 2005, **56**:171–184.
36. Jolles DD, Grol MJ, Van Buchem MA, Rombouts SARB, Crone EA: **Practice effects in the brain: changes in cerebral activation after working memory practice depend on task demands.** *Neuroimage* 2010, **52**:658–668.
37. Mackey AP, Singley ATM, Bunge SA: **Intensive reasoning training alters patterns of brain connectivity at rest.** *J Neurosci* 2013, **33**:4796–4803.
38. Valenzuela MJ, Sachdev P: **Brain reserve and dementia: a systematic review.** *Psychol Med* 2006, **36**:441–454.
39. Chou YH, Chen NK, Madden DJ: **Functional brain connectivity and cognition: effects of adult age and task demands.** *Neurobiol Aging* 2013, **34**:1925–1934.
40. Liu YW, Julkunen V, Paajanen T, Westman E, Wahlund LO, Aitken A, Sobow T, Mecocci P, Tsolaki M, Vellas B, Muehlboeck S, Spenger C, Lovestone S, Simmons A, Soininen H: **Education increases reserve against Alzheimer's disease-evidence from structural MRI analysis.** *Neuroradiology* 2012, **54**:929–938.
41. Bartres-Faz D, Sole-Padulles C, Junque C, Rami L, Bosch B, Bargallo N, Falcon C, Sanchez-Valle R, Molinuevo JL: **Interactions of cognitive reserve with regional brain anatomy and brain function during a working memory task in healthy elders.** *Biol Psychol* 2009, **80**:256–259.
42. Bastin C, Yakushev I, Bahri MA, Fellgiebel A, Eustache F, Landeau B, Scheurich A, Feyers D, Collette F, Chetelat G, Salmon E: **Cognitive reserve impacts on inter-individual variability in resting-state cerebral metabolism in normal aging.** *Neuroimage* 2012, **63**:713–722.
43. Ansado J, Monchi O, Ennabil N, Deslauriers J, Jubault T, Faure S, Joanette Y: **Coping with task demand in aging using neural compensation and neural reserve triggers primarily intra-hemispheric-based neurofunctional reorganization.** *Neurosci Res* 2013, **75**:295–304.
44. Fries JF, Bruce B, Chakravarty E: **Compression of morbidity 1980-2011: a focused review of paradigms and progress.** *J Aging Res* 2011, **261702**:1–10.
45. Conard MA, Matthews RA: **Modeling the stress process: personality eclipses dysfunctional cognitions and workload in predicting stress.** *Personal Individ Differ* 2008, **44**:171–181.
46. Epstein S, Katz L: **Coping ability, stress, productive load, and symptoms.** *J Pers Soc Psychol* 1992, **62**:813–825.

5

Work-related outcomes in randomized, double blind, placebo-controlled trials in osteoarthritis – are they adequately reported in journal publications?

Daniel Sowah, Flora Balat and Sebastian Straube*

Abstract

Background: Osteoarthritis (OA) has a high prevalence in Western societies and can affect an individual's life in a number of domains, including work. In our experience, treatment trials on OA, however, rarely report work-related outcomes. Here we conducted a systematic review to assess the reporting of work-related outcomes in randomized, double blind, placebo-controlled trials in OA. Our systematic review also compared two search strategies for identifying eligible publications, one where work-related terms were included in the database search string (A) and one where this was not the case and work-related outcomes were identified by searches of full text Portable Document Formats (PDFs) (B). Search strategy A would conventionally be used and would only identify publications where work-related terms were mentioned in the title or abstract. Search strategy B presents the innovation of full text PDF searching and would identify publications were work-related terms were reported in the full text, regardless of whether they are mentioned in the title and abstract or not. We hypothesize that search strategy B identifies more relevant publications than search strategy A.

Methods: Electronic database searching was performed in Medline (Pubmed) from database inception to February 23, 2017 to identify peer-reviewed articles of randomized, double blind, placebo-controlled treatment trials in OA of the hand, hip, or knee, available as full-text PDFs. For search strategy A, search terms to identify work-related outcomes were included in the database search string, while search strategy B did not have these terms included in the database search string, but instead involved full text PDF searching. We included English language articles only and only those articles where searchable PDFs were available, to enable a comparison between search strategies A and B. Additionally, included studies also needed to report on pain intensity in relation to the work-related outcomes.

Results: Search strategy A yielded 50 hits combined for hand, hip or knee OA that mentioned some work-related concept in the title or abstract; 12 articles had to be excluded because they were not available as searchable PDFs. Screening of the remaining 38 articles resulted in only two articles that satisfied our inclusion criteria. Search strategy B yielded 986 hits, out of which 201 articles were excluded because searchable full text PDFs were not available. PDF full text searching and further screening resulted in 10 articles that were considered eligible for our review.

(Continued on next page)

* Correspondence: straube@ualberta.ca
Division of Preventive Medicine, Department of Medicine, University of Alberta, 5-30 University Terrace, 8303-112 Street, Edmonton, AB T6G 2T4, Canada

(Continued from previous page)
Conclusions: Work-related outcomes are rarely reported in journal publication on randomized, double blind, placebo-controlled trials of hand, hip or knee OA. Searching full text PDFs yields more eligible articles than searching titles and abstracts only.

Keywords: Systematic review, Search strategies, Treatment trials, Osteoarthritis, Work-related health outcomes,

Background

Osteoarthritis (OA) is a very common condition among the aging population with a high incidence at age 50 years and older [1]. The prevalence estimates of OA vary depending on the specific joint that is affected and the characteristics of the population under study [2, 3]. A study by the World Health Organization (WHO) Scientific Group on Rheumatic Diseases estimated that 10% of the world's population who are 60 years or older are affected by some form of OA [4]. Based on x-ray imaging, the prevalence of knee OA among an adult cohort aged 56–84 years in Malmo, Sweden, was about 25%, while symptomatic knee OA had a prevalence of 15% [5]. Of the 978 subjects in the Framingham Study Community [6], it was estimated that hip OA was present in 20% of the cohort based on imaging and about 4% had symptomatic OA.

OA is typically characterized by pain, impairment of mobility and stiffness [7]. The pain is related to loss of cartilage, which may lead to joint failure [8, 9]. Factors identified that are associated with OA include inflammation, obesity, weak muscles, cartilage defects and genetic factors [9]. Joints commonly affected by OA include the knee, hips, hand and wrist. Osteoarthritic pain and other accompanying symptoms may lead to a reduction in patients' quality of life and may also interfere with productivity at the workplace [9]. Indeed, it has been shown that moderate to severe chronic painful conditions may lead to lack of productivity at work [10], work absenteeism as well as substantial financial costs imposed on the healthcare system [10, 11].

For the present review, we refer to outcomes that speak to a person's ability to work or to productivity at work as 'work-related outcomes'. Data on such work-related outcomes, which are commonly captured as time lost from work or interference with work ability, are often collected in pain trials – typically as answers to component questions of commonly used questionnaires. However, these work-related outcomes are only infrequently reported in publications on such pain trials [12]. How work-related outcomes in trials on OA specifically have been reported in the scientific literature is not known; this is the subject of the present review.

In this systematic review, we therefore investigated the reporting of work-related outcomes in randomized, double blind, placebo-controlled trials on the treatment of hand, hip or knee OA. Additionally, we had aimed to analyze pain intensity as an outcome in OA trials and to link this pain intensity to work-related outcomes informative of work ability and productivity; however, the data we found did not enable us to conduct dependable analyses on these issues. While there is evidence that work-related outcomes are not frequently reported in journal article abstracts [12], they could conceivably still be reported more often in the full journal articles.

In systematic reviews, electronic database searching involves the use of search terms to identify different concepts and combination of these different concepts. This is followed by screening of the search results based on title and abstract, then full text articles are further assessed, and relevant articles that satisfy the eligibility criteria are included in the review. One major objective of systematic reviews is to capture all (or as large a proportion as possible) of the relevant publications regarding a subject through the database search [13, 14].

The aim of the present publication was to conduct a systematic review employing two distinct search strategies: one where work-related terms were included in the database search string (A) and one where this was not the case and work-related outcomes were identified instead by searches of full text Portable Document Formats (PDFs) (B). Search strategy A would conventionally be used and would only identify publications where work-related terms were mentioned in the title or abstract. Search strategy B presents the innovation of full text PDF searching and would identify publications were work-related terms were reported in the full text, regardless of whether they are mentioned in the title and abstract or not. We hypothesize that search strategy B identifies more relevant publications than search strategy A.

Methods

Literature search

Electronic database searches were performed in Medline (Pubmed) from database inception to February 23, 2017. We did not search in a second database, nor did we complement the electronic database search by manual searching. We are aware that this means potentially relevant material was not found, but, to address to aim of the present study, a convenience sample as it was produced by our single database search was deemed sufficient. For search strategy A, search terms to identify work-related outcomes were included in the database search string, while search strategy B did not have these terms included in the database search string, but involved full text PDF searching for work-related terms. The overall approach to searching is shown in Fig. 1.

To be eligible for inclusion in this systematic review, articles must be randomized, double blind, placebo-controlled trials on the treatment of OA of the hand, hip or knee. The publications must be written in English, must report on work-related outcomes, and must be available as searchable PDFs, to enable a comparison between search strategies A and B. Included studies also needed to report on pain intensity in relation to the work-related outcomes.

The search results from search strategy A were screened as abstracts, and publications that did not mention work-related terms were excluded at that stage. The remaining full-text PDFs were further screened to identify articles that satisfied our inclusion criteria. The pathway for search strategy B involved identification of full text PDFs from the search results without restriction to those mentioning work-related terms in the title or abstract, and excluding all abstracts for which the full-text publication could not be found as searchable PDFs. To enable a comparison between search strategies A and B, the articles deemed eligible for inclusion via either search strategy needed to be available to us as searchable PDFs.

When screening the full text journal publication, we searched for the following words, parts of words or phrases in the searchable PDFs to identify those articles that reported work-related outcomes: *work, employ, job, labor, labour, sick leave* or *sick listed*. The screening of the full text articles and selection of included studies was performed by one investigator (FB) and was independently confirmed by another investigator (DS). Discrepancies were resolved by the senior investigator (SS).

Analysis

Simple proportions of articles reporting outcomes of interest were calculated. No meta-analysis was undertaken as we did not find data suitable for this approach. Had we found such data, we would have used a random effects model or fixed effect model for meta-analysis, as determined by between study heterogeneity (I-squared statistic). We would have calculated odds ratios for dichotomous data and standardized mean differences for continuous data.

Results

Search strategy A yielded 50 hits combined for hand, hip or knee OA, all mentioning some work-related concept in the title or the abstract (Fig. 1). Full text PDFs were not available for 12 papers (24% of the total) and these were therefore excluded. Of the remaining 38 full text PDFs that were screened, only two satisfied our inclusion criteria as shown in Fig. 2.

Search strategy B generated 986 articles of which there were no duplicates. Of these, 201 records (20% of the total) were excluded because the full text PDFs were not available to us. The remaining 785 full-text articles were screened by electronically searching the PDFs for the work-related terms and verifying the other study characteristics needed for inclusion. This resulted in 722 articles being excluded mainly because the articles did not mention any work-related concept or the articles were not randomized, double blind, placebo-controlled trials. The remaining 63 articles, which mentioned some work-related concept, were further screened to determine which articles actually evaluated and reported work-related concepts associated with OA in the respective study. As shown in Fig. 3, 51 studies were excluded at this stage resulting in 12 studies being retained. Furthermore, two studies [15, 16] did not report on pain intensity in relation to the reported work-related outcomes and were therefore excluded, leading to ten studies that were included in this systematic review. As a tool for assessing the degree of pain associated with the respective OA, six of the included studies [17–22] employed a visual analogue scale (VAS). These studies, however, varied in the work-related outcome measures reported. The work-related outcome measures reported included resumption of work, number of days on sick leave, work performance, pain interference with work and work limitation. Of the four remaining included studies, one study [23] assessed pain intensity using a self-administered, validated questionnaire adopted from the McGill pain questionnaire, the SF-36 Health Survey, and the Medical College of Wisconsin noncancer pain questionnaire. Two of the studies [24, 25] employed the Brief Pain Inventory to assess pain, while one study [26] used a five-point pain scale.

Further comparison between the hits identified with search strategies A and B showed that the ten eligible articles that resulted from search strategy B also included the two eligible articles obtained from search strategy A. Additionally, all the available 38 full text PDFs resulting from search strategy A were also captured by results from search strategy B.

Table 1 lists the 51 excluded articles assessed as full text PDFs and the reasons for their exclusion. Of these 51 excluded articles, five concerned hand OA, 13 hip OA, and 33 knee OA.

Although 18 of the 51 excluded studies mentioned some work-related concept in the 'Introduction' section of the respective article, they subsequently did not report on any work-related outcome measure of the study participants. The work-related concepts mentioned in the 'Introduction' section of the respective article

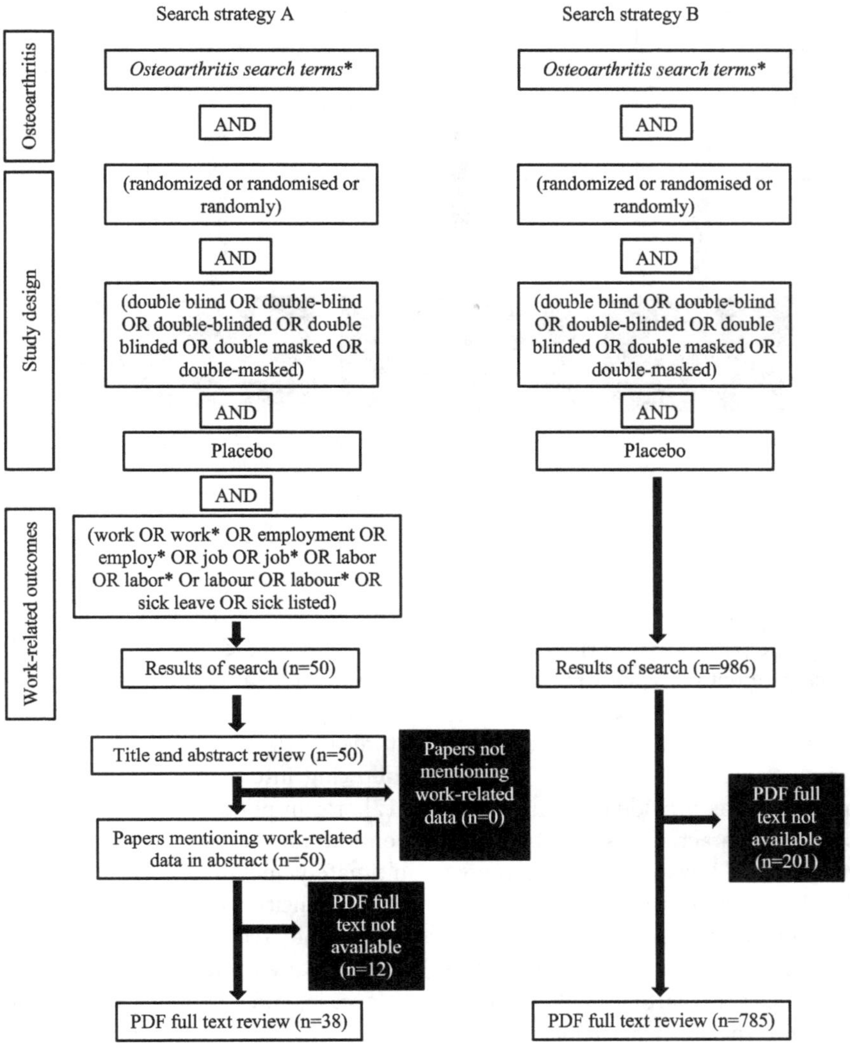

*: Represents the various search terms for osteoarthritis based on site of OA as shown in the table below.

Site	Osteoarthritis search terms
Hand	(osteoarthritis OR osteoarthrosis OR degenerative arthritis OR OA) AND (hand OR wrist OR carpal OR finger OR thumb OR digit OR digital OR interphalangeal OR metacarpophalangeal)
Hip	(((osteoarthritis OR osteoarthrosis OR degenerative arthritis OR OA) AND hip) OR coxarthritis OR coxarthrosis)
Knee	(((osteoarthritis OR osteoarthrosis OR degenerative arthritis OR OA) AND knee) OR gonarthritis OR gonarthrosis)

Fig. 1 Search strategy and screening of records resulting from two distinct search strategies

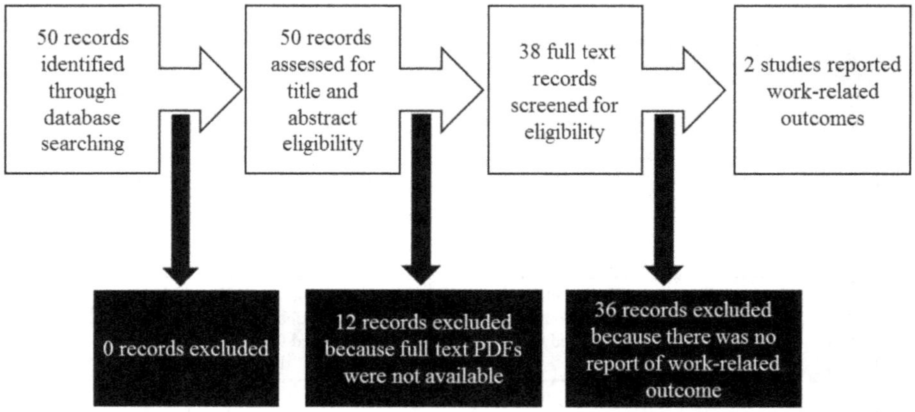
50 records identified through database searching
50 records assessed for title and abstract eligibility
38 full text records screened for eligibility
2 studies reported work-related outcomes
0 records excluded
12 records excluded because full text PDFs were not available
36 records excluded because there was no report of work-related outcome

Fig. 2 Screening and selection of full text PDF articles of trials reporting work-related outcomes of hand, hip or knee osteoarthritis based on search strategy A. An electronic database search was conducted in Medline (Pubmed) to identify full text articles of randomized, double blind, placebo-controlled trials that reported on work-related outcomes. All articles in which full text PDFs were not available were excluded. The rest were screened and articles that met the requirement for inclusion were selected

included work disability, inability to work, absenteeism from work, reduced participation in work, decreased work performance, lost productive work time and cost associated with lost work time. None of these work-related concepts were assessed in the participants of the respective studies.

Employment or job status was provided as part of the study participants' baseline characteristics in 12 studies. The authors of these studies, however, did not report further on any work-related outcomes of the trials. Although some of the excluded studies made mention of some work-related concepts in the 'Discussion' and other sections of the articles (21 articles), these were, again, not directly related to the study participants.

Overall, 12 studies reported on the impact of OA and treatments for OA on work-related outcomes related to the study participants (Table 2). One study was on hand OA, two were on hip OA and nine were on knee OA. The particular type of work-related outcomes reported included 'number of days on sick leave' (one study) [18], decreased work performance (three studies) [22], limitation of work (four studies) [20–22], pain interference with normal work (five studies) [20–22], and improvement in normal work following intervention (two studies) [22]. In one study [17], resumption of work following therapeutic intervention for hand OA was reported. The ten studies ultimately included in our review (Table 2) reported pain intensity as well as work interference or time off work. The treatments investigated in the ten included studies varied and included naproxen, acetaminophen, celecoxib, rofecoxib, tramadol, duloxetine, soy protein, avocado/soybean unsaponifiables and glycosaminoglycan polysulphate.

These ten included articles demonstrated a considerable degree of variability in their reporting of both the work-related outcome measure and pain intensity. This prevented further analysis to determine the correlation

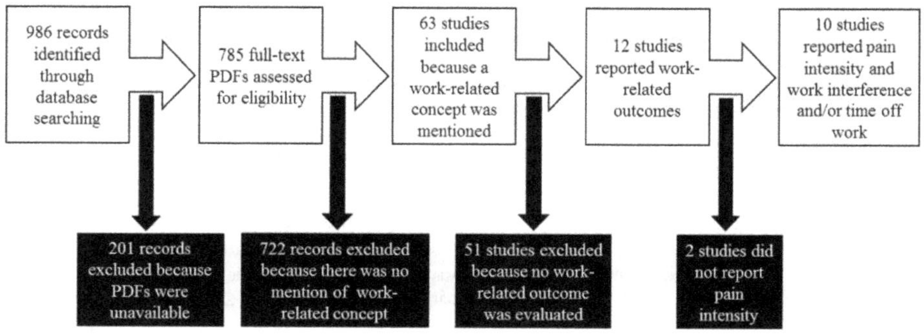

Fig. 3 Screening and selection of full text PDF articles of trials reporting work-related outcomes of hand, hip or knee osteoarthritis based on search strategy B. An electronic database search was conducted in Medline (Pubmed) to identify full text articles of randomized, double blind, placebo-controlled trials. All articles in which full text PDFs were not available were excluded. The rest were screened and articles where the full text PDFs mentioned work-related outcome and that met our other requirement were included

Table 1 Articles not reporting work-related outcomes in osteoarthritis (excluded after review of full text PDF publications)

Reference	Reason for exclusion
Hand osteoarthritis	
Barthel 2010 [32]	Impact of hand OA mentioned in 'Discussion' section, but no work-related outcome was reported
Nieman 2013 [33]	Work disability and inability to work due to knee OA were mentioned in 'Background' section, but no work-related outcome was reported
Pope 2004 [34]	Though job status (% working full time, part-time, retired, homemaker) was reported, no work-related outcomes were reported
Richmond 2013 [35]	Number of patients in paid employment reported as part of subjects' baseline characteristics, but no work-related outcome was reported
Taibi 2009 [36]	Number of patients working mentioned as a part of patients' baseline characteristics but no work-related outcome measure was reported
Hip osteoarthritis	
Cheras 2010 [37]	'Work disability' mentioned in 'Introduction' section but no work-related outcome measure was reported for study subjects
Ernst 2003 [38]	Systematic review
Florete 2008 [39]	'Leading cause of disability; 'cost' estimated as 'lost productive work time'; mentioned as effects of OA in 'Introduction' section, but no work-related outcome measure was reported for study subjects
Gana 2006 [40]	'Leading cause of disability; 'cost' estimated as 'lost productive work time'; mentioned as effects of OA in 'Introduction' section, but no work-related outcome measure was reported for study subjects
Jabbari 2011 [41]	Review article
Lambert 2007 [42]	No work-related outcome measure was reported
Maheu 1998 [43]	'Number or percent of patients' included in the study and still working was mentioned as a baseline characteristic but no work-related outcome measure was reported
Moskowitz 2003 [44]	Study was a pooled analysis and not a randomized controlled trial
Plosker 2011 [45]	Review article
Pope 2004 [34]	Though job status (% working full time, part-time, retired, homemaker) was mentioned as subjects' baseline characteristics, no work-related outcome was reported separately
Rozendaal 2005 [46]	Randomized controlled trial study protocol design
Turan 2014 [47]	Loss of labor force mentioned in 'Introduction' section only, but no work-related outcome measure was reported
Willich 2010 [48]	Employment status (full/part-time) mentioned as part of patients' baseline characteristic, but no work-related outcome measure was reported
Knee osteoarthritis	
Alfredo 2011 [49]	Absenteeism due to OA was mentioned in 'Introduction' section, but no work-related outcome measure was reported
Auw Yang 2008 [50]	Cost due to loss of productivity at work mentioned in 'Discussion' section, but no work-related outcome measure was reported
Babul 2004 [51]	Lost work days due to OA mentioned in 'Introduction' section, but no work-related outcome measure was reported
Brown 2013 [52]	Review article
Burch 2007 [53]	Cost due to lost productive work time mentioned in 'Introduction' section, but no work-related outcome measure was reported
Cheras 2010 [37]	Costs associated with OA and work disability mentioned in 'Introduction' section, but no work-related outcome measure was reported
Cibere 2005 [54]	Work disability and costs associated with knee OA mentioned in 'Introduction' section, but no work-related outcome measure was reported
Florete 2008 [39]	'Leading cause of disability'; 'cost' estimated as 'lost productive work time'; mentioned as effects of OA in 'Introduction' section, but no work-related outcome measure was reported
Frakes 2011 [55]	Normal work mentioned as a part of secondary assessment questionnaire due to pain, but no work-related outcome measure was reported separately
Gana 2006 [40]	'Leading cause of disability'; 'cost' estimated as 'lost productive work time'; mentioned as effects of OA in 'Introduction' section, but no work-related outcome measure was reported

Table 1 Articles not reporting work-related outcomes in osteoarthritis (excluded after review of full text PDF publications) *(Continued)*

Reference	Reason for exclusion
Hsieh 2012 [56]	Work status mentioned as a baseline characteristic but no work-related outcome measure was reported
Hsieh 2012 [57]	Work status mentioned as a baseline characteristic but no work-related outcome measure was reported
Hsieh 2012 [58]	Work status mentioned as a baseline characteristic but no work-related outcome measure was reported
Ilan 2004 [59]	Delay in return to work mentioned in 'Introduction' section and not reported elsewhere
Jia 2016 [60]	'Patients maintaining their work activities' was mentioned in the 'Discussion' session, but no outcome measure was reported
Kannus 1992 [61]	Ability to work mentioned as part of assessment of pain due to OA, but no outcome measure was reported
Maheu 1998 [43]	'Number or percent of patients' included in the study and still working was mentioned, but no outcome measure was reported
Magrans-Courtney 2011 [62]	Ability to work mentioned as part of assessment of pain due to OA, but no outcome measure was reported
Mata 2015 [63]	'Reduced participation in work' mentioned in 'Introduction' section, but no outcome measure was reported
Möller 2010 [64]	Work mentioned as part of patients' assessment tool, but no outcome measure was reported
Mazzuca 2004 [65]	Employment status mentioned as a part of patients' baseline characteristics, but no outcome measure was reported
Pavelka 1995 [66]	Employment status mentioned as a part of patients' baseline characteristics, but no outcome measure was reported
Pincus 2001 [67]	Employment status mentioned as a part of patients' baseline characteristics, but no outcome measure was reported
Pope 2004 [34]	Though job status (% of patients working full time, part-time, retired, homemaker) was mentioned as subjects' baseline characteristics, no work-related outcome was reported
Sanghi 2013 [68]	Disability leading to work loss mentioned in 'Introduction' section, but no outcome measure was reported
Schauss 2012 [69]	Inability to work mentioned in the 'Methods' section, but no outcome measure was reported
Segal 2001 [70]	'Hampers work' mentioned in 'Introduction' section, but no outcome measure was reported
Sihvonen 2013 [71]	Work mentioned as part of patients' baseline characteristics, but no outcome measure was reported
Singer 2011 [72]	'Work activities' mentioned as part of questionnaire to assess quality of life, but no outcome measure was reported
Taverner 2010 [73]	'Usual work' mentioned as part of outcome measurement tool, but no outcome measure was reported separately
van der Weegen 2015 [74]	Effect of OA pain on work was mentioned in 'Introduction' section; work activities mentioned as part of assessment tool, but no outcome measure was reported separately
Zhao 1999 [75]	Work mentioned as part of quality of life assessment tool, but no outcome measure was reported separately

between pain intensity and work-related outcome measures, which we had originally planned to do.

In summary, out of the 785 articles that could have reported on work-related outcomes in relation to pain intensity, only 1.3% (10/785) did so.

Discussion

OA can place a substantial burden on an individual's life and may lead to reduced productivity at work, interference with work, absenteeism and cost associated with lost work time [27, 28]. Trials on therapies for OA rarely consider the impact of the condition on work-related outcomes. The present systematic review aimed to evaluate the extent to which these work-related outcomes are reported in publications on randomized, double blind, placebo-controlled trials of hand, hip or knee OA. Our systematic review showed that only 1.3% (10/785) of full text articles reported on both, pain intensity (measured mostly by the visual analogue scale) and work interference or time off work.

This finding is consistent with other research, which demonstrated that work-related outcomes in pain trials are infrequently reported based on a database search of abstracts [12]. Chronic pain has been shown to negatively impact work-related outcomes by interfering with productivity and performance at the workplace [29], but this impact is often not captured in the outcomes reported in publications on intervention trials.

In the present review, two different search strategies, strategy A and strategy B, were compared. As described, strategy A followed the conventional search approach, which yielded two articles out of 50 possible identified

Table 2 Articles reporting work-related outcomes

Reference	Work-related outcomes reported
Hand osteoarthritis	
Pastinen 1988 [17]	Resumption of work mentioned following treatment of hand OA
Hip osteoarthritis	
Lequesne 2002 [18]	Number of days on sick leave
Smugar 2006 [19]	Decreased work performance
Knee osteoarthritis	
Arjmandi 2004 [23]	Limitation of work due to pain; improvement of work performance and productivity
Chappell 2009 [24]	Pain interference with normal work
Chappell 2011 [25]	Pain interference with normal work
Essex 2012 [20]	Pain interference and work limitation
Golden 2004 [26]	Impact of intervention on work
Hochberg 2011 [21]	Pain interference with normal work
Schein 2008 [22]	Degree of pain interference with work; improvement in work limitation; difficulty in performing work
Schiff 2004 [15]	Improvement in quality of life with regards to work
Wang 2012 [16]	Effect of knee OA on work

All but the final two table entries (Schiff 2004 [15] and Wang 2012 [16]) were included in our systematic review

records, which satisfied our inclusion criteria. By contrast, strategy B, which involved full text PDF searching, generated 986 records out of which ten articles were ultimately eligible. This demonstrates that full text PDF searching may be a useful strategy in circumstances when outcomes of interest are expected to not be reported in abstracts.

The ten included articles demonstrated a high degree of heterogeneity in the reporting of the pain assessment scale employed and the work-related outcome measures reported. Thus, it was not possible to perform any further analysis to determine the association between the pain intensity and work-related outcome measures, which we had originally planned to do. If future studies on OA were to follow similar approaches to assess pain intensity and work-related outcomes, this would enable meta-analysis of data from different studies. Standardization of the outcomes reported would therefore be of benefit.

Although some of the publications collected data on job or employment status of the study participants, the impact on work ability of the pain resulting from OA, and the treatments studied, is most often not reported. We suggest that future trials should put more emphasis on reporting such work-related outcomes in journal publications.

Our findings are limited by the fact that the search was conducted in only one database; potentially relevant articles may therefore have been missed. Stevinson et al. [13] demonstrated that searching only one database was not adequate to capture all possible publications on a given subject. Nonetheless, for our purposes in this systematic review, the results allow us to estimate the extent of under-reporting of work-related outcomes in randomized, double blind, placebo-controlled trials in OA, which is substantial.

Since reduction in pain intensity may lead to an improvement in an individual's work ability [12], we recommend that treatment trials of OA should routinely report on the work-related outcomes of the study participants. This is in keeping with a recent publication to define an international standard set of outcome measures for patients with hip or knee osteoarthritis, which recommended the reporting of a patient's work status at baseline and a regular follow-up to evaluate the impact of OA [30]. The recommendations also included various standardized instruments for evaluating pain and impact on overall quality of life. Further, a recent review suggested that core outcomes in OA trials should include time off work (sick leave), employment status, work productivity and work interference [31]. Although most of the included articles in the present review measured either one or more of the above work-related outcomes, the reporting of a particular outcome was inconsistent between the studies. As mentioned above, a standard for work-related outcome measures and reporting that adheres to the same would be goals for the future.

Conclusions

Work-related outcomes are inadequately reported in journal publication on randomized, double blind, placebo-controlled trials of hand, hip and knee OA. This is an area where future studies can do better.

Abbreviations

OA: Osteoarthritis; PDF: Portable Document Format; VAS: Visual analogue scale; WHO: World Health Organization

Funding

This study was supported by institutional funds from the University of Alberta's Faculty of Medicine and Dentistry and Department of Medicine provided to Sebastian Straube.

Authors' contributions

SS conceived of the study and supervised it. FB performed the database search and selected eligible articles. DS confirmed study selection, qualitatively synthesized the data and drafted the manuscript. All authors read and approved the final manuscript.

Competing interests

The authors declare that they have no competing interests.

References

1. Lawrence JS, Bremner JM, Bier F. Osteo-arthrosis. prevalence in the population and relationship between symptoms and x-ray changes. Ann Rheum Dis. 1966;25(1):1–24.
2. Zhang Y, Jordan JM. Epidemiology of osteoarthritis. Clin Geriatr Med. 2010; 26(3):355–69.
3. Cho HJ, Morey V, Kang JY, Kim KW, Kim TK. Prevalence and risk factors of spine, shoulder, hand, hip, and knee osteoarthritis in community-dwelling koreans older than age 65 years. Clin Orthop Relat Res. 2015;473(10):3307–14. https://doi.org/10.1007/s11999-015-4450-3.
4. Woolf AD, Pfleger B. Burden of major musculoskeletal conditions. Bull World Health Organ. 2003;81(9):646–56.
5. Turkiewicz A, de Verdier M G, Engstrom G, et al. Prevalence of knee pain and knee OA in southern sweden and the proportion that seeks medical care. Rheumatology (Oxford). 2015;54(5):827–35. https://doi.org/10.1093/rheumatology/keu409.
6. Kim C, Linsenmeyer KD, Vlad SC, et al. Prevalence of radiographic and symptomatic hip osteoarthritis in an urban United States community: the Framingham osteoarthritis study. Arthritis Rheumatol. 2014;66(11):3013–7. https://doi.org/10.1002/art.38795.
7. Felson DT. Clinical practice. osteoarthritis of the knee. N Engl J Med. 2006; 354(8):841–8.
8. Hunter DJ, Felson DT. Osteoarthritis. BMJ. 2006;332(7542):639–42.
9. Sharma AR, Jagga S, Lee SS, Nam JS. Interplay between cartilage and subchondral bone contributing to pathogenesis of osteoarthritis. Int J Mol Sci. 2013;14(10):19805–30. https://doi.org/10.3390/ijms141019805.
10. Andrew R, Derry S, Taylor RS, Straube S, Phillips CJ. The costs and consequences of adequately managed chronic non-cancer pain and chronic neuropathic pain. Pain Pract. 2014;14(1):79–94. https://doi.org/10.1111/papr.12050.
11. Langley P, Muller-Schwefe G, Nicolaou A, Liedgens H, Pergolizzi J, Varrassi G. The impact of pain on labor force participation, absenteeism and presenteeism in the European Union. J Med Econ. 2010;13(4):662–72. https://doi.org/10.3111/13696998.2010.529379.
12. Wolf I, Friede T, Hallier E, Straube S. Work-related outcomes in randomised placebo-controlled pain trials: a systematic review and meta-analysis. J Occup Med Toxicol. 2014;9:25–6673-9-25. eCollection 2014. https://doi.org/10.1186/1745-6673-9-25.
13. Stevinson C, Lawlor DA. Searching multiple databases for systematic reviews: added value or diminishing returns? Complement Ther Med. 2004;12(4):228–32.
14. Egger M, Smith GD, O'Rourke K. Introduction: rationale, potentials, and promise of systematic reviews - systematic reviews in health care: meta-analysis in context, second edition - egger - wiley online library. In: Egger M, Smith GD, Altman DG, editors. Systematic reviews in health care: Meta-analysis in context. Vol 2018. Second Edition ed. London: BMJ Publishing Group; 2008. p. 3–19. Accessed 2 Sept 2018. https://doi.org/10.1002/9780470693926.ch1.
15. Schiff M, Minic M. Comparison of the analgesic efficacy and safety of nonprescription doses of naproxen sodium and ibuprofen in the treatment of osteoarthritis of the knee. J Rheumatol. 2004;31(7):1373–83.
16. Wang X, Cao Y, Pang J, et al. Traditional Chinese herbal patch for short-term management of knee osteoarthritis: a randomized, double-blind, placebo-controlled trial. Evid Based Complement Alternat Med. 2012;2012(171706):1–9.
17. Pastinen O, Forsskahl B, Marklund M. Local glycosaminoglycan polysulphate injection therapy in osteoarthritis of the hand. A placebo-controlled clinical study. Scand J Rheumatol. 1988;17(3):197–202.
18. Lequesne M, Maheu E, Cadet C, Dreiser RL. Structural effect of avocado/soybean unsaponifiables on joint space loss in osteoarthritis of the hip. Arthritis Rheum. 2002;47(1):50–8. https://doi.org/10.1002/art1.10239.
19. Smugar SS, Schnitzer TJ, Weaver AL, Rubin BR, Polis AB, Tershakovec AM. Rofecoxib 12.5 mg, rofecoxib 25 mg, and celecoxib 200 mg in the treatment of symptomatic osteoarthritis: results of two similarly designed studies. Curr Med Res Opin. 2006;22(7):1353–67. https://doi.org/10.1185/030079906X104876.
20. Essex MN, O'Connell M, Bhadra BP. Response to nonsteroidal anti-inflammatory drugs in african americans with osteoarthritis of the knee. J Int Med Res. 2012;40(6):2251–66.
21. Hochberg MC, Fort JG, Svensson O, Hwang C, Sostek M. Fixed-dose combination of enteric-coated naproxen and immediate-release esomeprazole has comparable efficacy to celecoxib for knee osteoarthritis: two randomized trials. Curr Med Res Opin. 2011;27(6):1243–53.
22. Schein JR, Kosinski MR, Janagap-Benson C, Gajria K, Lin P, Freedman JD. Functionality and health-status benefits associated with reduction of osteoarthritis pain. Curr Med Res Opin. 2008;24(5):1255–65. https://doi.org/10.1185/030079908X291912.
23. Arjmandi BH, Khalil DA, Lucas EA, et al. Soy protein may alleviate osteoarthritis symptoms. Phytomedicine. 2004;11(7–8):567–75.
24. Chappell AS, Ossanna MJ, Liu-Seifert H, et al. Duloxetine, a centrally acting analgesic, in the treatment of patients with osteoarthritis knee pain: a 13-week, randomized, placebo-controlled trial. Pain. 2009;146(3):253–60. https://doi.org/10.1016/j.pain.2009.06.024.
25. Chappell AS, Desaiah D, Liu-Seifert H, et al. A double-blind, randomized, placebo-controlled study of the efficacy and safety of duloxetine for the treatment of chronic pain due to osteoarthritis of the knee. Pain Pract. 2011; 11(1):33–41. https://doi.org/10.1111/j.1533-2500.2010.00401.x.
26. Golden HE, Moskowitz RW, Minic M. Analgesic efficacy and safety of nonprescription doses of naproxen sodium compared with acetaminophen in the treatment of osteoarthritis of the knee. Am J Ther. 2004;11(2):85–94.
27. Goetzel RZ, Long SR, Ozminkowski RJ, Hawkins K, Wang S, Lynch W. Health, absence, disability, and presenteeism cost estimates of certain physical and mental health conditions affecting U.S. employers. J Occup Environ Med. 2004;46(4):398–412.
28. Muchmore L, Lynch WD, Gardner HH, Williamson T, Burke T. Prevalence of arthritis and associated joint disorders in an employed population and the associated healthcare, sick leave, disability, and workers' compensation benefits cost and productivity loss of employers. J Occup Environ Med. 2003;45(4):369–78.
29. Patel AS, Farquharson R, Carroll D, et al. The impact and burden of chronic pain in the workplace: A qualitative systematic review. Pain Pract. 2012;12(7):578–89. https://doi.org/10.1111/j.1533-2500.2012.00547.x.
30. Rolfson O, Wissig S, van Maasakkers L, et al. Defining an international standard set of outcome measures for patients with hip or knee osteoarthritis: Consensus of the international consortium for health outcomes measurement hip and knee osteoarthritis working group. Arthritis Care Res (Hoboken). 2016;68(11):1631–9. https://doi.org/10.1002/acr.22868.
31. Fan X, Straube S. Reporting on work-related low back pain: data sources, discrepancies and the art of discovering truths. Pain Manag. 2016;6(5):553–9.

32. Barthel HR, Peniston JH, Clark MB, Gold MS, Altman RD. Correlation of pain relief with physical function in hand osteoarthritis: Randomized controlled trial post hoc analysis. Arthritis Res Ther. 2010;12(1):R7. https://doi.org/10.1186/ar2906.
33. Nieman DC, Shanely RA, Luo B, Dew D, Meaney MP, Sha W. A commercialized dietary supplement alleviates joint pain in community adults: a double-blind, placebo-controlled community trial. Nutr J. 2013; 12(1):154–2891-12-154. https://doi.org/10.1186/1475-2891-12-154.
34. Pope JE, Prashker M, Anderson J. The efficacy and cost effectiveness of N of 1 studies with diclofenac compared to standard treatment with nonsteroidal antiinflammatory drugs in osteoarthritis. J Rheumatol. 2004; 31(1):140–9.
35. Richmond JS, Gunadasa S, Bland M, MacPherson H. Copper bracelets and magnetic wrist straps for rheumatoid arthritis – analgesic and anti-inflammatory effects: a randomised double-blind placebo controlled crossover trial. PLoS One. 2013;8(9):e71529.
36. Taibi DM, Bourguignon C, Gill TA. A feasibility study of valerian extract for sleep disturbance in person with arthritis. Biol Res Nurs. 2009;10(4):409–17. https://doi.org/10.1177/1099800408324252.
37. Cheras PA, Myers SP, Paul-Brent PA, Outerbridge KH, Nielsen GV. Randomized double-blind placebo-controlled trial on the potential modes of action of SheaFlex70 in osteoarthritis. Phytother Res. 2010;24(8):1126–31. https://doi.org/10.1002/ptr.3075.
38. Ernst E. Avocado-soybean unsaponifiables (ASU) for osteoarthritis - a systematic review. Clin Rheumatol. 2003;22(4–5):285–8. https://doi.org/10.1007/s10067-003-0731-4.
39. Florete OG, Xiang J, Vorsanger GJ. Effects of extended-release tramadol on pain-related sleep parameters in patients with osteoarthritis. Expert Opin Pharmacother. 2008;9(11):1817–27. https://doi.org/10.1517/14656566.9.11.1817.
40. Gana TJ, Pascual ML, Fleming RR, et al. Extended-release tramadol in the treatment of osteoarthritis: a multicenter, randomized, double-blind, placebo-controlled clinical trial. Curr Med Res Opin. 2006;22(7):1391–401. https://doi.org/10.1185/030079906X115595.
41. Jabbari B, Machado D. Treatment of refractory pain with botulinum toxins--an evidence-based review. Pain Med. 2011;12(11):1594–606. https://doi.org/10.1111/j.1526-4637.2011.01245.x.
42. Lambert RG, Hutchings EJ, Grace MG, Jhangri GS, Conner-Spady B, Maksymowych WP. Steroid injection for osteoarthritis of the hip: A randomized, double-blind, placebo-controlled trial. Arthritis Rheum. 2007; 56(7):2278–87. https://doi.org/10.1002/art.22739.
43. Maheu E, Mazieres B, Valat JP, et al. Symptomatic efficacy of avocado/soybean unsaponifiables in the treatment of osteoarthritis of the knee and hip: a prospective, randomized, double-blind, placebo-controlled, multicenter clinical trial with a six-month treatment period and a two-month followup demonstrating a persistent effect. Arthritis Rheum. 1998; 41(1):81–91. https://doi.org/10.1002/1529-0131(199801)41:13.0.CO;2-9.
44. Moskowitz RW, Sunshine A, Brugger A, Lefkowith JB, Zhao WW, Geis GS. American pain society pain questionnaire and other pain measures in the assessment of osteoarthritis pain: a pooled analysis of three celecoxib pivotal studies. Am J Ther. 2003;10(1):12–20.
45. Plosker GL, Lyseng-Williamson KA. Buprenorphine 5, 10 and 20 µg/h transdermal patch: A guide to its use in chronic non-malignant pain. CNS Drugs. 2012;1((26(4))):367–73.
46. Rozendaal RM, Koes BW, Weinans H, et al. The effect of glucosamine sulphate on osteoarthritis: design of a long-term randomised clinical trial [ISRCTN54513166]. BMC Musculoskelet Disord. 2005;6:20.
47. Turan Y, Bayraktar K, Kahvecioglu F, et al. Is magnetotherapy applied to bilateral hips effective in ankylosing spondylitis patients? a randomized, double-blind, controlled study. Rheumatol Int. 2014;34(3):357–65. https://doi.org/10.1007/s00296-013-2941-7.
48. Willich SN, Rossnagel K, Roll S, et al. Rose hip herbal remedy in patients with rheumatoid arthritis - a randomised controlled trial. Phytomedicine. 2010;17(2):87–93. https://doi.org/10.1016/j.phymed.2009.09.003.
49. Alfredo PP, Bjordal JM, Dreyer SH, et al. Efficacy of low level laser therapy associated with exercises in knee osteoarthritis: A randomized double-blind study. Clin Rehabil. 2012;26(6):523–33. https://doi.org/10.1177/0269215511425962.
50. Auw Yang KG, Raijmakers NJ, van Arkel ER, et al. Autologous interleukin-1 receptor antagonist improves function and symptoms in osteoarthritis when compared to placebo in a prospective randomized controlled trial. Osteoarthr Cartil. 2008;16(4):498–505.
51. Babul N, Noveck R, Chipman H, Roth SH, Gana T, Albert K. Efficacy and safety of extended-release, once-daily tramadol in chronic pain: A randomized 12-week clinical trial in osteoarthritis of the knee. J Pain Symptom Manage. 2004;28(1):59–71. https://doi.org/10.1016/j.jpainsymman.2003.11.006 .
52. Brown JP, Boulay LJ. Clinical experience with duloxetine in the management of chronic musculoskeletal pain. A focus on osteoarthritis of the knee. Ther Adv Musculoskelet Dis. 2013;5(6):291–304. https://doi.org/10.1177/1759720X13508508.
53. Burch F, Fishman R, Messina N, et al. A comparison of the analgesic efficacy of tramadol contramid OAD versus placebo in patients with pain due to osteoarthritis. J Pain Symptom Manag. 2007;34(3):328–38.
54. Cibere J, Thorne A, Kopec JA, et al. Glucosamine sulfate and cartilage type II collagen degradation in patients with knee osteoarthritis: randomized discontinuation trial results employing biomarkers. J Rheumatol. 2005;32(5): 896–902.
55. Frakes EP, Risser RC, Ball TD, Hochberg MC, Wohlreich MM. Duloxetine added to oral nonsteroidal anti-inflammatory drugs for treatment of knee pain due to osteoarthritis: results of a randomized, double-blind, placebo-controlled trial. Curr Med Res Opin. 2011;27(12):2361–72.
56. Hsieh RL, Lo MT, Liao WC, Lee WC. Short-term effects of 890-nanometer radiation on pain, physical activity, and postural stability in patients with knee osteoarthritis: a double-blind, randomized, placebo-controlled study. Arch Phys Med Rehabil. 2012;93(5):757–64.
57. Hsieh R, Liao W, Lee W. Local and systemic cardiovascular effects from monochromatic infrared therapy in patients with knee osteoarthritis: A double-blind, randomized, placebo-controlled study. Evid Based Complement Alternat Med. 2012;2012(583016):eCAM.
58. Hsieh RL, Lo MT, Lee WC, Liao WC. Therapeutic effects of short-term monochromatic infrared energy therapy on patients with knee osteoarthritis: a double-blind, randomized, placebo-controlled study. J Orthop Sports Phys Ther. 2012;42(11):47–56.
59. Ilan DI, Liporace FA, Rosen J, Cannavo D. Efficacy of rofecoxib for pain control after knee arthroscopy: a prospective, randomized, double-blinded clinical trial. Arthroscopy. 2004;20(8):813–8.
60. Jia L, Wang Y, Chen J, Chen W. Efficacy of focused low-intensity pulsed ultrasound therapy for the management of knee osteoarthritis: A randomized, double blind, placebo-controlled trial. Sci Rep. 2016;6:35453. https://doi.org/10.1038/srep35453.
61. Kannus P, Natri A, Niittymäki S, Järvinen M. Effect of intraarticular glycosaminoglycan polysulfate treatment on patellofemoral pain syndrome. A prospective, randomized double-blind trial comparing glycosaminoglycan polysulfate with placebo and quadriceps muscle exercises. Arthritis Rheum. 1992;35(9):1053–61.
62. Magrans-Courtney T, Wilborn C, Rasmussen C, et al. Effects of diet type and supplementation of glucosamine, chondroitin, and MSM on body composition, functional status, and markers of health in women with knee osteoarthritis initiating a resistance-based exercise and weight loss program. J Int Soc Sports Nutr. 2011;8(1):8.
63. Mata J, Cabrera S, Sanchis P, et al. Electro-acupuncture for treatment of knee pain from osteoarthritis and the possible endocrinology changes: a study protocol for a randomized controlled trial. Trials. 2015;16:248–015–0766-2. https://doi.org/10.1186/s13063-015-0766-2.
64. Möller I, Pérez M, Monfort J, et al. Effectiveness of chondroitin sulphate in patients with concomitant knee osteoarthritis and psoriasis: A randomized, double-blind, placebo-controlled study. Osteoarthr Cartil. 2010;Suppl 1:S32–40.
65. Mazzuca SA, Page MC, Meldrum RD, Brandt KD, Petty-Saphon S. Pilot study of the effects of a heat-retaining knee sleeve on joint pain, stiffness, and function in patients with knee osteoarthritis. Arthritis Rheum. 2004;51(5): 716–21. https://doi.org/10.1002/art.20683.
66. Pavelka K Jr, Sedlackova M, Gatterova J, Becvar R, Pavelka KS. Glycosaminoglycan polysulfuric acid (GAGPS) in osteoarthritis of the knee. Osteoarthr Cartil. 1995;3(1):15–23.
67. Pincus T, Koch GG, Sokka T, et al. A randomized, double-blind, crossover clinical trial of diclofenac plus misoprostol versus acetaminophen in patients with osteoarthritis of the hip or knee. Arthritis Rheum. 2001;44(7):1587–98.
68. Sanghi D, Mishra A, Sharma AC, et al. Does vitamin D improve osteoarthritis of the knee: A randomized controlled pilot trial. Clin Orthop Relat Res. 2013; 471(11):3556–62. https://doi.org/10.1007/s11999-013-3201-6.

69. Schauss AG, Stenehjem J, Park J, Endres JR, Clewell A. Effect of the novel low molecular weight hydrolyzed chicken sternal cartilage extract, BioCell collagen, on improving osteoarthritis-related symptoms: a randomized, double-blind, placebo-controlled trial. J Agric Food Chem. 2012;60(16):4096–101.
70. Segal NA, Toda Y, Huston J, et al. Two configurations of static magnetic fields for treating rheumatoid arthritis of the knee: a double-blind clinical trial. Arch Phys Med Rehabil. 2001;82(10):1453–60.
71. Sihvonen R, Paavola M, Malmivaara A, et al. Arthroscopic partial meniscectomy versus sham surgery for a degenerative meniscal tear. N Engl J Med. 2013;369(26):2515–24. https://doi.org/10.1056/NEJMoa1305189.
72. Singer BJ, Silbert PL, Song S, Dunne JW, Singer KP. Treatment of refractory anterior knee pain using botulinum toxin type a (dysport) injection to the distal vastus lateralis muscle: a randomised placebo controlled crossover trial. Br J Sports Med. 2011;45(8):640–5.
73. Taverner MG, Ward TL, Loughnan TE. Transcutaneous pulsed radiofrequency treatment in patients with painful knee awaiting total knee joint replacement. Clin J Pain. 2010;26(5):429–32. https://doi.org/10.1097/AJP.0b013e3181d92a87.
74. van der Weegen W, Wullems JA, Bos E, Noten H, van Drumpt RA. No difference between intra-articular injection of hyaluronic acid and placebo for mild to moderate knee osteoarthritis: A randomized, controlled, double-blind trial. J Arthroplast 30(5):754–7. 2015;30(5):754–7. https://doi.org/10.1016/j.arth.2014.12.012.
75. Zhao SZ, McMillen JI, Markenson JA, et al. Evaluation of the functional status aspects of health-related quality of life of patients with osteoarthritis treated with celecoxib. Pharmacotherapy. 1999;19(11):1269–78.

6

Simultaneous measurement of formic acid, methanol and ethanol in vitreous and blood samples of postmortem by headspace GC-FID

Hamideh Ghorbani[1], Alireza Nezami[2], Behjat Sheikholeslami[3], Arya Hedjazi[1] and Mahnaz Ahmadimanesh[1,2*]

Abstract

Background: Formic acid (formate) is the main reason for toxicity and death through methanol poisoning. The simultaneous determination of methanol, ethanol, and formate in the body can help to discover the cause of death and is useful in the diagnosis of acute methanol poisoning. The measurement of formate is not yet available in Iran. With regard to the increasing rate of methanol poisoning and its related mortality in Iran, as well as the main role of formate in methanol poisoning, this study was designed to set up an analytical method for the concurrent determination of ethanol, methanol, and formate.

Methods: Following the modification of a previously developed gas chromatography method, vitreous and blood samples of 43 postmortem cases with a history of methanol intoxication were collected over a period of 2 years at the Legal Medicine Organization of Mashhad. Thereafter, ethanol, methanol, and formate concentrations were measured by headspace GC/FID. Formate esterification was performed by the methylation of formate with sulfuric acid and methanol. In order to confirm the esterification method for the production of methyl formate, we used gas chromatography with a mass detector (GC/MS) because of its higher sensitivity and accuracy. Furthermore, the correlations between formate and methanol concentrations in blood and vitreous samples, and between formate and methanol were investigated.

Results: A significant relationship was found only between methanol concentrations in blood and vitreous samples ($P < 0.03$).

Conclusions: In postmortems, with the passage of time since alcohol ingestion, the measurement of only methanol concentration cannot determine the degree of toxicity or the cause of death. Therefore, using the present analytical method and measurement of formic acid, we can estimate the degree of toxicity and cause of death.

Keywords: Methanol, Formic acid, Methyl formate, Postmortem, Poisoning, Measurement

* Correspondence: Ahmadimm931@mums.ac.ir; Mahnaz_Ahmadimanesh@yahoo.com
[1]Legal Medicine Research Center, Legal Medicine Organization, Tehran, Iran
[2]Department of Pharmacodynamics & Toxicology, Mashhad University of Medical Science, School of Pharmacy, P. O. Box: 91388-13944, Mashhad, Iran
Full list of author information is available at the end of the article

Background

Methanol (wood spirits) is a widely used commercial and industrial alcohol. It is also found in the production process of non-standard alcoholic beverages using grape twigs [1]. In the human body, it is first metabolized to formaldehyde by alcohol dehydrogenase in the liver. Then it is converted to formate, which, in turn, is transformed to CO_2 and H_2O [1–3]. Methanol itself has low toxicity, and there is a relatively negligible correlation between toxicity or mortality and methanol blood or serum concentrations [4, 5]. Formaldehyde is very toxic but it has a short half-life and does not accumulate; hence, no considerable formaldehyde concentrations are found in body fluids and tissues following the administration of methanol [6]. Formic acid is considered to be the main toxic compound produced in the course of methyl alcohol metabolism. Formic acid accumulates in the body and is the main reason for toxic effects and death through methanol poisoning [6–8]. Commonly reported adverse effects related to high serum concentrations of formic acid include visual damage, optical nerve injury, abdominal problems, nausea, and headache. Subsequently, high formic acid concentrations result in respiratory problems, renal failure, and finally lead to coma and death [9]. Therefore, it seems necessary to determine the serum concentrations of methanol and especially of formic acid, in order to evaluate the causes of these observed adverse effects.

The measurement of formate is not yet available in Iran. With regard to the increasing rate of methanol poisoning and its related mortality in Iran, and also to the role of formate in methanol poisoning and the importance of its measurement in determining the causes of poisoning and death [10], this study was designed to set up an analytical method for the detection of formic acid in human samples. While flame ionization detectors (FIDs) are commonly used to measure methyl and ethyl alcohol, they are almost unable to determine formate concentration [9, 11, 12]. An esterification step is needed for formic acid detection [11, 12]. Enzymatic methods have also been used to determine the formate concentration [13]. Headspace gas chromatography (HSGC) has been utilized for the detection of formic acid using sodium propionate as an internal standard [14]. Also, the GC/MS has recently been used for the detection of formic acid [15, 16].

In the present study, using a previously developed gas chromatography method with some modification [11], we simultaneously measured formic acid, methanol, and ethanol concentrations in 43 postmortems of vitreous and blood samples by headspace GC/FID. Furthermore, we investigated the relationship between concentrations of analytes in blood and vitreous samples.

Methods

Methyl formate, formic acid (95%), sulfuric acid (97%), ethanol (96%), methanol, acetonitrile (99.9%), dichloromethane, and distilled water were purchased from Merck Company (analytical grade).

Sample collection and storage

In the present study, 43 victims who died of methanol poisoning were investigated from April 2014 to April 2016. This work was approved by Tehran Legal Medicine Research Center Ethics Committee. All bodies were transferred to the Mashhad Legal Medicine Organization (LMO) within 24 h of death. For all cases, the interval of time between death and sampling was less than 24 h. Also, the interval of time between sampling and the analyses of the samples was less than 2 h. All autopsies of major organs were studied together with a review of clinical histories. Blood and vitreous samples were analyzed to determine methanol, formic acid, and ethanol concentrations. Blood samples were taken from the femoral region and stored in tubes containing sodium fluoride (NaF). All the blood and vitreous (without preservatives) samples were stored at −4 °C. Moral consent was taken from the family of the deceased before the experiment.

Headspace GC/FID was used in the sample analysis for the simultaneous determination of ethanol, methanol, and formic acid. The GC/MS was also used to confirm the results of GC/FID. The detailed conditions of these devices were listed as follows:

GC/FID headspace conditions

The 7890A Headspace GC/FID model was provided by Agilent. Data analysis was performed using Agilent chemstation REV.B.04.03. Nitrogen carrier gas (purity 99.9992%) was supplied by nitrogen cylinders. Hydrogen gas was supplied from a Chebios hydrogen generator. The complete details of the GC/FID procedure are presented in Table 1.

GC/MS conditions

The GC/MS was from the Agilent Company (6890 N-5978B). Helium carrier gas was supplied by helium cylinders. The scan mode was used for the GC/MS analysis. Data analysis was performed using MSD chemstation G1701EA E.02.01.1177. The full details of the GC/MS are shown in Table 2.

Derivatization

Since gas chromatography cannot detect formic acid, it is necessary to convert it to methyl formate by esterification (derivatization) before its quantification in blood and vitreous samples. The following steps were performed for the derivatization of formic acid: 1 mL samples containing formic acid were transferred to headspace vials (Restek)

Table 1 Parameter values for HS GC/FID

Parameter	Type	Value
Carrier gas	Nitrogen	Nitrogen cylinders
Column:	Capillary column of the Restek Corporation (J & W RTX-BAC1 Model)	Dimensions = 30 m * 530 μm * 3 μm Flow = 1.5 ml/min Pressure = 1.2 psi
Detector:	FID	Heater = 250 °C H_2 Flow = 40 ml/min Air Flow = 400 ml/min
Oven:	Gradient	Initial temperature = 60 °C Hold time = 5 min Rate = 10 °C Final temperature = 130 °C Run time = 12 min
Inlet:		Temperature = 90 °C Total flow = 79.5 ml/min Septum Purge Flow = 3 ml/min Gas Saver = on
Injector	Headspace split (1:20)	200 °C
Headspace:		Zone temperature = 40 °C Event time = 15 min

coated with a microfilm; 500 μl of concentrated sulfuric acid (97%) was added as a catalyst and then mixed; the samples were incubated for 20 min at room temperature; 30 μl of pure methanol (99.9%) for the conversion of formic acid to methyl formate and 30 μl acetonitrile (0.197 M was prepared from pure acetonitrile (99.99%) by diluting with water) as an internal standard were added; the resultant was shaken; and finally, following a 20-min incubation at room temperature, the samples were prepared for injection [11, 12].

Preparation of stock solutions and calibration curve

At first, pure methyl formate was injected into the GC/MS to ensure that detection by GC/FID and the determined retention time were properly conducted [15, 16]. Thereafter, standard samples of methyl formate were prepared from formic acid according to the literature [9, 11, 12].

Table 2 Parameter values for GC/MS

Parameter	Type	Value
Carrier gas	Helium	Helium cylinders
Column:	capillary column (19,091 F) - General	Size 5 mm Flow = 0.5 ml/min
Detector:	Mass	
Oven:	Gradient	Initial temperature = 65 °C Rate = 5 °C Final temperature = 90 °C Run time = 7.5 min
Inlet:		Temperature = 90 °C Total flow = 79.5 ml/min Septum Purge Flow = 3 ml/min Gas Saver = on
Injector	split less	90 °C

After this, liquid–liquid extraction was done using a mixture of water and di-chloromethane (1:1, *v*/v), and organic layers were infused to the device. Figures of pure methyl formate were compared with those produced from formic acid in samples, in order to ensure the accuracy of the derivatization process.

In the next step, separate standard aqueous samples of ethanol, methanol, and formic acid were prepared and then, after the derivatization of formic acid using the procedure mentioned above, injected to HSGC/FID to define their retention times. To draw the calibration curve, 10 concentrations of ethanol, methanol, and formic acid were prepared in concentration ranges of 20 to 200 mg/dL, 50 to 500 mg/dL, and 0.5 to 150 mg/dL, respectively. All bioanalytical method validation procedures for calculating accuracy, precision, recovery, and limit of quantitation (LOQ) were done according to the Food and Drug Administration (FDA) guidance for industry [17].

Application of method in biologic matrices

The blank samples (blood and vitreous) were mixed with a certain amount of ethanol and methanol and injected into the device (Fig. 1). In the second step, they were mixed with a certain amount of formic acid and injected into the device following derivatization to methyl formate (Fig. 2). In order to confirm the retention time of methyl formate, 20 μl of pure methyl formate was added to the samples and the samples were spiked (Fig. 3). This work was performed three times in 3 days and the mean values were compared with the desired values. Since ethanol and methanol may affect the process of derivatization, we analyzed methanol and ethanol concentrations in all samples before derivatization.

Pearson correlation

Relationships between the blood and vitreous concentrations of methanol and formic acid were evaluated using the Pearson correlation tool.

Statistical analysis

Statistical analysis was performed using SPSS version 22. Appropriate parametric tests were used. Two tailed tests with a *P* value less than 0.05 were considered statistically significant.

Results

Analytical method

The retention time for methyl formate in the GC/MS was 1.85 min. The retention time in GC/FID for methyl formate, methanol, and ethanol were 6.2, 5.3, and 6.7 min, respectively.

The calibration curves for all analytes were made in a previously mentioned range of concentrations. The

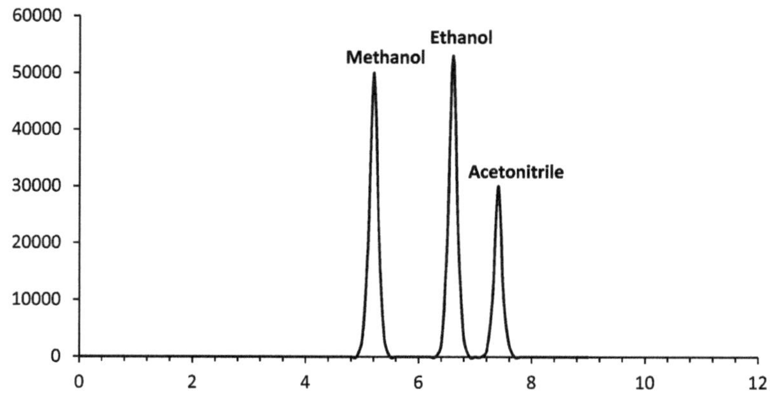

Fig. 1 HSGC/FID chromatogram of blank human vitreous spiked with methanol (200 mg/dl), ethanol (150 mg/dl) and acetonitrile (0.197 M) as an internal standard

correlation coefficients (R2) for formic acid, methanol, and ethanol were 0.992, 0.999, and 0.999, respectively. In this study, a recovery rate of over 89% was calculated. For all analytes involving the blood and vitreous samples, the limit of detection (LOD) and the LOQ were 0.5 mg/dL and 1.5 mg/dL, respectively. The mentioned bioanalytical method provided an accuracy of 97.3–102.4%, and the precision, relative standard deviation (RSD %) was better than 9.6% for control samples (Table 3).

Demographic data

The age range of the deceased persons was 23–81 years, with the average being 42.11 years (six females and 37 males). The dose and the time of ingestion, and the history of consumption were unknown. Therefore, the time interval between ingestion and death was unclear, and it was not possible to find a correlation between dosage, ingestion time, and incidence of death.

Clinical finding

Measured concentrations in both blood and vitreous samples are shown in Table 4. Also, the minimum and maximum concentrations for ethanol, methanol, and formic acid in the blood and vitreous samples are shown in Table 4. The mean and median values of concentrations, and correlations between mean concentrations were analyzed. A real sample chromatogram is displayed in Fig. 4.

In some cases, where methanol concentrations were under the limit of detection, formic acid concentrations were detected and vice versa. Considering the values of the Pearson correlation coefficient for methanol and formic acid, it appears that there is a very strong linear relation between the blood and vitreous concentrations of methanol (correlation coefficient: 0.987; significance: 0.00). However, no significant correlations were found between concentrations of formate in the blood and vitreous samples. Moreover, formate and methanol concentrations in both the blood and vitreous samples showed weak correlations (correlation coefficient: < 0.2).

Discussion

The incidence of methanol poisoning and related mortality has increased worldwide in the last decade [10].

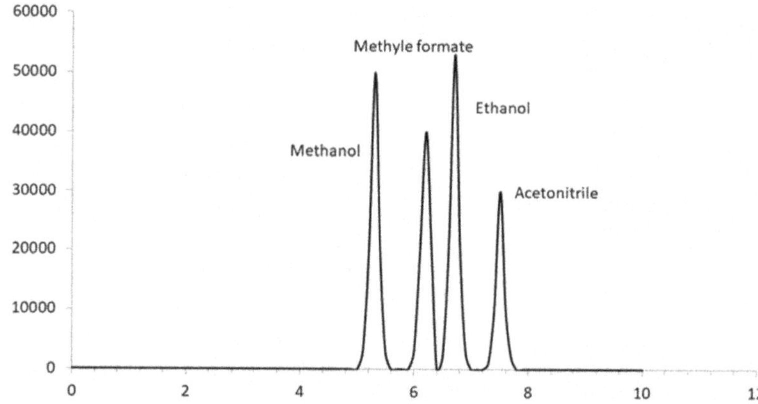

Fig. 2 HSGC/FID chromatogram of blank human vitreous spiked with methanol (200 mg/dl), methyl formate (65 mg/dl), ethanol (150 mg/dl) and acetonitrile (0.197 M) as an internal standard

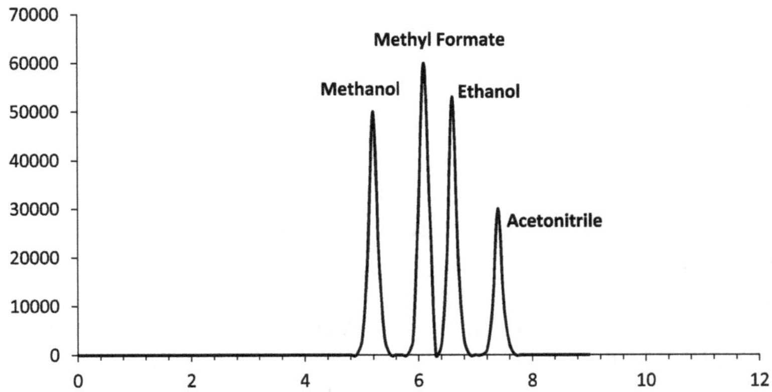

Fig. 3 HSGC/FID chromatogram of blank human vitreous spiked with methanol (200 mg/dl), methyl formate (65 mg/dl plus 20 μl of pure methyl formate), ethanol (150 mg/dl) and acetonitrile (0.197 M) as an internal standard

Also, owing to the consumption of contaminated beverages, its rate has increased in Iran [10]. In a methanol-poisoning outbreak in Mashhad in May 2009, 11 out of 25 patients referred to Imam Reza Hospital died [10].

With regard to the prohibition of alcohol consumption in Iran, alcoholic beverages are usually produced using illegal and non-standard (contaminated) methods [10]. In most cases, due to the existence of wood during fermentation, methanol concentration is considerable in

Table 3 Determination of accuracy and precision for formic acid, methanol and ethanol in human vitreous and whole blood

Concentration (mg/dl)	Within-day (n = 3)			Between-day (*n* = 3)		
	Mean ± SD	Accuracy	Precision	Mean ± SD	Accuracy	Precision
Formica acid (blood)						
0.5	0.49 ± 0.02	98.0	4.08	0.49 ± 0.01	99.3	2.32
75	75.6 ± 1.5	100.8	2.01	73 ± 1	97.3	1.37
150	153.6 ± 6.1	102.4	3.97	153.6 ± 7.7	102.4	5.01
Methanol (blood)						
50	54.2 ± 4.7	101.8	3.75	48.8 ± 1.04	97.6	2.13
250	248.6 ± 7.6	99.4	3.09	247.5 ± 8.4	99.1	3.41
500	491.6 ± 47.2	98.3	9.61	503.3 ± 35.4	100.6	7.04
Ethanol (blood)						
20	20.4 ± 0.9	102.0	4.67	20.2 ± 0.8	101.2	4.12
100	97.5 ± 7.6	97.5	7.89	98.8 ± 9.2	98.8	9.3
200	199.3 ± 18.1	99.6	9.10	203.3 ± 16.6	101.6	8.19
Formica acid (vitreous)						
0.5	0.5 ± 0.01	101.1	3.34	0.5 ± 0.01	100.8	3.37
75	76.5 ± 0.7	102.0	0.98	76.1 ± 3.5	101.5	4.69
150	148.7 ± 4.1	99.2	2.77	150.5 ± 4.8	100.3	3.20
Methanol (vitreous)						
50	49.2 ± 1.6	98.5	3.32	50.3 ± 2.7	100.7	5.47
250	251.2 ± 14.4	100.5	5.73	255.8 ± 12.3	102.3	4.82
500	499.1 ± 35.5	99.8	7.12	506.6 ± 33.2	101.4	6.57
Ethanol (vitreous)						
20	19.5 ± 0.4	97.7	2.13	19.8 ± 0.7	98.9	2.87
100	99.5 ± 5.07	99.5	5.09	100.2 ± 4.36	100.2	4.36
200	204.3 ± 12.6	102.2	6.19	200.6 ± 11.01	100.3	5.48

Table 4 Mean and median of methanol, ethanol and formic acid concentrations in vitreous and blood

Analytes	Methanol mg/dL		Formic acid mg/dL		Ethanol mg/dL
Matrix	Vitreous	Blood	Vitreous	Blood	Vitreous
Mean ± SD	162.3 ± 179.5	131.9 ± 146.5	68.7 ± 37.5	79.6 ± 39.5	21.5 ± 48.2
Median (Min-Max)	80 (0–591)	59 (0–507.3)	73 (0–132.8)	84 (0–157)	1.2 (0–227.5)

the final product. Since handmade beverages have low concentrations of ethanol, consumers usually drink large amounts of liquor to reach the desired mood and effective blood concentrations. Therefore, the amount of methanol intake increases. This can be associated with an increased risk of poisoning. As a matter of fact, the incidence of deliberate poisoning or suicide by methanol is very low in Iran; methanol poisoning is generally accidental and unintentional [10, 18]. In unintentional poisoning, especially in a case of contaminated beverage consumption, simultaneous determination of methanol, ethanol, and formic acid in the body can help to discover the cause of death; it is also useful in the diagnosis of acute methanol poisoning [19–22]. Nowadays, GC/FID is an appropriate quantifying device available in most laboratories [9, 11, 12].

Given that the GC/FID device is often used for alcohol detection at the LMO in Iran, this study could provide a suitable method for the simultaneous determination of alcohol and formic acid. In this study, we also used the GC/MS to guarantee the sensitivity and accuracy of the mentioned GC/FID method since it is more sensitive and accurate than GC/FID [23, 24]. Compared with the GC/FID method developed by Bursova et al. [9], the present method provided smaller values for LOD and LOQ. Also, Bursova et al. [9], utilized two different columns in the GC/FID to validate the method, but we used two different chromatographic devices, GC/MS and GC/FID. We used the general column of the GC/MS (used to identify all materials) without headspace. As direct injection of samples containing sulfuric acid may cause damage in the column, a liquid–liquid extraction step was used to prevent such damage [15, 16]. In order to rule out the influence of methanol and ethanol on derivatization, we first analyzed their concentrations before derivatization. Even if other derivatization agents (like isopropanol) are used [9], it is possible to have the same effect in cases of methanol and ethanol presence in patient samples; then the reported final concentration would be false. Therefore, it is better that methanol and ethanol concentrations are detected before derivatization.

According to methanol kinetics and the late occurrence of methanol toxicity symptoms, there is a time interval between consumption and death [1, 8, 25]. Variations in dose, genetic factors, physical conditions like weight and sex, and history of alcohol consumption affect the metabolism of methanol; they also have an impact on the severity of its toxicity, and the time gap between its consumption and death [3, 5, 25]. Hence, information regarding corpse history can be useful for detecting the cause of death. However, since we collected samples from the Department of Forensic Medicine, the complete detailed information was not available as the family of the deceased, in most cases, refused to answer such questions. Generally, in this study, the dose, elapsed time, concurrent use of other substances, and history of the poisoned person remained unknown. This was the most important limitation of this work. Consequently, it was very difficult to

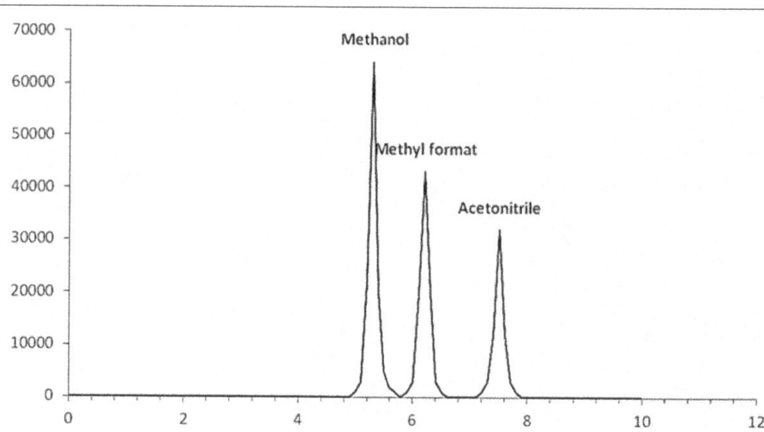

Fig. 4 HSGC/FID chromatogram of a human vitreous sample of post-mortem containing, methanol (310.5 mg/dl), methyl formate (70.08 mg/dl) and acetonitrile (0.197 M) as an internal standard

correlate the observed methanol concentrations to the incidence of death.

Following the investigation of relationships between the observed concentrations, we found a strong correlation between methanol concentration in the blood and vitreous samples, similar to the finding of Graham R. Jones et al. [22]. Moreover, like the mentioned study, we found poor correlations between methanol and formic acid concentrations in both the blood and vitreous samples. Also, there was a weak correlation between the vitreous and blood concentrations of formic acid [22]. This can happen due to different circumstances in the metabolism of methanol and formic acid production including genetics, simultaneous use of other substances and dosage, and received medical treatment [25]. These issues can explain the difference between formic acid formation and methanol metabolism. Since there was a weak negative correlation between the blood concentrations of methanol and formic acid in our study, formic acid concentration increased alongside the decrease of methanol blood concentration.

Cytochrome oxidase was inhibited by format in concentrations of 5–30 mmol/L and/or above 20 mg/dl [1]. In previous reports, poisoning and death happened following a wide range of methanol doses [12]. According to numerous studies in this field, there are considerable differences between individuals and reports stating concentrations that may cause poisoning and death [12]. In the study by Graham R. Jones et al. [22], it was shown that the majority of vitreous and blood samples from postmortems had formic acid in concentrations around 0.5 g/L or above. They also stated that the lowest methanol concentration in blood associated with death was 70 mg/dl. In the present study, lower concentrations associated with death were observed. This was due to different genetic conditions in metabolism, which resulted in different concentrations. In cases involving the simultaneous detection of ethanol (more than 20 μg/dl) and methanol or formic acid, poisoning by contaminated beverages was confirmed. With regard to this, in cases of methanol or formic acid detection (without ethanol observation), only poisoning by methanol was confirmed.

Conclusion

In this study, we could confirm methanol poisoning by the determination of formic acid in each sample (vitreous or blood), even in cases where there was a considerable time gap between the use of methanol and death (despite methanol negative); but we did not find a new relationship between concentrations. Also, in cases with high concentration of formic acid, the cause of death was confirmed. Therefore, using this method for the measurement of formic acid, the degree of toxicity and the cause of death can be estimated.

Abbreviations

FID: Flame Ionization Detector; Formate: Formic acid; GC/MS: Gas Chromatography with Mass Detector; HSGC: Headspace Gas Chromatography

Acknowledgements

Special thanks to the personnel of Mashhad Legal Medicine Organization.

Funding

This study was financially supported by grants from Legal Medicine Research Center, Tehran, Iran and Legal Medicine of Razavi Khorasan, Mashhad, Iran.

Authors' contributions

MA designed the experiments; AN performed the experiments; HG analyzed the data; AH contributed reagents; MA and BS wrote the manuscript. All of the authors gave final approval and agreed to be accountable for all aspects of the work in ensuring that questions relating to the accuracy or integrity of any part of the work are appropriately investigated and resolved.

Competing interests

The authors declare that they have no competing interests.

Author details

[1]Legal Medicine Research Center, Legal Medicine Organization, Tehran, Iran. [2]Department of Pharmacodynamics & Toxicology, Mashhad University of Medical Science, School of Pharmacy, P. O. Box: 91388-13944, Mashhad, Iran. [3]Faculty of Pharmacy, Lorestan University of Medical Sciences, Khorramabad, Iran.

References

1. Haddad LM, Winchester JF. Clinical management of poisoning and drug overdose. 4th edition. Philadelphia: WB Saunders company; 2007.
2. Lanigan S. Final report on the safety assessment of methyl alcohol. Int J Toxicol. 2000;20:57–85.
3. Wiener S, et al. Toxic alcohols. Gold frank's Toxicologic Emergencies, 2006.
4. Kostic MA, Dart RC. Rethinking the toxic methanol level. J Toxicol Clin Toxicol. 2003;41(6):793–800.
5. Fraser AD, Coffin L, Worth D. Drug and chemical metabolites in clinical toxicology investigations: the importance of ethylene glycol, methanol and cannabinoid metabolite analyses. Clin Biochem. 2002;35(7):501–11.
6. Jacobsen D, et al. Methanol and formate kinetics in late diagnosed methanol intoxication. Med Toxicol Adverse Drug Exp. 1988;3(5):418–23.
7. Treichel JL, et al. Formate, the toxic metabolite of methanol, in cultured ocular cells. Neurotoxicology. 2003;24(6):825–34.
8. Kerns W, et al. Formate kinetics in methanol poisoning. J Toxicol Clin Toxicol. 2002;40(2):137–43.
9. Bursová M, Hložek T, Čabala R. Simultaneous determination of methanol, ethanol and formic acid in serum and urine by headspace GC-FID. J Anal Toxicol. 2015;39(9):741–5.
10. Afshari R. Epidemics/outbreaks of methanol poisoning. Asia Pac J Med Toxicol. 2014;3:24.
11. Abolin C, et al. Gas chromatographic head-space assay of formic acid as methyl formate in biologic fluids: potential application to methanol poisoning. Biochem Med. 1980;23(2):209–18.
12. Ferrari LA, et al. Post-mortem analysis of formic acid disposition in acute methanol intoxication. Forensic Sci Int. 2003;133(1):152–8.
13. Mori H, Ohmori R. Determination of formate using immobilized formate dehydrogenase in a flow system and its application to analyze the formate content of foodstuffs. J Health Sci. 2008;54(2):212–5.

14. Fraser AD, MacNeil W. Gas chromatographic analysis of methyl formate and application in methanol poisoning cases. J Anal Toxicol. 1989;13(2):73–6.
15. Kage S, et al. Simultaneous determination of formate and acetate in whole blood and urine from humans using gas chromatography–mass spectrometry. J Chromatogr B. 2004;805(1):113–7.
16. del Barrio M-A, et al. Simultaneous determination of formic acid and formaldehyde in pharmaceutical excipients using headspace GC/MS. J Pharm Biomed Anal. 2006;41(3):738–43.
17. Food and Drug Administration. Guidance for industry: Quality systems approach to pharmaceutical cGMP regulations. Pharmaceutical CGMPs. 2006.
18. Afshari R. Preclinical toxicology and emergency treatment of poisoning. 2014, iran: Mashhad University of Medical Sciences and Health Services.
19. Lukasik-Głębocka M, et al. Usefulness of blood formic acid detection in the methanol poisoning in the practice of clinical toxicology department-preliminary assessment. Przeglad lekarski. 2013;71(9):475–8.
20. Zakharov S, et al. Is the measurement of serum formate concentration useful in the diagnostics of acute methanol poisoning? A prospective study of 38 patients. Basic Clin Pharmacol Toxicol. 2015;116(5):445–51.
21. Morikawa G, et al. Study of blood concentration analysis for formate in acute methanol poisoning. Chudoku kenkyu. 2015;28(3):243–6.
22. Jones GR, Singer PP, Rittenbach K. The relationship of methanol and formate concentrations in fatalities where methanol is detected. J Forensic Sci. 2007;52(6):1376–82.
23. Sloan KM, Mustacich RV, Eckenrode BA. Development and evaluation of a low thermal mass gas chromatograph for rapid forensic GC–MS analyses. Field Anal Chem Technol. 2001;5(6):288–301.
24. Krone N, et al. Gas chromatography/mass spectrometry (GC/MS) remains a pre-eminent discovery tool in clinical steroid investigations even in the era of fast liquid chromatography tandem mass spectrometry (LC/MS/MS). J Steroid Biochem Mol Biol. 2010;121(3):496–504.
25. Hantson P, Haufroid V, Wallemacq P. Formate kinetics in methanol poisoning. Hum Exp Toxicol. 2005;24(2):55–9.

7

Occupational contact dermatitis from protein in sea products: who is the most affected, the fisherman or the chef?

B. Loddé[1,2,3,5*], P. Cros[4], A. M. Roguedas-Contios[4], R. Pougnet[1,2,3,5], D. Lucas[5], JD. Dewitte[1,2,3,5] and L. Misery[4,5]

Abstract

Background: Protein contact dermatitis has frequently been reported in case studies (usually in cases involving contact with seafood products), but there are very few descriptive series.
The objectives of this present study were firstly to determine the incidence of protein contact dermatitis among fishermen in France and compare it with data from onshore work involving seafood exposure. Second, to discover what factors could explain any differences.
In order to answer these questions we analysed data from the French national occupational disease surveillance and prevention network (RNV3P) and occupational diseases declared to the French National Network for Monitoring and Prevention of Occupational Disease. This retrospective study was done for a 13 year period.

Case presentation: Between 2000 and 2012, we only found eight cases of protein contact dermatitis in the French network. There were no cases of protein contact dermatitis in the seafaring population. The eight cases from the French network are essentially allergies to different fish and chefs are the professionals most affected. Atopy is present in half of these cases.
In the seafaring population we found several cases of allergic delayed-time contact dermatitis due to bryozoans and to gloves but no protein contact dermatitis.

Conclusions: Chefs who have to cook seafood are more at risk of occupational protein contact dermatitis than fishermen. We think that skin protection (that is to say glove wearing) is better implemented in the fishing sector than in the catering profession on shore in France.

Keywords: Maritime, Seafood, Contact dermatitis

Bakcground

Protein contact dermatitis is an allergic dermatitis first described in 1976 by Hjorth and Roed-Petersen [1]. It is likely to be under-recorded, as the diagnosis requires the association of the presence of specific clinical signs (which can appear in different forms) with a protein-type trigger factor examined by a specific dermato-allergological evaluation.

Its physiopathology involves a type 1 allergic reaction mediated by IgE, and in some cases an associated delayed type 4 hypersensitivity reaction (according to the Gell and Coombs classification) [2]. The delayed reaction is the subject of controversy, however, because of the frequent negative results of delayed-reading tests and the clinical symptoms that occur immediately following contact with the allergen [3, 4]. Hence, the reaction is mainly considered as an immediate hypersensitivity reaction caused by high molecular weight proteins penetrating the epidermis. This penetration is facilitated by the alteration of the epidermis due to, for example, previous atopic dermatitis or irritant contact dermatitis [5–7].

Protein contact dermatitis is characterised by clinical lesions resembling chronic or recurrent eczema. There may be exacerbations in the form of an urticarial or blistering rash that becomes itchy after contact with a

* Correspondence: Brice.lodde@chu-brest.fr
[1]Université Européenne de Bretagne, Rennes, France
[2]Université de Brest, EA 4686 – CS 93837 – 29238, Brest Cedex 3, France

product containing proteins. The lesions are located in the contact areas, hence often on the hands but also extending up to the wrists and forearms [5, 7]. There can be non-cutaneous signs, especially among atopic subjects (respiratory signs indicating rhinitis or associated asthma). There are rarely digestive signs when the allergen [2] is ingested, and there are very rarely any systemic reactions [8].

These manifestations are often triggered by contact with plant or animal proteins present in food. When the exposure is intense, which is to say repeated, they can often be considered to be an occupational disease [7]. Protein contact dermatitis was first described in this way in 1976 in sandwich preparers [1].

In France, where employees are compensated in cases of confirmed occupational diseases, the frequency of occupational allergic contact dermatitis is of the order of 7 to 8 cases for 10,000 employees/year, where over 90% are eczemas [5].

From an etiologic standpoint, cases of protein contact dermatitis have frequently been reported in case studies (namely in cases where there is contact with seafood products), but there are very few descriptive series [9, 10]. Hence, we sought to determine the frequency of these specific cases of dermatitis amongst those in professions where they are most likely to handle such products.

Being at the start of the distribution chain, professional fishermen seemed, at first glance, to be the group most exposed to such proteins.

The main objective of this study was to determine the frequency of protein contact dermatitis linked to seafood products within the group of the working population that appeared to be the most exposed.

The secondary objectives were to compare the data obtained with data from cases reported during professional activities on land, to research differences between them and to determine what factors could explain these.

In order to carry out this study, which was both descriptive and retrospective, we selected two populations in which we could find indicators of occupational pathologies. The first group consisted of a population of professional French fishermen, and the other of all those who had sought medical advice at a French centre for occupational diseases. There are 31 of these centres in teaching hospitals spread across the nation.

All of the patient consultation records obtained from these occupational disease centres, which are specialised units in hospitals, are entered and coded by senior doctors in the French National Network for Monitoring and Prevention of Occupational Disease (RNVPPP) [11]. This network identifies all the occupational health problems that have been referred for expert advice within a hospital centre. The resulting files are often complex as they describe cases that have not been resolved by an urban general medicine practice.

For each case, the disease code (the International Classification of Diseases, 10th edition), the (occupational) substance, company's activity, and patient's occupation are recorded during the consultation. The case record is concluded by a clinical summary.

This allowed us to research, within the RNVPPP, all of the cases in which the disease code (CIM-10) corresponded to an allergic contact dermatitis and for which the substance code was fish, crustacean, mollusc or seaweed. We then asked each centre where the cases had been coded for the patients' medical files in order to analyse them. These files were then anonymised and archived. A file had to contain at least one detailed history of the disease, one clinical exam, and one allergological evaluation done by means of a skin prick test and/or a patch test and/or specific IgE testing. The patients had to have seen a senior doctor in order to establish the diagnosis. The patients with typical delayed-time allergic contact dermatitis and/or irritant contact dermatitis (related to soaps, detergents, etc.), or imprecise or questionable clinical histories were excluded from our study. The focus of the study was on occupational protein contact dermatitis.

For comparison, we also researched all cases of occupational skin disease declared under the ENIM (the social security scheme for maritime professions). This retrospective national study focused on illnesses reported over a 13-year period. The files were analysed by ENIM, which compensates professional seafarers who are officially affected by an occupational maritime disease.

Case presentation

Among the 145,293 medical cases registered in the RNVPP between 2000 and 2012, 8 patients were declared as being affected by protein contact dermatitis caused by fish or crustaceans or sea product. Moreover 2 other cases appeared imprecise and seemed to be irritant contact dermatitis to sea products (and to other irritants). Because there was no mention of positive prick-test or positive IgE these 2 cases were excluded from our description.

There were no reported cases of protein contact dermatitis in the population of seafarers (there being an average of about 35,000 registered seafarers per year). Within this population, 25 cases of occupational skin disease caused by allergies were found in 13 years. These were all cases of typical allergic delayed-time contact dermatitis. The allergens were mercaptobenzothiazole, thiuram (a component of protective gloves), bryozoans, and even seaweeds, but there was no mention of occupational dermatitis caused by fish or crustacean proteins.

Description of the eight cases of occupational protein contact dermatitis

Seventy-five percent of patients ($n = 6$) were men. The average age at the time of diagnosis was 26 years (range = 19–50 years). The latency of the diagnosis was, on average, 36 months, with significant deviations ranging from 4 months to 13 years.

Seven out of the eight patients were chefs or worked in the catering sector (that is to say about 900, 000 employees (with seasonable variations) per year in France, 200, 000 of whom are chefs); one patient was a pet shop employee. Four patients had a prior history of skin problems (eczema) and one patient was asthmatic (Table 1).

In every case, the diagnosis was made by a senior doctor and included a skin prick test. The pricks were made with extracts of foods usually handled for each patient (food extracts were prepared by cutting pieces of fish or crustacean flesh which were then crushed into a solution with physiologic serum then put into contact with patient skin to be pricked through), and also with commercial extracts for five foods (salmon, hake, bass, shrimp and lobster).

For negative control prick test, physiologic serum was used. For positive control prick test, 9% concentration of codeine phosphate solution was used. These solutions and commercial extracts of fish allergens solutions can be purchased at ALK® laboratories (55 271 Varennes en Argonne Cedex, France).

The mean-size of the positive control test was 2 mm for the wheal and 30 mm for the erythema (0/0 for the negative one). A positive test was at least the same size as the wheal of the positive control test with at least the same size of the erythema in comparison with the positive control test.

Reactions to salmon were the most frequent. They were reported for five patients (Table 1).

Patch testing was also carried out for these 8 patients. The patch test procedure was the same for all of them. Concerning patch tests, 8 mm diameter aluminium round finn chambers on Scanpor were used to perform the exploration. In France these devices are essentially provided by Stallergenes® (6, rue Alexis de Tocqueville 92160 Antony, France). Stallergenes® is commercializing the products of SmartPractice® 3400 E. McDowell Rd, Phoenix, AZ 850008 USA.

At the time of second appointment (48 h later) patch tests were removed and third appointment was given 96 h later. There were Standard European batteries, which showed sensitivity to nickel in one case. The patch tests carried out with the fish and crustacean flesh were prepared by cutting little pieces of native sea product and put in the chamber. They were all negative.

No scratch tests were performed, and none of the specific IgE testing came back positive for proteins of any type (parvalbumin) or for any species of fish. The concurrence of the clinical history and positivity of the skin prick tests hence confirmed the diagnosis.

None of the patients showed local or systemic reactions during ingestion of the substances in question for seafood-based protein dermatitis. No urticarial reaction to seafood were reported by the patients. By contrast, four out of eight patients reported skin lesions that had been diagnosed as irritant contact dermatitis in the preceding months.

Finally, none of the eight patients mentioned using gloves when handling fish.

Discussion

The risk of occupational seafood-based protein contact dermatitis appears to be low in the populations that we studied. It is therefore difficult to draw statistical conclusions with so few occurrences.

The social security agency for professional seafarers has no recorded cases of protein contact dermatitis. Within this population, the occurrence of occupational allergic dermatitis entitling the sufferer to compensation

Table 1 Description of the population affected by seafood-based protein contact dermatitis

Case	Age	Sex	Occupation	Diagnostic latency	Atopy	Allergen positive testing	Allergen negative testing
1	50	male	chef	14 months	+	Salmon	Crustaceans, trout, pollock, whiting, hake, seabass, scallop
2	23	male	chef	3 years	+	Salmon, whiting	Crustaceans, hake, pollock, scallop
3	19	female	chef	4 months	-	Pollock	Shrimp, salmon, whiting, hake, scallop
4	20	male	chef	6 months	+	Crustaceans	Pollock, whiting, hake, seabass, scallop
5	25	male	chef	4 months	-	Salmon	Crustaceans, trout, pollock, whiting, hake, seabass, scallop
6	33	male	chef	13 years	-	Salmon, monkfish, scallops	Shrimp, trout, pollock, whiting, hake, seabass,
7	19	male	chef	-	+	Salmon	Crustaceans, trout, pollock, whiting, hake, seabass, scallop
8	21	female	Pet shop employee	7 months	-	Daphnia	Shrimp, food for fish

is also low since, over the last 13 years, reports of occupational dermatological diseases have only occurred 0 to 5 times per year (25 in 13 years). These were always related to allergic contact dermatitis based on a delayed-type contact allergy rather than being related to protein contact dermatitis [12–14].

The simplest explanation could be that the disease did not occur during the study period (13 years), although a number of articles do in fact indicate a low prevalence of this disease. Moreover, having been described for the first time in 1976, protein contact dermatitis is still a little-known disease and is hence probably underdiagnosed [1, 15]. Additionally, our study is retrospective as it uses the registry for the compensation of occupational diseases. The registry is non-exhaustive in its overview of skin diseases present in the fishing profession (infectious, cancerous and other non-allergic skin diseases having been left out of the search). As such, the study selects only the patients who chose to have their skin problem diagnosed as well as to claim for compensation.

It is indeed possible that some fishermen, aware of their condition, hide their dermatitis out of fear of the seafarer's doctor revoking their medical clearance to embark. It is therefore possible that the fear of losing one's job (for medical reasons) may often make people reluctant to talk about their health problems with their regular doctor, and even more so with the doctor in charge of determining their medical fitness for work.

In a fish preparation plant, Aasmoe et al. found over 50% of workers had clinical occupational dermatitis but only 2.6% of the employees said they felt hindered by their condition [16]. The study sheds light on the fact that, in a population of workers such as fishermen, who are accustomed to difficult working conditions, there is a relative trivialization of skin problems that are considered minor. Such skin problems are therefore never mentioned to a health professional.

Another explanation that needs to be considered is a healthy worker effect: affected workers may have left the industry of their own accord so as to prevent their health problem from worsening rather than gone to see a doctor about their dermatitis or gone as far as to declare the condition. Their positions are then filled exclusively by healthy individuals. This hypothesis is frequently put forward to explain the rarity of this pathology in occupations that are particularly at risk [16, 17]. Nonetheless, we could also investigate the question of the positive protective influence of the maritime environment with regard to sensitivity to seafood proteins.

Additionally, glove protection may limit exposure sufficiently to avoid triggering sensitivity. In this context, fishermen seem very diligent in wearing skin protection gear while carrying out their professional tasks, during which the risk of injury is also high [12].

Furthermore, atopy, which was frequent in the second population of professionals affected by protein contact dermatitis, is very infrequent in the seafaring population [13]. Certain atopic pathologies, such as unstable atopic asthma, make it difficult for sufferers to do these jobs, resulting in the exclusion of a population at risk of developing protein contact dermatitis.

Among the other people working with seafood, the population of workers in seafood processing companies would logically be expected to be the most affected. Among employees of seafood processing companies in France, however, no cases of protein contact dermatitis were recorded, in contrast with results in a number of publications [16–18]. When compared to major fish-producing countries such as Norway and South Africa, this result is surprising.

As is the case for fishermen, the explanation may be that primary protection, such as wearing gloves and other protective clothing in factories may be sufficiently well applied so as to limit the occurrence of these diseases, in addition to a strict medical aptitude filter, which may exclude the more at-risk workers with atopic symptoms.

Given the employment statistics in France, fish processing jobs are often seasonal ones. Frequently, these professions see a significant turnover in the labour force and a rapid shift in career orientation when an employee isn't satisfied with the type of work. Kalogermitros showed that the intensity and, more importantly, the duration of exposure are risk factors in fish processing companies, which perhaps explains the absence of cases among French workers since they frequently change jobs or careers [19]. Furthermore, the population of seasonal workers often bypasses occupational medical examinations, and thus workers under-report the occupational diseases that could subsequently be of harm to them.

The population of chefs is the most affected population in our study. They often handle fish bare-handed, which may explain the prevalence of protein contact dermatitis in our study. Moreover, there are other factors that influence the increased risk for protein contact dermatitis. Halkier et al. showed that skin reactions particularly increased with the post-mortem age of the fish [20]. In addition, the liquid from fish, which has a high protein content, has been recognised as a risk factor in several studies [16, 21]. In a study by Aasmoe, those doing jobs involving filleting and (bare-handed) shrimp peeling were the most at risk among 883 employees of a seafood processing plant [16]. Given the preparation techniques, it appears logical that chefs would be the most affected occupation.

With salmon, there may be an added risk of protein contact dermatitis. The question of whether salmonid proteins are more sensitizing than proteins from other ocean fish warrants further investigation. Additionally, because the species can also be fished in fresh water and produced in aquaculture, it may be less often caught by fishermen at sea leading to a lower prevalence of associated skin problems in this population and a greater incidence in other groups.

Ultimately, the rarity of this dermatitis even among at-risk occupations can be explained, as is the case for fishermen, by the specificity of the files from occupational disease centres. Indeed, only the most complicated cases seek medical attention in these hospital centres, leading the population to be made up of all the "worst" cases, which could not be solved in general medical practices. In order to corroborate this information, we can say that over a 6-year period in Nancy (France), four cases of seafood protein contact dermatitis were reported among chefs by means of a local awareness network (both within and between hospitals), while we have seen eight cases throughout France in 13 years, including one chef from Nancy in the RNVPPP [22].

Finally, this skin disease is perhaps under-diagnosed because of the recentness of its description and complex and unresolved aetiology. Many indeed believe that it may be triggered by a combination of type 1 and 4 reactions from the Gell and Coombs classification. Arguments to support this are the existence of positive patch tests with more moderate reactions [23], the positive nature of scratch tests (which allow for a better penetration of the allergen) [24], the efficiency of corticoids as opposed to antihistamines, and the cutaneous symptoms with rare or minimal urticarial reactions [25]. Moreover, we were amazed by the absence in our population, as well as in the literature, of a description of systemic reactions during the ingestion of raw or cooked seafood by affected patients [7]. Only two cases were reported, and both were in patients with a filaggrin mutation, which is a known risk factor for allergic disease [26, 27]. The physiopathology is therefore complex and needs to be clarified in order to gain a better understanding and make a better diagnosis of this pathology.

Nevertheless in our study none of the patients with positive prick test results to seafood had corresponding specific IgE in the serum. Perhaps because the explored allergen is not the same for the prick-test and the specific IgE and/or the time of the blood testing (sometimes very later after the beginning of the disease) was not at the maximum synthesize of these specific IgE.

Conclusion

Chefs (specifically those who work with seafood) appear to be at higher risk of occupational protein contact dermatitis than fishermen. The influence of glove protection during fishing activities as compared to the bare-handed work of many chefs warrants further investigation. Furthermore, atopy that seems to be a risk factor among chefs is infrequent among fishermen. Indeed, the condition is frequently a reason for medical unfitness for onboard work, especially when the person has already suffered from unstable atopic asthma.

Abbreviations

CIM-10: Classification Internationale des Maladies 10ème version (International classification of diseases 10th edition); ENIM: Etablissement National des Invalides de la Marine (the social security scheme for maritime professions); IgE: Immunoglobulin E; RNV3P: Réseau National de Vigilance et de Prévention des Pathologies Professionnelles (French national occupational disease surveillance and prevention network)

Acknowledgments

Grant support: This network was supported by funds from French Agency for Food, Environmental and Occupational Health & Safety (Anses), the National Health Insurance system for employees (CNAM-TS), the French Occupational Medicine Society (SFMT), the Grenoble university hospital, the National health insurance system for agricultural workers (CCMSA) and the French Institute for Public Health Surveillance (InVS).
The authors would like to thank the rnv3p members: Angers (Roquelaure Y., Petit A.), Amiens (Doutrellot-Philippon C.), Bobigny-Avicenne (Guillon F.), Besançon (Aptel M., Thiebaut A.), Bordeaux (Rinaldo M., Verdun-Esquer C.), Brest (Dewitte J.D., Lodde B.), Caen (Clin B., Marquignon M.F.), Cherbourg (Marquignon M.F.), Clermont-Ferrand (Chamoux A., Dutheil F.), Créteil (Pairon J.C., Andujar P.), Dijon (Smolik H.J.), Garches (Ameille J., d'Escatha A.), Grenoble (de Gaudemaris R., Bonneterre V.), Le Havre (Gislard A., Rollin L.), Lille (Frimat P., Nisse C.), Limoges (Druet-Cabanac M.), Lyon (Pilonchéry-Massardier A., Bergeret A.), Marseille (Lehucher-Michel M.P.), Montpellier (Roulet A.), Nancy (Paris C., Penven E.), Nantes (Géraut C., Dupas D.), Paris-Cochin (Choudat D., Bensefa-Colas L.), Paris-Hôtel-Dieu (Léger D., Prévot-Balensi E.), Paris-Fernand Widal (Garnier R., Villa A.), Poitiers (Ben-Brik E., Berson C.), Reims (Deschamps F., Lesage F.X.), Rennes (Caubet A., Gouyet T.), Rouen (Gehanno J.F.), Saint-Etienne (Fontana L., Pélissier C.), Strasbourg (Gonzalez M., Nourry N.), Toulouse (Soulat J.M., Hérin F.), Tours (Lasfargues G., Haguenoer K.).

Funding

The RNVPPP is a national institution and no funding were necessary to obtain data from it.

Authors' contributions

BL had the idea of the study and collected data. He wrote the first manuscript. PC improved the manuscript. AMRC, RP and DL participated in the design of the study. JDD helped us for the methodology. LM helped to draft the manuscript and corrected the final version. All authors read and approved the final manuscript.

Competing interests

The authors declare that they have no competing interests.

Author details

[1]Université Européenne de Bretagne, Rennes, France. [2]Université de Brest, EA 4686 – CS 93837 – 29238, Brest Cedex 3, France. [3]Service de Santé au Travail et Maladies liées à l'environnement, CHRU Morvan, 2 avenue FOCH, Brest Cedex 29609, France. [4]Service de dermato-vénéréologie CHRU Morvan, 2 avenue FOCH, Brest Cedex 29609, France. [5]Société Française de Médecine Maritime, 22, Avenue Camille Desmoulins, Brest 29200, France.

References

1. Hjorth N, Roed-Petersen J. Occupational protein contact dermatitis in food handlers. Contact Dermatitis. 1976;2:28–42.
2. Janssens V, Morren M, Dooms-Goossens A, et al. Protein contact dermatitis: myth or reality? Br J Dermatol. 1995;132:1–6.
3. Wuthrich B. Protein contact dermatitis. Br J Dermatol. 1996;135:332–3.
4. Jappe U, Bonnekoh B, Hausen BM, et al. Garlic-related dermatoses: case report and review of the literature. Am J Contact Dermat. 1999;10:37–9.
5. Doutre MS. Occupational contact urticaria and protein contact dermatitis. Eur J Dermatol. 2005;15:419–24.
6. Vocanson M, Hennino A, Chavagnac C, et al. Contribution of CD4(+) and CD8(+) T-cells in contact hypersensitivity and allergic contact dermatitis. Expert Rev Clin Immunol. 2005;1:75–86.
7. Amaro C, Goossens A. Immunological occupational contact urticaria and contact dermatitis from proteins: a review. Contact Dermatitis. 2008;58:67–75.
8. Rycroft RJG, Menné T, Frosh PJ, Lepoittevin JP. Chapter 5 Immediate contact reactions written by Lahti A and Basketter D in Textbook of contact dermatitis. Springer-Verlag Berlin Heidelberg Edition; 2001. p. 1114. ISBN 978-3-662-10304-3.
9. Barata AR, Conde-Salazar L. Protein contact dermatitis—case report. An Bras Dermatol. 2013;88:611–3.
10. Hernández-Bel P, De La Cuadra J, García R, Alegre V. Protein contact dermatitis: review of 27 cases. Actas Dermosifiliogr. 2011;102(5):336–43.
11. Bonneterre VFL, Bicout D. Programmed health surveillance and detection of emerging diseases in occupational health: contribution of the French national occupational disease surveillance and prevention network (RNV3P). Occup Environ Med. 2010;67(3):178–86.
12. Loddé B, Roguedas-Contios AM, Pougnet R, Paris P, Jegaden D, Misery L, Dewitte JD. Prevalence of Occupational Contact Dermatitis to Mercaptobenzothiazole in a Population of Seamen and Prognosis after 3-Year Evaluation. J Allergy Ther. 2013;139. doi:10.4172/2155-6121.1000139.
13. Loddé B, Jegaden D, Dewitte JD. Maladies professionnelles cutanées maritimes. Nouv Dermatol. 2004;23:458–64.
14. Jegaden D, Dewitte JD, Loddé B. Maritime medicine in France. Int Marit Health. 2004;55:131–6.
15. Loddé B, Roguedas-Contios AM. Dermatoses professionnelles. EMC-Dermatologie. 2014;9(3):1–14. Article 98-800-A-10.
16. Aasmoe L, Bang B, Andorsen GS, et al. Skin symptoms in the seafood-processing industry in north Norway. Contact Dermatitis. 2005;52:102–7.
17. Halkier-Sorensen L, Heickendorff L, Dalsgaard I, et al. Skin symptoms among workers in the fish processing industry are caused by high molecular weight compounds. Contact Dermatitis. 1991;24:94–100.
18. Lopata AL, Baatjies R, Thrower SJ, et al. Occupational allergies in the seafood industry—a comparative study of Australian and South African workplaces. Int Marit Health. 2004;55:61–73.
19. Kalogeromitros D, Makris M, Gregoriou S, et al. IgE-mediated sensitization in seafood processing workers. Allergy Asthma Proc. 2006;27:399–403.
20. Halkier-Sorensen L, Thestrup-Pedersen K. Skin irritancy from fish is related to its postmortem age. Contact Dermatitis. 1989;21:172–8.
21. Halkier-Sorensen L, Thestrup-Pedersen K. Skin physiological changes in employees in the fish processing industry immediately following work. A field study. Contact Dermatitis. 1991;25:19–24.
22. Poreaux CWJ, François F, Paris C, Barbaud A. Caractéristiques des dermatites de contact aux protéines d'origine professionnelle. Paris: JDP; 2013.
23. Scharer L, Hafner J, Wuthrich B, et al. Occupational protein contact dermatitis from shrimps. A new presentation of the crustacean-mite syndrome. Contact Dermatitis. 2002;46:181–2.
24. Saloga J, Knop J. Does sensitization through the skin occur? Allergy. 2000; 55:905–9.
25. Lachapelle JM. Allergic contact dermatitis: clinical aspects. Rev Environ Health. 2014;29:185–94.
26. Kaae J, Menne T, Thyssen JP. Severe occupational protein contact dermatitis caused by fish in 2 patients with filaggrin mutations. Contact Dermatitis. 2013;68:319–20.
27. Irvine AD, McLean WH, Leung DY. Filaggrin mutations associated with skin and allergic diseases. N Engl J Med. 2011;365:1315–27.

8

Work-related outcomes in randomised placebo-controlled pain trials

Ingmar Wolf[1,2], Tim Friede[1], Ernst Hallier[2] and Sebastian Straube[2*]

Abstract

Background: Chronic painful conditions have an important influence on the ability to work. Work-related outcomes, however, are not commonly reported in publications on trials investigating the treatment of chronic painful conditions. We aim to provide an overview of the reporting of work-related outcomes in such trials and investigate the relationship between work-related outcomes and pain outcomes.

Methods: We conducted a systematic literature search in PubMed with the aim of identifying randomised placebo-controlled clinical trials investigating treatments for chronic painful conditions or rheumatic diseases that also reported on work-related outcomes. Methodological study quality was assessed with the Oxford Quality Scale (OQS). Meta-analyses were conducted for the outcomes of interference with work and number of patients with at least 30% reduction in pain intensity (30% pain responders). The correlation between work-related and pain outcomes was investigated with regression analyses.

Results: We included 31 publications reporting on 27 datasets from randomised placebo-controlled trials (with a total of 11,434 study participants) conducted in chronic painful or rheumatic diseases and reporting on work-related outcomes. These 31 publications make up only about 0.2% of all publications on randomised placebo-controlled trials in such conditions. The methodological quality of the included studies was high; only nine studies scored less than four (out of a maximum five) points on the OQS. Sixteen different work-related outcomes were reported on in the studies. Of 25 studies testing for the statistical significance of changes in work-related outcomes over the course of the trials, 14 (56%) reported a significant improvement; the others reported non-significant changes. Eight studies reported data on both interference with work and 30% pain responders: meta-analyses demonstrated similar, statistically significant improvements in both these outcomes with active therapy compared to placebo and regression analysis showed that these outcomes were correlated.

Conclusions: Despite the importance of pain as a reason for decreased ability to work, work-related outcomes are reported in substantially less than 1% of publications on placebo-controlled trials in chronic painful and rheumatic diseases. Work-related outcomes and pain responder outcomes are closely related.

Keywords: Chronic painful conditions, Rheumatic diseases, Randomised controlled trials, Work-related outcomes

* Correspondence: sebastian.straube@gmail.com
[2]Institute of Occupational, Social and Environmental Medicine, University Medical Center Göttingen, Waldweg 37 B, 37073 Göttingen, Germany
Full list of author information is available at the end of the article

Background

Chronic painful conditions are very common as a recent systematic review of prevalence studies has demonstrated [1]. For example, a large survey found that about one fifth of European adults suffered from pain of at least six months' duration and a third of those pain sufferers had severe pain [2]. Patients affected by a chronic painful disease experience the adverse effects of their condition on a number of domains of life, including work. In different studies 13% to 76% of chronic pain patients experienced loss of employment or were unable to undertake employment [1]. Those with moderate and, especially, severe pain are particularly affected [3]. Targeting inability to work and interference with work due to chronic pain therefore is important both from an individual as well as a societal, economic, perspective. It would be informative to know how work ability is affected by common pain treatments.

However, work-related outcomes are not commonly reported in publications on randomised controlled trials investigating the treatment of chronic painful conditions or rheumatic diseases (where pain typically is a prominent symptom). Where such data have been analysed, there is good evidence that those patients experiencing substantial improvements in pain outcomes in the context of clinical trials also experience a substantial improvement in their ability to work [4]. The question is how generalisable this agreement between work-related and pain-related study outcomes is.

With this publication we aim to, firstly, provide an overview of the reporting of work-related outcomes in chronic pain trials and, secondly, investigate the relationship between work-related outcomes and pain-related outcomes across different studies. Because for pain intensity the reporting as 'responder outcomes', such as the proportion of study participants experiencing at least 30%, or 50%, reduction in pain intensity over the course of a trial (30% or 50% pain responders), is more informative than treatment group average data, we focus on pain responder outcomes; this is in agreement with recent guidance on performing systematic reviews in the chronic pain field [5].

Methods

Literature search, study quality assessment, and data extraction

We conducted a systematic literature search in Medline (PubMed) with the aim of identifying randomised controlled clinical trials investigating treatments for chronic painful conditions or rheumatic diseases that reported on any work-related study outcomes. We limited ourselves to placebo-controlled (or sham-controlled) studies to ensure some basic comparability between the studies and to be able to compare active treatments vs. placebo for work-related and pain-related study outcomes.

Our search strategy is shown in Figure 1 and included search terms to identify work-related outcomes, search terms to identify chronic painful conditions or rheumatic diseases, and search terms to identify placebo or sham controlled studies. We did not activate any filters in PubMed but limited ourselves to articles published as full papers in English or German. The date of the last search was 13 June 2013. To estimate the total number of publications that could potentially have reported on work-related outcomes, we also performed our search without the work-related terms.

For inclusion in our systematic review studies needed to be single or double blind, use a placebo or sham control, include patients suffering from chronic pain (of at least 3 months' duration) or with a rheumatic disease, and report on any work-related outcomes. We anticipated that a variety of work-related measures would be reported in the studies. In order to be inclusive we accepted any outcome measure that specifically addresses work or any aspect of work and were work-related effects were reported separately (i.e. not only as a summary score covering work and other domains of life). Studies investigating children or experimentally induced pain were excluded.

We assessed the methodological study quality with the Oxford Quality Scale, a standard and very widely used instrument for evaluating clinical trials that assesses the domains of randomisation, blinding and withdrawals/dropouts, and grades study quality on a scale of zero to five points [6].

Data were extracted on the publication details, the conditions studied, the treatments investigated, study size and duration, as well as work-related and pain-related study outcomes.

Data analysis

We assessed means (and standard deviations [SDs]) of differences in work-related outcomes between trial beginning and end. If a study did not report SDs for mean differences between baseline and end of study values, SDs were estimated from p-values from hypothesis tests on the baseline to trial end differences. Studies reporting medians and interquartile ranges only had their data transformed to means and SDs by assuming the median to be the mean and the interquartile range to be 1.35 SDs.

Meta-analysis of data was performed with Review Manager (RevMan) [7]. Meta-analyses were conducted for the outcomes of 'interference with work' and 30% pain responders. Data for 'interference with work' were from component questions of the Brief Pain Inventory (question on pain interfering with normal work, including both work outside the home and housework), the Fibromyalgia Impact Questionnaire (question on how much pain or other symptoms of fibromyalgia interfered with the ability

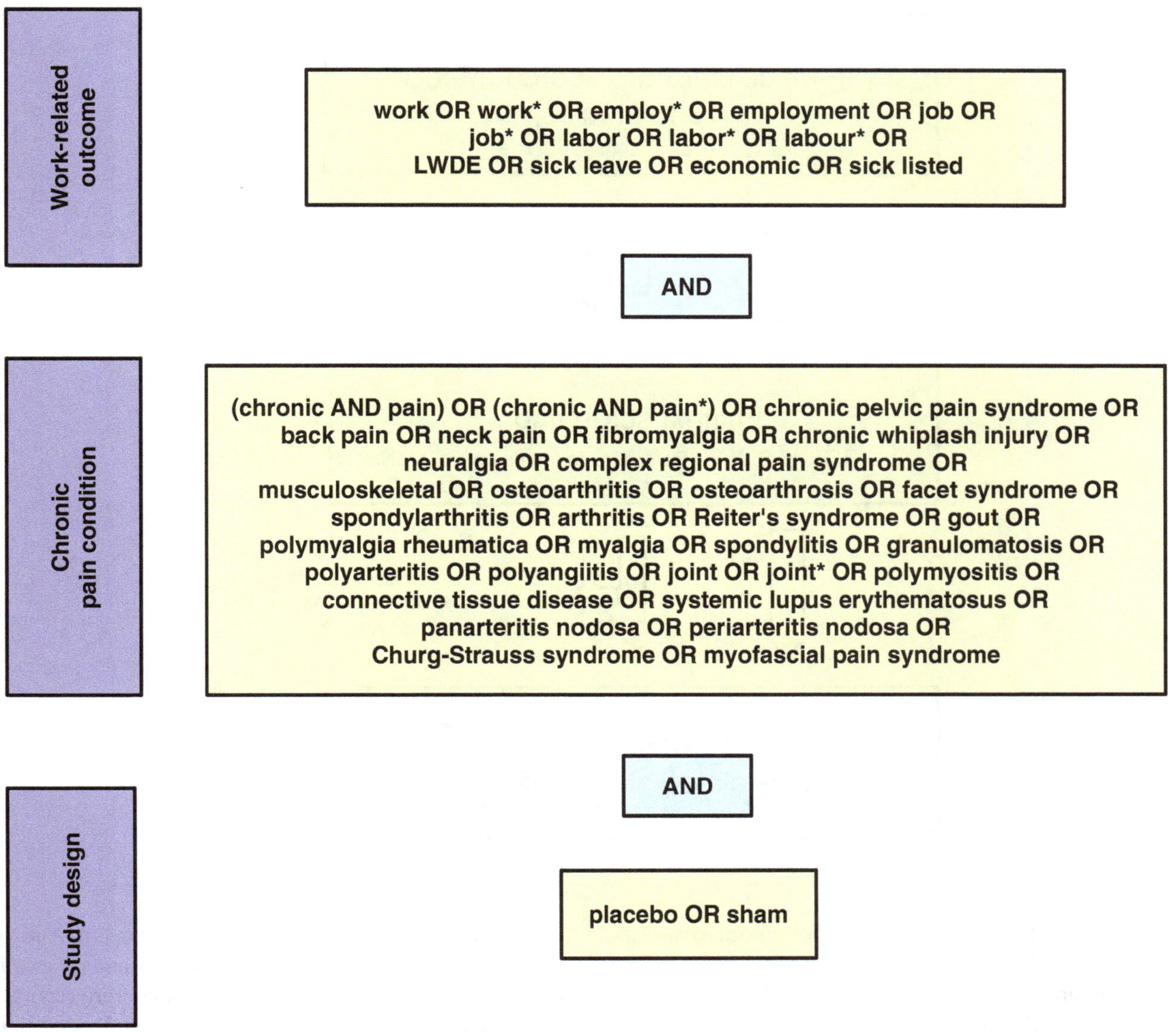

Figure 1 Search strategy. LWDE – lost workday equivalents.

to do work, including housework) and the Sheehan Disability Scale (question on how much the symptoms have disrupted work or school work). These three questions were all assessed on scales of 0–10 points.

For meta-analyses the random effects model was used. If the between study heterogeneity was estimated to be zero (i.e. $I^2 = 0$), the analysis is equivalent to a fixed effect meta-analysis.

The relationships between the outcomes of interference with work and 30%, or 50%, pain responders were investigated with regression analyses.

A further regression analysis was conducted for work-related and pain-related outcomes expressed as mean differences. In order to utilise all available data, which were expressed as different outcomes, we standardised the mean differences of the work-related and pain-related endpoints, as described by Hedges [8], before performing linear regression analysis.

All regression analyses were conducted in R [9]. The weights for the included studies were assigned according to the inverse variances of their work-related endpoints.

Results

Reporting of work-related outcomes

Our systematic literature search (Figure 2) yielded 1063 potentially relevant hits of which 948 were excluded as not relevant on the basis of study titles and abstracts. One hundred and fifteen remaining articles and one additional study from the references of a meta-analysis were examined as full texts. Eighty five of these full texts needed to be excluded. Additional file 1 details the excluded studies with reasons for their exclusion.

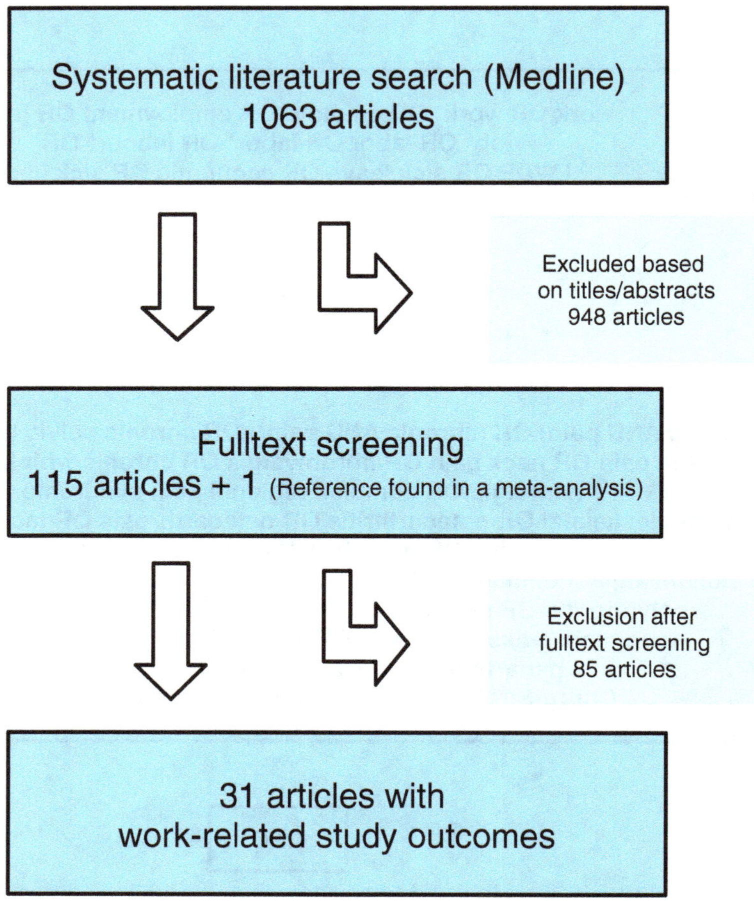

Figure 2 Study selection.

We identified as suitable for inclusion in our systematic review 31 publications [4,10-39] reporting on 27 datasets from randomised placebo-controlled trials in chronic painful diseases or rheumatic diseases (Table 1). Typically such a dataset corresponds to data from one clinical trial. Arnold et al. [12] and Bradley et al. [18] are meta-analyses that incorporated the same four clinical trials [11,20,40,41]. Two of these published work-related data [11,20]. In order to avoid counting the same patients more than once, all these studies were treated as one dataset. Bennett et al. [16] and Bennett et al. [17] were also treated as one dataset, because they both reported on the same trial. Furthermore, Straube et al. [4] reported an individual patient meta-analysis of work-related data from four trials but was counted as one dataset because the work-related data had not been published separately for those trials.

The 31 publications reporting on work-related outcomes comprised only 0.23% of all publications on randomised placebo-controlled trials in chronic painful or rheumatic conditions (13,754 hits when searching as in Figure 1 but without the work-related search terms). The 31 studies that reported on work-related outcomes included a total of 11,434 patients (mean ages in the studies ranged from 34 to 63 years; overall 76% of patients were women). Among the 31 studies, the reporting of work-related outcomes was diverse: 16 different work-related outcomes were reported on (Table 1). The methodological study quality was generally high; only nine studies scored less than four (out of a maximum five) points on the OQS (Table 1).

Of 25 studies testing for the statistical significance of changes in work-related outcomes over the course of the trials, 14 (56%) reported a significant improvement; the others reported non-significant changes (Table 2).

Relationship between work and pain outcomes

We wanted to examine the relationship between work-related outcomes and pain-related outcomes. As elaborated above we primarily used responder outcomes for pain intensity and as regards work-related outcomes we used the outcome of 'interference with work' as estimated from the answers to similar questions about interference with work (or disruption of work) from three commonly used questionnaires. There were eight studies [4,12,21,22,32,34-36] that reported data on both interference with work and 30% pain responders; these studies were included in meta-analyses for the outcomes

Table 1 Details of the included studies

Data sets	Articles	Conditions	Active interventions	Patients	Work-related outcomes	Study duration (in weeks)	OQS score
1	Albert et al. 2013 [10]	Chr. back pain	Amoxicillin–Clavulanate	162	Time lost from work	52	5
2	Baron et al. 2010 [14]	Chr. back pain	Pregabalin	217	WPAI	5	4
3	Carlsson & Sjölund 2001 [19]	Chr. back pain	Acupuncture, electroacupuncture	51	Employment status	32	5
4	Jarzem et al. 2005 [25]	Chr. back pain	TENS	350	McGill Work Scale	12	5
5	Lehmann et al. 1986 [29]	Chr. back pain	TENS, electroacupuncture	54	Employment status	3	4
6	Licciardone et al. 2003 [30]	Chr. back pain	Osteopathic manipulative treatment	91	Time lost from work	20	3
7	Skljarevski et al. 2009 [34]	Chr. back pain	Duloxetine	404	BPI-I	13	5
8	Skljarevski et al. 2010a [35]	Chr. back pain	Duloxetine	236	BPI-I, WPAI	13	4
9	Skljarevski et al. 2010b [36]	Chr. back pain	Duloxetine	401	BPI-I, WPAI	12	3
10	He et al. 2005 [24]	Chr. neck pain	Body acupuncture + body electrostimulation + ear acupressure	24	Activity impairment at work	4	2
11	Manchikanti et al. 2010 [31]	Chr. neck pain	Bupivacaine and steroid injection	120	Employability, employment status	96	5
12	Bennett et al. 2003 + 2005 [16,17]	Fibromyalgia	Tramadol-Acetaminophen	315	FIQ, time lost from work, SF-36	8	3
13	Bradley et al. 2010 [18] + Arnold et al. 2009 [12] (Arnold et al. 2005 [11] + Chappell et al. 2008 [20])	Fibromyalgia	Duloxetine	1332	Bradley 2010 [18]: FIQ, Arnold 2009 [12]: SDS (Arnold 2005 [11]: BPI, Chappell 2008 [20]: SDS)	12-28	Review (Arnold et al. 2005 [11]: 5, Chappell et al. 2008 [20]: 3)
14	Straube et al. 2011 [4]	Fibromyalgia	Pregabalin	2757	FIQ, time lost from work, SF-36, SDS, MAF	8-14	Review
15	Chappell et al. 2009 [21]	Osteoarthritis (knee)	Duloxetine	231	BPI-I	13	5
16	Chappell et al. 2011 [22]	Osteoarthritis (knee)	Duloxetine	256	BPI-I	13	5
17	Markenson et al. 2005 [32]	Osteoarthritis	Oxycodone	109	BPI-I	12	4
18	Kavanaugh et al. 2006 [26]	Psoriatic arthritis	Infliximab	200	SF-36, employment status, employability, impact on productivity at work (VAS), time lost from work	22	3
19	Kavanaugh et al. 2013 [28]	Psoriatic arthritis	Golimumab	405	Impact on productivity at work (VAS)	24	4
20	Egsmose et al. 1997 [23]	Reactive arthritis	Sulphasalazine	83	Time lost from work	24	3
21	Bejarano et al. 2008 [15]	Rheumatoid arthritis	Adalimumab + MTX	148	Employment status, WIS, Time lost from work	56	5
22	Kavanaugh et al. 2009 [27]	Rheumatoid arthritis	Certolizumab pegol + MTX	1601	WPS, time lost from work	24 + 52	3
23	Meireles et al. 2010 [33]	Rheumatoid arthritis	Low-level laser therapy	82	DASH	8	5

Table 1 Details of the included studies *(Continued)*

24	Smolen et al. 2006 [37]	Rheumatoid arthritis	Infliximab + MTX	1004	Employability, time lost from work	54	5
25	Strand et al. 1999 [38]	Rheumatoid arthritis	Leflunomide, MTX	482	Productivity at work	48	4
26	Barkham et al. 2010 [13]	Ankylosing spondylitis	Entanercept	40	WIS, time lost from work	12	3
27	van der Heijde et al. 2006 [39]	Ankylosing spondylitis	Infliximab	279	SF-36, impact on productivity at work (VAS), time lost from work	24	4

BPI-I – Brief Pain Inventory: Interference with normal work; chr. – chronic; DASH – Disabilities of the Arm, Shoulder and Hand Questionnaire; FIQ – Fibromyalgia Impact Questionnaire; MAF – Multidimensional Assessment of Fatigue; MTX – methotrexate; OQS – Oxford Quality Scale; SDS – Sheehan Disability Scale; SF-36 – Short Form 36 Health Survey; TENS – transcutaneous electrical nerve stimulation; VAS – visual analogue scale; WIS – Work Instability Scale; WPAI – Work Productivity and Activity Impairment Questionnaire; WPS – Work Productivity Survey. For reviews, information in brackets refers to the primary publications on which the reviews were based.

Table 2 'Vote count' of studies investigating work-related outcomes with statistical methods

Significant improvement	Non-significant changes
Bejarano et al. 2008 [15]	Albert et al. 2013 [10]
Bennett et al. 2003 [16]	Barkham et al. 2010 [13]
Bradley et al. 2010 [18]	Baron et al. 2010 [14]
Chappell et al. 2011 [22]	Chappell et al. 2009 [21]
He et al. 2005 [24]	Egsmose et al. 1997 [23]
Kavanaugh et al. 2006 [26]	Jarzem et al. 2005 [25]
Kavanaugh et al. 2009 [27]	Lehmann et al. 1986 [29]
Kavanaugh et al. 2013 [28]	Licciardone et al. 2003 [30]
Meireles et al. 2010 [33]	Skljarevski et al. 2009 [34]
Markenson et al. 2005 [32]	Straube et al. 2011 [4]
Skljarevski et al. 2010a [35]	van der Heijde et al. 2006 [39]
Skljarevski et al. 2010b [36]	
Smolen et al. 2006 [37]	
Strand et al. 1999 [38]	

The results of active treatment groups were pooled. Studies reported either significant improvements or non-significant changes; no study reported a significant worsening in work-related outcomes.

of interference with work (Figure 3) and 30% pain responders (Figure 4). For Straube et al. [4] data about pain responders was taken from Straube et al. [42].

These meta-analyses demonstrated statistically significant improvements in both outcomes with active therapy compared to placebo and also demonstrated that both outcomes behaved in a roughly similar manner, in individual studies and overall.

To assess the degree of similarity between these outcomes formally, we performed regression analyses (Figure 5); these showed that the outcomes were significantly correlated when the 30% responder rates were expressed as risk differences (p = 0.012) as well as when they were expressed as risk ratios (p = 0.015). For the 50% responder rates we found a significant correlation when the responder rates were expressed as risk ratios (p = 0.038), but significance was narrowly missed when they were expressed as risk differences (p = 0.053). As the study of Skljarevski et al. [34] did not report 50% pain responder rates, it did not contribute to those analyses.

Nine studies reported mean differences of different pain-related and work-related outcomes. Six trials assessed interference with work and pain severity with questions from the Brief Pain Inventory [21,22,32,34-36]. Arnold et al. [12] reported data on disruption of work from the Sheehan Disability Scale and data on pain from the Brief Pain Inventory. Two studies used visual analogue scales to evaluate productivity at work and pain [26,39]. The data for the pain-related outcomes for these two studies, Kavanaugh et al. [26] and van der Heijde et al. [39], were taken from Antoni et al. [43] and van der Heijde et al. [44]. Because of the multiple outcomes reported across the papers we standardised the reported mean differences before performing linear regression. Again, a statistically significant correlation emerged (p = 0.035).

Discussion

We were able to confirm our impression that work-related outcomes are indeed reported only very infrequently in chronic pain and rheumatology trials. This is somewhat surprising, given the importance of pain as a reason for decreased ability to work and given that a number of questionnaires that are commonly used in pain and rheumatology trials contain component questions addressing work-related outcomes [4]. The problem very likely is not one of the collection of work-related data but of the reporting of such data in publications.

This means two things. Firstly, that raising awareness of the importance of work-related outcomes among people and institutions involved in conducting trials in chronic pain and rheumatology is worthwhile and may lead to such data being reported more commonly for future trials and, secondly, that re-analysis of existing datasets could be informative, as long as access to work-related data can

Study or Subgroup	Active Mean	Active SD	Active Total	Control Mean	Control SD	Control Total	Weight	Mean Difference IV, Fixed, 95% CI
Arnold 2009	1.46	2.51	628	1.09	2.45	417	36.2%	0.37 [0.06, 0.68]
Chappell 2009	2.75	2.35	104	2.24	2.39	118	8.7%	0.51 [-0.11, 1.13]
Chappell 2011	2.16	2.49	128	1.31	2.38	128	9.5%	0.85 [0.25, 1.45]
Markenson 2005	1.9	2.99	56	0.6	2.83	50	2.8%	1.30 [0.19, 2.41]
Skljareveski 2009	2.46	2.69	271	1.95	2.76	113	9.4%	0.51 [-0.09, 1.11]
Skljareveski 2010a	2.25	2.71	109	1.5	2.68	115	6.8%	0.75 [0.04, 1.46]
Skljareveski 2010b	2.17	2.09	195	1.66	2.12	199	19.7%	0.51 [0.09, 0.93]
Straube 2011	1.27	7.63	1666	1.2	7.22	556	6.9%	0.07 [-0.63, 0.77]
Total (95% CI)			**3157**			**1696**	**100.0%**	**0.50 [0.32, 0.68]**

Heterogeneity: $Chi^2 = 5.94$, df = 7 (P = 0.55); $I^2 = 0\%$
Test for overall effect: Z = 5.31 (P < 0.00001)

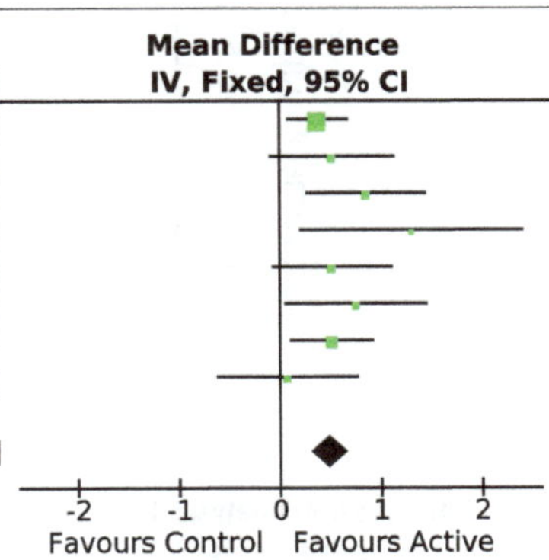

Figure 3 Interference with work. Meta-analysis of the improvement in interference with work over the duration of the studies. CI – confidence interval, Fixed – fixed effect model, IV – inverse variance, SD – standard deviation.

Study or Subgroup	Active Events	Active Total	Control Events	Control Total	Weight	Risk Ratio IV, Random, 95% CI
Arnold 2009	369	774	169	526	16.1%	1.48 [1.28, 1.71]
Chappell 2009	63	107	52	116	11.9%	1.31 [1.02, 1.70]
Chappell 2011	84	128	56	128	12.8%	1.50 [1.19, 1.89]
Markenson 2005	21	56	9	51	3.6%	2.13 [1.07, 4.21]
Skljareveski 2009	151	287	51	117	12.8%	1.21 [0.96, 1.52]
Skljareveski 2010a	59	111	46	116	11.0%	1.34 [1.01, 1.78]
Skljareveski 2010b	111	195	97	199	14.5%	1.17 [0.97, 1.41]
Straube 2011	759	1936	269	689	17.4%	1.00 [0.90, 1.12]
Total (95% CI)		**3594**		**1942**	**100.0%**	**1.29 [1.12, 1.49]**
Total events	1617		749			

Heterogeneity: Tau² = 0.03; Chi² = 25.90, df = 7 (P = 0.0005); I² = 73%
Test for overall effect: Z = 3.48 (P = 0.0005)

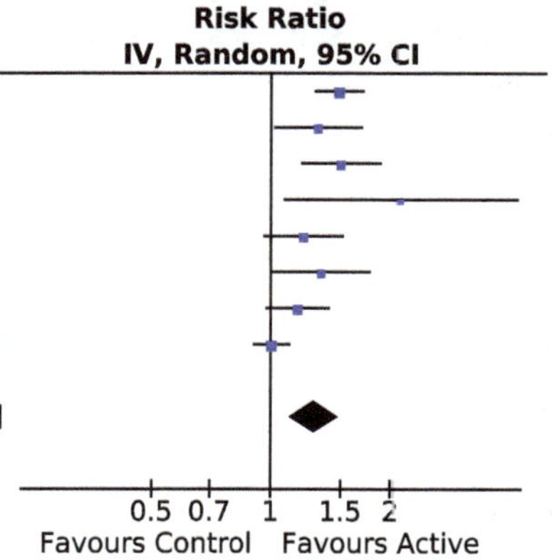

Figure 4 30% pain responders. Meta-analysis of the proportion of study participants attaining at least 30% reduction in pain intensity over the duration of the studies. CI – confidence interval, IV – inverse variance, Random – random effects model, SD – standard deviation.

be obtained, preferably at the level of the individual patient.

Some limitations of our analysis need to be discussed: we based our systematic review on searching only one database and were limited (due to the linguistic skills of the authors, or lack thereof) to papers published in English or German. It is quite possible that we missed relevant studies published in journals not indexed in Medline, published in languages other than English or German, or published after our search had closed. We do not claim, therefore, to have identified all placebo-controlled trials conducted in chronic pain or rheumatologic diseases and reporting on work related outcomes. What we have, however, should be a fairly good and representative sample, including important trials published recently and in high impact journals.

We have confidence in our conclusion, therefore, that work-related outcomes are indeed reported very infrequently in journal publications resulting from chronic pain and rheumatology trials.

Chronic pain significantly interferes with work. A recent large systematic review of observational studies demonstrated the negative impact of chronic pain on work related outcomes [45]. It is therefore logical to suspect that pain relief will be associated with an improvement in the ability to work. Based on the evidence included in our systematic review (eight studies, with 5726 participants, conducted in fibromyalgia, back pain and osteoarthritis,

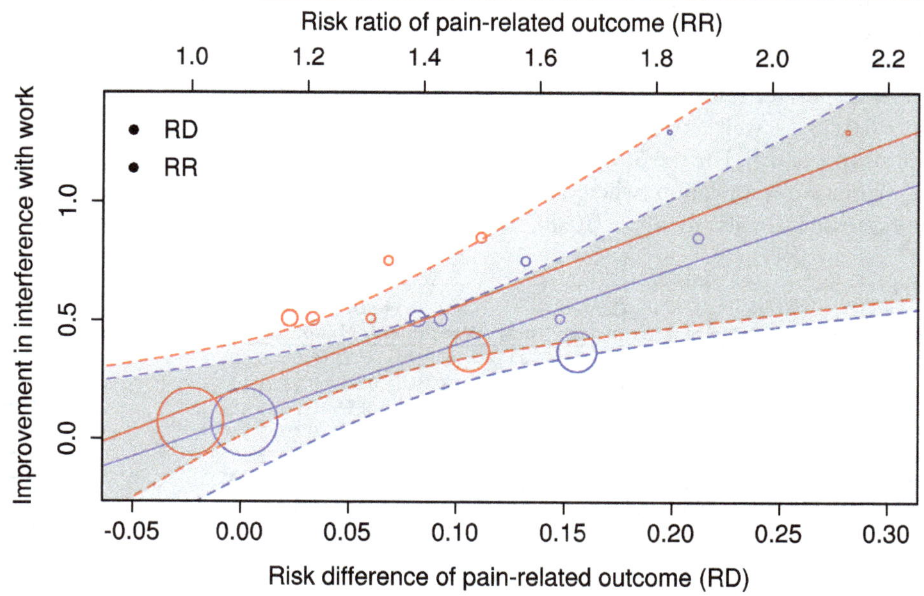

Figure 5 Regression analysis. Regression analysis of the improvement in interference with work from study beginning to end and '30% pain responders', expressed as risk ratios [RR, red colour] or risk differences [RD, blue colour]. Interference with work was measured on a scale of 0–10 points. The size of the symbols represents the weights of the individual studies in the regression analysis (inverse variance). Regression lines are solid; broken lines mark the 95% confidence intervals.

investigating as treatments duloxetine, pregabalin, and oxicodone, and lasting eight to 28 weeks) we conclude that the outcome of improvement in interference with work is indeed closely related to the outcome of attaining at least 30% reduction in pain intensity over the course of the studies. Future work, in other painful conditions and assessing different treatments, needs to assess how robust this relationship is and whether pain-related outcomes (such as 30% pain responders) can perhaps be used to estimate interference with work. If they can, then this would open the door to using pain responder outcomes for evaluations of the impact of pain treatments also on work ability, which might be an important consideration for the assessment of pain treatments.

Conclusions

Firstly, work-related outcomes are reported very infrequently, in substantially less than 1% of the publications we identified in our search for placebo-controlled trials in chronic painful and rheumatic diseases.

Secondly, work-related outcomes and pain responder outcomes are closely related. Future studies, perhaps based on individual patient analyses and meta-analyses of existing datasets, should address whether pain responder outcomes can be used to assess ability to work.

Competing interests

SS has participated in grants from Pfizer and Reckitt-Benckiser and has received a lecture fee and an honorarium from Oxford Medical Knowledge for work on data from pain trials. TF is a consultant to Novartis Pharma AG, Biogen Idec, Phamalog and Grünenthal.

Authors' contributions

IW did the searching, data extraction, and study quality assessment, performed the analyses, and made the figures and tables. SS conceived of the study, supervised IW for his doctoral dissertation on this subject, and drafted the manuscript. TF provided statistical advice for the analysis and also supervised IW for his doctoral dissertation. All authors contributed to revising the manuscript and approved the final version of the manuscript.

Author details

[1]Department of Medical Statistics, University Medical Center Göttingen, Humboldtallee 32, 37073 Göttingen, Germany. [2]Institute of Occupational, Social and Environmental Medicine, University Medical Center Göttingen, Waldweg 37 B, 37073 Göttingen, Germany.

References

1. Moore RA, Derry S, Taylor RS, Straube S, Phillips CJ: **The costs and consequences of adequately managed chronic non-cancer pain and chronic neuropathic pain.** *Pain Pract* 2014, **14**:79–94.
2. Breivik H, Collett B, Ventafridda V, Cohen R, Gallacher D: **Survey of chronic pain in Europe: prevalence, impact on daily life, and treatment.** *Eur J Pain* 2006, **10**:287–333.
3. Langley P, Müller-Schwefe G, Nicolaou A, Liedgens H, Pergolizzi J, Varrassi G: **The impact of pain on labor force participation, absenteeism and presenteeism in the European Union.** *J Med Econ* 2010, **13**:662–672.
4. Straube S, Moore RA, Paine J, Derry S, Phillips CJ, Hallier E, McQuay HJ: **Interference with work in fibromyalgia: effect of treatment with pregabalin and relation to pain response.** *BMC Musculoskelet Disord* 2011, **12**:125.
5. Moore RA, Eccleston C, Derry S, Wiffen P, Bell RF, Straube S, McQuay H, ACTINPAIN Writing Group of the IASP Special Interest Group on Systematic Reviews in Pain Relief; Cochrane Pain, Palliative and Supportive Care Systematic Review Group Editors: **"Evidence" in chronic pain–establishing best practice in the reporting of systematic review.** *Pain* 2010, **150**:386–389.
6. Jadad AR, Moore RA, Carroll D, Jenkinson C, Reynolds DJ, Gavaghan DJ, McQuay HJ: **Assessing the quality of reports of randomized clinical trials: is blinding necessary?** *Control Clin Trials* 1996, **17**:1–12.
7. *Review Manager (RevMan) [Computer program]. Version 5.2.* Copenhagen: The Nordic Cochrane Centre, The Cochrane Collaboration; 2012.
8. Hedges LV: **Distribution theory for glass's estimator of effect size and related estimators.** *J Educ Behav Stat* 1981, **6**:107–128.
9. R: A language and environment for statistical computing: *Version 3.0.3. The R Foundation for Statistical Computing, R Core Team.* Vienna, Austria: R Foundation for Statistical Computing; 2014. URL http://www.R-project.org/.
10. Albert HB, Sorensen JS, Christensen BS, Manniche C: **Antibiotic treatment in patients with chronic low back pain and vertebral bone edema (Modic type 1 changes): a double-blind randomized clinical controlled trial of efficacy.** *Eur Spine J* 2013, **22**:697–707.
11. Arnold LM, Rosen A, Pritchett YL, D'Souza DN, Goldstein DJ, Iyengar S, Wernicke JF: **A randomized, double-blind, placebo-controlled trial of duloxetine in the treatment of women with fibromyalgia with or without major depressive disorder.** *Pain* 2005, **2005**(119):5–15.
12. Arnold LM, Clauw DJ, Wohlreich MM, Wang F, Ahl J, Gaynor PJ, Chappell AS: **Efficacy of duloxetine in patients with fibromyalgia: pooled analysis of 4 placebo-controlled clinical trials.** *Prim Care Companion J Clin Psychiatry* 2009, **11**:237–244.
13. Barkham N, Coates LC, Keen H, Hensor E, Fraser A, Redmond A, Cawkwell L, Emery P: **Double-blind placebo-controlled trial of etanercept in the prevention of work disability in ankylosing spondylitis.** *Ann Rheum Dis* 2010, **69**:1926–1928.
14. Baron R, Freynhagen R, Tölle TR, Cloutier C, Leon T, Murphy TK, Phillips K, A0081007 investigators: **The efficacy and safety of pregabalin in the treatment of neuropathic pain associated with chronic lumbosacral radiculopathy.** *Pain* 2010, **150**:420–427.
15. Bejarano V, Quinn M, Conaghan PG, Reece R, Keenan AM, Walker D, Gough A, Green M, McGonagle D, Adebajo A, Jarrett S, Doherty S, Hordon L, Melsom R, Unnebrink K, Kupper H, Emery P, Yorkshire Early Arthritis Register Consortium: **Effect of the early use of the anti-tumor necrosis factor adalimumab on the prevention of job loss in patients with early rheumatoid arthritis.** *Arthritis Rheum* 2008, **59**:1467–1474.
16. Bennett RM, Kamin M, Karim R, Rosenthal N: **Tramadol and acetaminophen combination tablets in the treatment of fibromyalgia pain: a double-blind, randomized, placebo-controlled study.** *Am J Med* 2003, **114**:537–545.
17. Bennett RM, Schein J, Kosinski MR, Hewitt DJ, Jordan DM, Rosenthal NR: **Impact of fibromyalgia pain on health-related quality of life before and after treatment with tramadol/acetaminophen.** *Arthritis Rheum* 2005, **53**:519–527.
18. Bradley LA, Bennett R, Russell IJ, Wohlreich MM, Chappell AS, Wang F, D'Souza DN, Moldofsky H: **Effect of duloxetine in patients with fibromyalgia: tiredness subgroups.** *Arthritis Res Ther* 2010, **12**:R141.
19. Carlsson CP, Sjölund BH: **Acupuncture for chronic low back pain: a randomized placebo-controlled study with long-term follow-up.** *Clin J Pain* 2001, **17**:296–305.
20. Chappell AS, Bradley LA, Wiltse C, Detke MJ, D'Souza DN, Spaeth M: **A six-month double-blind, placebo-controlled, randomized clinical trial of duloxetine for the treatment of fibromyalgia.** *Int J Gen Med* 2008, **1**:91–102.
21. Chappell AS, Ossanna MJ, Liu-Seifert H, Iyengar S, Skljarevski V, Li LC, Bennett RM, Collins H: **Duloxetine, a centrally acting analgesic, in the treatment of patients with osteoarthritis knee pain: a 13-week, randomized, placebo-controlled trial.** *Pain* 2009, **146**:253–260.

22. Chappell AS, Desaiah D, Liu-Seifert H, Zhang S, Skljarevski V, Belenkov Y, Brown JP: **A double-blind, randomized, placebo-controlled study of the efficacy and safety of duloxetine for the treatment of chronic pain due to osteoarthritis of the knee.** *Pain Pract* 2011, **11**:33–41.
23. Egsmose C, Hansen TM, Andersen LS, Beier JM, Christensen L, Ejstrup L, Peters ND, van der Heijde DM: **Limited effect of sulphasalazine treatment in reactive arthritis. A randomised double blind placebo controlled trial.** *Ann Rheum Dis* 1997, **56**:32–36.
24. He D, Høstmark AT, Veiersted KB, Medbø JI: **Effect of intensive acupuncture on pain-related social and psychological variables for women with chronic neck and shoulder pain–an RCT with six month and three year follow up.** *Acupunct Med* 2005, **23**:52–61.
25. Jarzem PF, Harvey EJ, Arcaro N, Kaczorowski J: **Transcutaneous Electrical Nerve Stimulation [TENS] for chronic low back pain.** *J Musculoskelet Pain* 2005, **13**:3–9.
26. Kavanaugh A, Antoni C, Mease P, Gladman D, Yan S, Bala M, Zhou B, Dooley LT, Beutler A, Guzzo C, Krueger GG: **Effect of infliximab therapy on employment, time lost from work, and productivity in patients with psoriatic arthritis.** *J Rheumatol* 2006, **33**:2254–2259.
27. Kavanaugh A, Smolen JS, Emery P, Purcaru O, Keystone E, Richard L, Strand V, van Vollenhoven RF: **Effect of certolizumab pegol with methotrexate on home and work place productivity and social activities in patients with active rheumatoid arthritis.** *Arthritis Rheum* 2009, **61**:1592–1600.
28. Kavanaugh A, McInnes IB, Krueger GG, Gladman D, Beutler A, Gathany T, Mack M, Tandon N, Han C, Mease P: **Patient-reported outcomes and the association with clinical response in patients with active psoriatic arthritis treated with golimumab: findings through 2 years of a phase III, multicenter, randomized, double-blind, placebo-controlled trial.** *Arthritis Care Res* 2013, **65**:1666–1673.
29. Lehmann TR, Russell DW, Spratt KF, Colby H, Liu YK, Fairchild ML, Christensen S: **Efficacy of electroacupuncture and TENS in the rehabilitation of chronic low back pain patients.** *Pain* 1986, **26**:277–290.
30. Licciardone JC, Stoll ST, Fulda KG, Russo DP, Siu J, Winn W, Swift J Jr: **Osteopathic manipulative treatment for chronic low back pain: a randomized controlled trial.** *Spine (Phila Pa 1976)* 2003, **28**:1355–1362.
31. Manchikanti L, Singh V, Falco FJ, Cash KA, Fellows B: **Comparative outcomes of a 2-year follow-up of cervical medial branch blocks in management of chronic neck pain: a randomized, double-blind controlled trial.** *Pain Physician* 2010, **13**:437–450.
32. Markenson JA, Croft J, Zhang PG, Richards P: **Treatment of persistent pain associated with osteoarthritis with controlled-release oxycodone tablets in a randomized controlled clinical trial.** *Clin J Pain* 2005, **21**:524–535.
33. Meireles SM, Jones A, Jennings F, Suda AL, Parizotto NA, Natour J: **Assessment of the effectiveness of low-level laser therapy on the hands of patients with rheumatoid arthritis: a randomized double-blind controlled trial.** *Clin Rheumatol* 2010, **29**:501–509.
34. Skljarevski V, Ossanna M, Liu-Seifert H, Zhang Q, Chappell A, Iyengar S, Detke M, Backonja M: **A double-blind, randomized trial of duloxetine versus placebo in the management of chronic low back pain.** *Eur J Neurol* 2009, **16**:1041–1048.
35. Skljarevski V, Desaiah D, Liu-Seifert H, Zhang Q, Chappell AS, Detke MJ, Iyengar S, Atkinson JH, Backonja M: **Efficacy and safety of duloxetine in patients with chronic low back pain.** *Spine (Phila Pa 1976)* 2010a, **35**:E578–E585.
36. Skljarevski V, Zhang S, Desaiah D, Alaka KJ, Palacios S, Miazgowski T, Patrick K: **Duloxetine versus placebo in patients with chronic low back pain: a 12-week, fixed-dose, randomized, double-blind trial.** *J Pain* 2010b, **11**:1282–1290.
37. Smolen JS, Han C, van der Heijde D, Emery P, Bathon JM, Keystone E, Kalden JR, Schiff M, Bala M, Baker D, Han J, Maini RN, St Clair EW: **Infliximab treatment maintains employability in patients with early rheumatoid arthritis.** *Arthritis Rheum* 2006, **54**:716–722.
38. Strand V, Tugwell P, Bombardier C, Maetzel A, Crawford B, Dorrier C, Thompson A, Wells G: **Function and health-related quality of life: results from a randomized controlled trial of leflunomide versus methotrexate or placebo in patients with active rheumatoid arthritis. Leflunomide Rheumatoid Arthritis Investigators Group.** *Arthritis Rheum* 1999, **42**:1870–1878.
39. van der Heijde D, Han C, DeVlam K, Burmester G, van den Bosch F, Williamson P, Bala M, Han J, Braun J: **Infliximab improves productivity and reduces workday loss in patients with ankylosing spondylitis: results from a randomized, placebo-controlled trial.** *Arthritis Rheum* 2006, **55**:569–574.
40. Arnold LM, Lu Y, Crofford LJ, Wohlreich M, Detke MJ, Iyengar S, Goldstein DJ: **A double-blind, multicenter trial comparing duloxetine with placebo in the treatment of fibromyalgia patients with or without major depressive disorder.** *Arthritis Rheum* 2004, **50**:2974–2984.
41. Russell IJ, Mease PJ, Smith TR, Kajdasz DK, Wohlreich MM, Detke MJ, Walker DJ, Chappell AS, Arnold LM: **Efficacy and safety of duloxetine for treatment of fibromyalgia in patients with or without major depressive disorder: results from a 6-month, randomized, double-blind, placebo-controlled, fixed-dose trial.** *Pain* 2008, **136**:432–444.
42. Straube S, Derry S, Moore RA, Paine J, McQuay HJ: **Pregabalin in fibromyalgia–responder analysis from individual patient data.** *BMC Musculoskelet Disord* 2010, **11**:150.
43. Antoni C, Krueger GG, deVlam K, Birbara C, Beutler A, Guzzo C, Zhou B, Dooley LT, Kavanaugh A: **Infliximab improves signs and symptoms of psoriatic arthritis: results of the IMPACT 2 trial.** *Ann Rheum Dis* 2005, **64**:1150–1157.
44. Van der Heijde D, Dijkmans B, Geusens P, Sieper J, DeWoody K, Williamson P, Braun J, Ankylosing Spondylitis Study for the Evaluation of Recombinant Infliximab Therapy Study Group: **Efficacy and safety of infliximab in patients with ankylosing spondylitis: results of a randomized, placebo-controlled trial (ASSERT).** *Arthritis Rheum* 2005, **52**:582–591.
45. Patel AS, Farquharson R, Carroll D, Moore A, Phillips CJ, Taylor RS, Barden J: **The impact and burden of chronic pain in the workplace: a qualitative systematic review.** *Pain Pract* 2012, **12**:578–589.

QFT-Plus: a plus in variability? – Evaluation of new generation IGRA in serial testing of students with a migration background in Germany

J. Knierer[1*], E. N. Gallegos Morales[1], A. Schablon[1], A. Nienhaus[1,2] and J. F. Kersten[1]

Abstract

Background: Currently available Interferon-gamma release assays (IGRAs) show a considerable variability in serial testing for latent tuberculosis infection (LTBI).
This study offers first results for the new generation IGRA QuantiFERON-TB Gold Plus (QFT-Plus) introduced in 2015 in comparison with its predecessor QuantiFERON-TB Gold In-Tube (QFT-GIT) from serial testing of students with a migration background at German universities.

Methods: Forty-one students were selected from a previous study. All students with a positive IGRA were asked and 11 agreed to participate in this cohort study. Additionally 30 students with negative IGRA results were selected by chance. Weekly testing with QFT-Plus and QFT-GIT was performed in all individuals over a 4-week period. IGRA variability was evaluated by calculating conversion and reversion rates.

Results: From 41 participants a total number of 163 serial measurements were analyzed for each IGRA, leading to 122 possible IGRA changes each. QFT-Plus had four conversions and two reversions leading to a conversion rate of 4.3% (4 of 93 possible conversions, 95% CI 1.4–11.3%) and reversion rate of 6.9% (2 of 29 possible reversions, 95% CI 1.2–24.2%). QFT-GIT had 2 conversions and 1 reversion causing slightly lower rates with 2.2% conversions (2 of 91, 95% CI 0.4–8.5%) and 3.2% reversions (1 of 31, 95% CI 0.2–18.5%). Inconsistent IGRA results occurred in 4 subjects for QFT-Plus (8 stable positives, 29 stable negatives) and in 2 subjects for QFT-GIT (9 stable positives, 30 stable negatives). Agreement between the two IGRAs was 95.1% ($\kappa = 0.89$). Variance attributed to the individuals was low (QFT-Plus: ICC = 0.88).

Conclusion: This study confirms occurrence of conversions and reversions for the new QFT-Plus in serial testing of a high-risk cohort in a low-incidence setting with improbable new TB contact during the study. QFT-Plus conversion and reversion rates were slightly higher than for the QFT-GIT but overall they were lower for both IGRAs than in other studies that investigated IGRA variability.

Keywords: Latent tuberculosis infection, QFT-Plus, Variability, Serial testing, Students

* Correspondence: jo.knierer@uke.de
[1]University Medical Center Hamburg-Eppendorf (UKE), Center of Excellence for Health Services Research in Nursing (CVcare), Hamburg, Germany
Full list of author information is available at the end of the article

Background

Since its first approval by the U.S. Food and Drug Administration (FDA) in 2001 [1] hopes were high for the Interferon-gamma release assay (IGRA) as a new method to test for latent tuberculosis infection (LTBI).

Meanwhile, for over a decade IGRAs have played an important role in global tuberculosis control as they offer a convenient way to screen for LTBI. They are increasingly used in high-income countries instead of the tuberculin skin test (TST) for LTBI-testing.

IGRAs have major advantages over the TST, such as delivering results after 24 h with no need for a second appointment, not being affected by the examiner's subjectivity that may influence TST interpretation, not struggling as an in vitro test with the problem of boosting in subsequent tests, using a positive control to facilitate interpretation in immunocompromised subjects and not cross-reacting with most nontuberculous mycobacteria (NTM) or BCG vaccine strains [2]. The latter improvement should lead to a higher specificity in BCG vaccinated subjects while maintaining a good sensitivity like that of the TST [3–5].

Beside their advantages over TST, IGRAs tend to show a high variability with high rates of conversions and reversions in serial testing, which was shown to be present in low as well as high TB incidence settings [6, 7]. Tagmouti et al. notice in a systematic review that IGRA test variability is higher than TST variability [8]. In settings where serial IGRA testing for LTBI is done, the elevated test variability leads to uncertainty whether chest X-ray or preventive chemotherapy is needed in the event of a positive test result with the knowledge that reversions tend to occur more frequently than conversions [8–11].

Following results from recent studies, several guidelines step back from promoting IGRAs as the standalone test for serial LTBI screening. Canada's 2013 guideline update recommends TST rather than IGRA for testing low-risk individuals, noting that IGRA is not recommended for serial testing for populations with ongoing exposure [12]. The 2010 updated U.S. guidelines allow either TST or IGRA as the method of choice for serial testing, pointing out that using IGRA might lead to higher conversion rates making it difficult to identify IGRA changes that truly represent a new infection [13]. In Europe the ECDC guidelines allow IGRA as a baseline test, likewise pointing out problems of increased test variability offering a two-step approach in order to increase specificity [14].

Pai et al. postulate the simple dichotomous definition of IGRA test results to be inappropriate as it causes higher conversion rates than what the annual TB infection risk in low-incidence settings would lead to expect [15]. Several studies suggest the use of a borderline zone in order to avoid unnecessary X-rays and preventive chemotherapy [9, 16–20].

Until recently two IGRAs were commercially available, QuantiFERON-TB Gold In-Tube (QFT-GIT) (Qiagen, Hilden, Germany) and T-SPOT.TB (Oxford Immunotec, Abingdon, UK) that have been subjects of interest for many studies. In 2015 Qiagen updated its IGRA lineup, now offering a new generation of QFT-GIT: QuantiFERON-TB Gold Plus (QFT-Plus). According to the manufacturer the QFT-Plus offers higher sensitivity and specificity in patients at highest risk for TB-infection and in immunocompromised patients [21]. The aim of this study was to see if this new generation IGRA offers a plus in areas where present IGRA products tend to struggle. We are aware of only one paper, published independently from the producer of QFT-Plus which investigates sensitivity and specificity of the new generation IGRA [22]. In particular, so far, no data is available on test variability of new generation QFT-Plus in serial testing. Therefore, the primary objective of our study was to evaluate QFT-Plus test variability in a direct head-to-head comparison of QFT-GIT and QFT-Plus in a cohort of students and young professionals with a migration background currently studying at a German university or technical college.

Methods

Study design and subjects

We recruited a total of 41 participants from our partner study in which students and young professionals with migration background were screened for LTBI using both IGRAs (QFT-GIT and QFT-Plus) (Gallegos Morales EN, Knierer J, Schablon A, Nienhaus A, Kersten JF: Prevalence of Latent Tuberculosis Infection among foreign students tested with QuantiFERON-TB Gold In-Tube and QuantiFERON-TB Gold Plus, submitted). All students that were screened positive in at least one of the two IGRAs at baseline were asked to participate in this cohort study. 11 out of 13 students with positive baseline results agreed to participate. Another 30 participants with negative baseline results in both IGRAs were selected by chance. The study was conducted at universities and technical colleges in Lübeck, Germany, between February 2016 and March 2016.

Inclusion criteria were an age of at least 18 years, student status or having completed studies at a German university, and a migration background. For fulfilling the migration background criteria, participants must have been foreign born in a country with a WHO-estimated tuberculosis incidence of at least 10 incident cases per 100,000 inhabitants per annum (hereinafter: ≥10:100,000). If born in a country with lower incidence, having a nationality of a country with a TB incidence of at least 10:100,000 allowed participation [23]. People without a migration background fulfilling the nationality criteria but only having that nationality because of their parents' nationality, were excluded.

Some IGRA studies tend to exclude people that have had a TST during the previous 3–6 months [17, 24]. In our study a recent TST application was not an exclusion criterion because many students, especially medicine students or students of natural sciences, do a TST during classes at the university. So the timeframe of the last TST application was queried in the questionnaire. None of the participants had a TST application during the ongoing study.

Exclusion criteria were withdrawal of consent, ongoing active TB infection or treatment for LTBI, insufficient Interferon-gamma (IFN-γ) production in the positive control at the first screening visit, and absence from more than one study visit.

Questionnaire items

The standardized questionnaire was offered in two languages: German and English. It covered information on the participants' study subject, work area, nationality and country of birth, time living in Germany permanently, immunosuppression caused by disease or current medication, information on contact with people with active tuberculosis, and specification of that contact. In detail we asked for: recent participation in tuberculosis screening and recent chest X-ray results; previous TST or IGRA results as well as BCG vaccination status (anamnestic and/ or verification by vaccination scars); own TB history and history of treatment for active TB or LTBI.

Diagnostic methods and data collection

The new generation IGRA QFT-Plus carries a lot of its predecessors' characteristics but uses two antigen tubes (TB1 and TB2) instead of one in the QFT-GIT. As in the QFT-GIT, T-lymphocyte secreted IFN-γ is quantitatively measured by ELISA technique after in vitro stimulation with antigens highly specific for Mycobacterium tuberculosis.

Both tubes contain the antigens ESAT-6 and CFP-10 (TB 7.7 additionally used in the QFT-GIT tube is no longer present in QFT-Plus tubes). The TB1 tube is designed to elicit cell-mediated immune (CMI) responses from $CD4^+$ T-helper lymphocytes whereas the TB2 tube additionally contains a set of peptides targeted to the induction of CMI responses from $CD8^+$ cytotoxic T-lymphocytes [25]. The latter might potentially help to distinguish active from latent TB and should improve sensitivity in immunocompromised patients e.g. children or HIV co-infected patients [21, 25].

Collection of all blood samples and care for participants were performed by two study physicians (JK, ENGM). Weekly testing (7 +/- 1 days) with QFT-Plus and QFT-GIT was performed in all individuals over a 4-week period. Participants were given individual appointments to make sure that the blood was taken at the same time of day on each visit.

As some studies suggest that variation of blood volume in the QFT tubes might be a reason for increased test variability [26], the blood was first collected in tubes with lithium heparin, expecting that a subsequent in-lab transfer of the blood in the QFT tubes would secure transfer of the accurate blood volume. The blood samples were transported to the laboratory within 8 h after blood collection. QFT tubes were then inoculated manually by professional medical technicians and directly incubated in strict adherence to the manufacturer's instructions within one hour after arrival of the samples at the laboratory.

IFN-γ ELISAs were performed directly after the incubation on all blood samples.

As suggested in the manufacturer's instructions QFT-GIT results were considered positive if the IFN-γ value was ≧ 0.35 IU/ml after correction for the negative control. QFT-Plus results were considered positive if the IFN-γ response after correction for the negative control was ≧ 0.35 IU/ml in one of the two TB antigen tubes (TB1 or TB2) or if both tubes (TB1 and TB2) showed ≧ 0.35 IU/ml.

Measurement resolution and laboratory restrictions led to a truncated interval of IFN-γ values: IFN-γ values > 10 IU/ml were leveled at 10 IU/ml; IFN-γ values <0.01 IU/ml or negative values were leveled at 0.00 IU/ml.

Conversion was defined as the change from a negative result (<0.35 IU/ml) in the previous visit to a positive result (≧0.35 IU/ml) in the next visit. In line with the above definition for QFT-Plus interpretation, it was sufficient if the change from negative results (<0.35 IU/ ml) in both TB antigen tubes to a positive result (≧0.35 IU/ml) was achieved in one of the two TB antigen tubes to count as a conversion. Reversion was defined as the change from a positive result to a negative result.

All participants were offered advice and explanation of their personal test results by the study physicians.

To rule out the possibility of active TB, participants with a positive test result in more than one study visit were advised to take a chest X-ray if not recently performed in context of TB screening. Participants with prior contact to a person with active TB during the last 2 years and positive results qualified for preventive chemotherapy. They were sent to pulmonary consultants for a second opinion and for planning and supervision of the therapy if suitable.

Statistical analysis

Categorical data is presented as counts and corresponding rates, continuous variables are presented as means, standard deviations (SD) and ranges where appropriate.

Agreement between the two test methods (QFT-GIT and QFT-Plus) was analyzed using Cohen's kappa coefficient. The variance attributed to the individuals, i.e. test reliability in the individual, was investigated for the QFT-Plus with the intraclass correlation coefficient

(ICC) in a 1-way design. An ICC of >0.8 is regarded as indicative for a high agreement and therefore a low intraindividual variance [27].

Data evaluation was performed using SPSS Version 22 (IBM Corp., Armonk, NY USA).

Results

Study population and risk factors for IGRA-positivity at baseline

The characteristics of our study population and baseline QFT-Plus results are presented in Table 1. Participants had a mean age of 25.5 ± 3.6 (range: 20 to 36) years, average time living in Germany was 3.8 ± 3.8 years (range: 4 months to 23.6 years), and 22 participants were born in a country with a TB incidence of ≧ 125:100,000. Participants' country of birth or country that allowed participation included all six WHO-regions: Africa (including: Cameroon, Ghana, Kenya, Nigeria, South Africa and United Republic of Tanzania), The Americas (including: Ecuador, Guatemala, Honduras and Mexico), South-East Asia (including: India, Indonesia and Nepal), Europe (including: Belarus, Lithunia, Russian Federation, Tajikistan and Ukraine), Eastern Mediterranean (including: Syrian Arab Republic and Yemen) and Western Pacific (including: China, Mongolia, Philippines, Republic of Korea and Vietnam).

Nineteen participants reported contact to a person with active TB of which 6 (32%) had a positive QFT-Plus at baseline with five out of six (83%) defining the TB contact as a family member. 11 participants declared a TST application, the average time since last TST was 5.7 years; two of these reported a TST application during the six months before inclusion in the study (in both cases one month beforehand). Both had consistent IGRA results on all four visits with full concordance between the two IGRAs; one had consistently negative and the other showed consistently positive IGRA results. Being consistently positive this participant was classified as true positive. 30 participants were never tested with TST.

One IGRA-positive participant had a personal history of active TB. On inclusion in our study this student was smear- and culturally negative after completion of anti-tuberculosis chemotherapy. None of the participants showed signs of ongoing active TB infection at the time of inclusion in the study.

IGRA positivity throughout the study and test intervals

All 41 participants turned up for their weekly appointments, resulting in 164 blood samples.

On visit 3, the laboratory was unable to analyze one blood sample. This led to a total of 163 valid IFN-γ values for each of the two IGRAs, i.e. four serial measurements at weekly intervals for 40 participants and three measurements for one participant.

Table 1 Description of study population and frequencies of QFT-Plus results at baseline

Variable	N (Col-%)	QFT-Plus positive[a] N (Row-%)	QFT-Plus negative[a] N (Row-%)
Gender			
Female	22 (53.7)	3 (13.6)	19 (86.4)
Male	19 (46.3)	6 (31.6)	13 (68.4)
Age			
20–25 years	26 (63.4)	3 (11.5)	23 (88.5)
26–36 years	15 (36.6)	6 (40.0)	9 (60.0)
Country of birth			
Classified by TB-incidence			
< 125:100 000	19 (46.3)	1 (5.3)	18 (94.7)
≥ 125:100 000	22 (53.7)	8 (36.4)	14 (63.6)
Classified by WHO-regions			
Africa	9 (22.0)	4 (44.4)	5 (55.6)
The Americas	6 (14.6)	0 (0.0)	6 (100.0)
South-East Asia	9 (22.0)	2 (22.2)	7 (77.8)
Europe	10 (24.4)	0 (0.0)	10 (100.0)
Eastern Mediterranean	2 (4.9)	0 (0.0)	2 (100.0)
Western Pacific	5 (12.2)	3 (60.0)	2 (40.0)
Time living in Germany			
< 2 years	15 (36.6)	3 (20.0)	12 (80.0)
2–10 years	25 (61.0)	6 (24.0)	19 (76.0)
> 10 years	1 (2.4)	0 (0.0)	1 (100.0)
Contact to TB			
Yes	19 (46.3)	6 (31.6)	13 (68.4)
No	22 (53.7)	3 (13.6)	19 (86.4)
Type of TB contact			
Relatives	8 (19.5)	5 (62.5)	3 (37.5)
Friends/acquaintances	3 (7.3)	0 (0.0)	3 (100.0)
Professional	6 (14.6)	0 (0.0)	6 (100.0)
Other type	2 (4.9)	1 (50.0)	1 (50.0)
TB in own history			
Yes	1 (2.4)	1 (100.0)	0 (0.0)
No	40 (97.6)	8 (20.0)	32 (80.0)
BCG-vaccination			
Yes	18 (43.9)	2 (11.1)	16 (88.9)
No	4 (9.8)	3 (75.0)	1 (25.0)
unknown	19 (46.3)	4 (21.1)	15 (78.9)
Previous TST			
Positive	3 (7.3)	2 (66.7)	1 (33.3)
Negative	5 (12.2)	0 (0.0)	5 (100.0)
Unknown	3 (7.3)	0 (0.0)	3 (100.0)
No TST	30 (73.2)	7 (23.3)	23 (76.7)

[a]QFT-Plus result at baseline

In one case (0.8%) the interval between tests was 6 days, 7-day interval in 107 cases (87.7%), 8-day interval in 13 cases (10.7%), and – because of the not analyzable blood sample – a 14-day interval in one case (0.8%).

All 11 recruited participants with initial IGRA positivity remained positive throughout the study in at least one of the two IGRAs. A 12th participant only showed one positive QFT-Plus result on visit 3 but reverted on the final visit. All 12 participants with IGRA positivity throughout the study had an LTBI risk due to their migration background: 11 participants with positive IGRA results were born in a country with a TB incidence of ≧125:100,000 and one positive participant was born in China which is classified as a high TB burden country by the WHO [28]. Over the whole study period nine participants showed stable positive QFT-GIT results and 30 had stable negative QFT-GIT results. For the QFT-Plus, eight participants were stable positive and 29 participants were stable negative. During the 4-week study period a total number of 42 positive results in the QFT-GIT and 40 positive results in the QFT-Plus were collected.

(Individual IGRA results and IFN-γ values for all participants throughout the study are shown in the table in the supplement [see Additional file 1]).

Reversions and conversions

Reversions and conversions occurred in four participants with inconsistent results, i.e. inconsistency of dichotomous IGRA test decisions during the study period (Table 2). All four showed inconsistent QFT-Plus results and only two of them also showed inconsistent QFT-GIT results.

For the QFT-GIT two conversions and one reversion were detected. One conversion was stable, the other conversion and reversion were caused by a fluctuating result: a reversion followed by a reconversion on the subsequent visit (pos-neg-pos-pos) (Fig. 1). The QFT-Plus had four conversions and two reversions of which one conversion and one reversion were based on fluctuating results (pos-neg-pos-pos and neg-neg-pos-neg) (Fig. 2). In the QFT-Plus two of the conversions and two reversions occurred only because of the IFN-γ measurement crossing the cutoff in tube TB2 (Fig. 3) and not in tube TB1 (Fig. 4).

All inconsistent results of the QFT-GIT occurred in the same participants that showed inconsistent QFT-Plus results during the study period.

The conversions and reversions in both IGRAs took place within a range close to the cutoff. For the QFT-GIT the lowest IFN-γ value that showed a conversion was 0.18 IU/ml, for QFT-Plus tube TB1 it was 0.11 IU/ml and tube TB2 0.09 IU/ml. The highest IFN-γ value that showed a reversion was 0.35 IU/ml for QFT-GIT and 0.64 IU/ml for tube TB2 of QFT-Plus. No QFT-Plus reversion was caused by crossing of the cutoff in tube TB1.

IGRA variability

For each participant four serial measurements at weekly intervals led to a possibility of reversions and conversions on three occasions. Overall, 163 valid IFN-γ values were collected for each IGRA. On the last visit 41 blood samples were analyzable, leaving 122 valid IFN-γ values for each IGRA that were followed by a subsequent result and therefore feasible for a change of the dichotomous IGRA test result. Total numbers for every visit with changes of IGRA results can be seen in the flow chart Fig. 5. With a total number of 42 positive QFT-GIT results of which 11 occurred on the final visit, 31 positive results were followed by a subsequent result and therefore feasible for reversion. Using the number of the above QFT-GIT reversions and conversions, a reversion rate of 3.2% (1 of 31 possible reversions, 95% CI 0.2–18.5%) and correspondingly calculated conversion rate of 2.2% (2 of 91 possible conversions, 95% CI 0.4–8.5%) was present in our study. The QFT-Plus had a reversion rate of 6.9% (2 of 29, 95% CI 1.2–24.2%) and a conversion rate of 4.3% (4 of 93, 95% CI 1.4–11.3%).

Concordance between the two IGRAs and Intraclass Correlation (ICC)

On visits 1 and 2, in 92.7% of results (38 of 41 subjects) of the two IGRAs were concordant, 95% on visit 3 (38 of 40) and on the final visit the IGRA results were concordant in

Table 2 Participants with inconsistent IGRA results in the weekly blood collections

Sex	No.	Age	IGRA	Visit 1	Visit 2	Visit 3	Visit 4	Overall trend
M	9	32	QFT-Plus	Neg. (0.15/0.19)	Neg. (0.17/0.14)	Neg. (0.14/0.09)	Pos. (0.34/0.40)	Inc.
			QFT-GIT	Pos. (0.40)	Pos. (0.62)	Pos. (0.66)	Pos. (0.65)	Pos.
M	10	20	QFT-Plus	Neg. (0.24/0.20)	Pos. (0.50/0.47)	Pos. (0.55/0.73)	Pos. (0.79/0.69)	Inc.
			QFT-GIT	Pos. (0.35)	Neg. (0.31)	Pos. (0.46)	Pos. (0.53)	Inc.
M	11	23	QFT-Plus	Pos. (0.32/0.64)	Neg. (0.11/0.12)	Pos. (0.46/0.40)	Pos. (0.56/0.61)	Inc.
			QFT-GIT	Neg. (0.18)	Pos. (0.52)	Pos. (0.47)	Pos. (0.63)	Inc.
M	12	25	QFT-Plus	Neg. (0.08/0.08)	Neg. (0.05/0.14)	Pos. (0.16/0.36)	Neg. (0.21/0.24)	Inc.
			QFT-GIT	Neg. (0.04)	Neg. (0.09)	Neg. (0.09)	Neg. (0.14)	Neg.

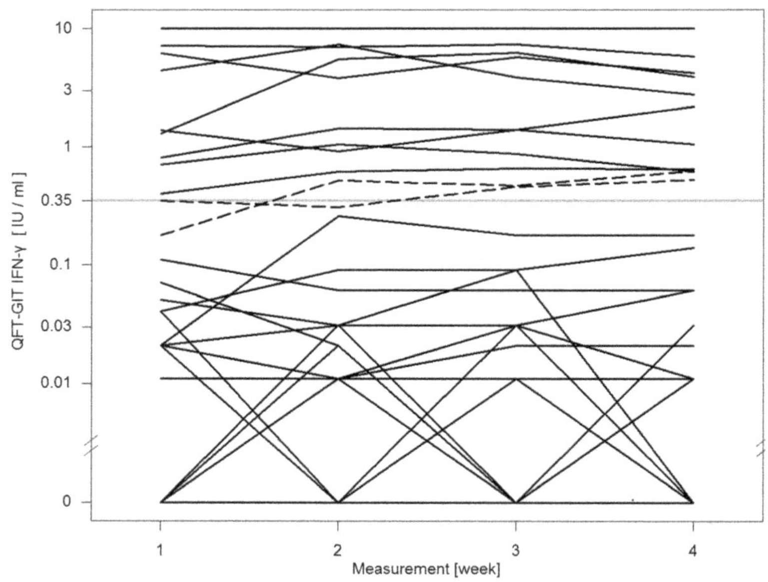

Fig. 1 QFT-GIT continuous IFN-γ courses of the individual participants during the four study weeks

all of the participants (41 of 41), leading to an overall agreement between the two IGRAs of 95.1% (155 of 163); Kappa: 0.89 (Table 3).

Figure 6 compares values of the two QFT-Plus tubes TB1 and TB2, showing that in three occasions QFT-Plus positivity was based on crossing of the manufacturers cutoff (0.35 IU/ml) only in tube TB2 whereas TB1 stayed under the cutoff. Figure 7 compares values of the QFT-GIT with QFT-Plus tube TB1 values. On six occasions the QFT-GIT showed values over the cutoff while the TB1 value was under the cutoff. Once the TB1 value was higher than the cutoff while QFT-GIT stayed under it. Figure 8 depicts the concordance between QFT-GIT and QFT-Plus Tube TB2. On five occasions the QFT-GIT had values over the cutoff while at the same time TB2 stayed under it. Three times TB2 was over the cutoff while QFT-GIT was under it.

The ICC for the QFT-Plus, representing the proportion of the variance that is attributed to the variation between individuals, was 0.88. This correspondingly indicates that variance in the individuals was low.

Active TB infection and chest X-ray results

None of the chest X-rays of participants with a positive IGRA-result showed signs of ongoing active TB. Despite

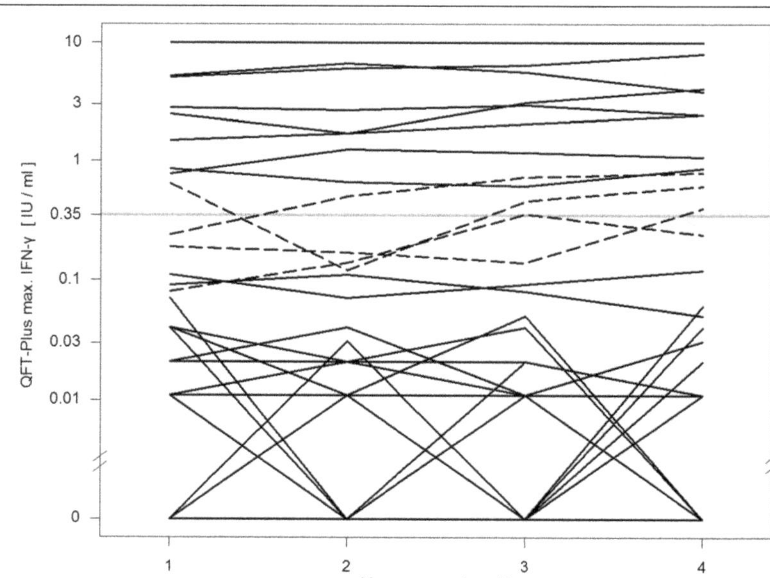

Fig. 2 QFT-Plus continuous IFN-γ courses using maximum IFN-γ value of the two antigen tubes

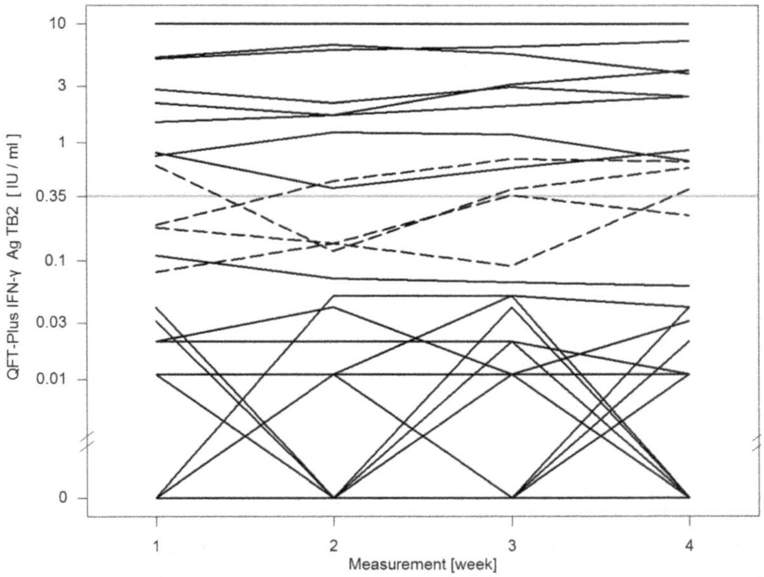

Fig. 3 QFT-Plus continuous IFN-γ courses during the four study weeks of TB Antigen Tube 2 (TB2)

the study physicians advice two of the participants refused to take their X-ray. As stated above, none of the participants showed clinical signs of ongoing active TB infection so it was assumed that no participant with active TB was taking part in the study.

The one participant formerly treated for active TB, but now being smear- and culturally negative, showed consistently positive results in both IGRAs.

Discussion

Our study confirms the occurrence of conversions and reversions in both the well studied QFT-GIT and the new generation IGRA QFT-Plus. The QFT-GIT had a reversion rate of 3.2% and a conversion rate of 2.2%. Both rates were slightly higher for the QFT-Plus: 6.9% reversions and 4.3% conversions. Due to the small number of blood samples evaluated, the confidence intervals for the variability rates of the two IGRAs compared are large and overlap each other.

The overall agreement between the two IGRAs of 95.1% (155/163) was good (κ = 0.89). Admittedly, one must take into account that a regression-to-the-mean phenomenon might have led to the increased concordance during the successive visits. This is caused by

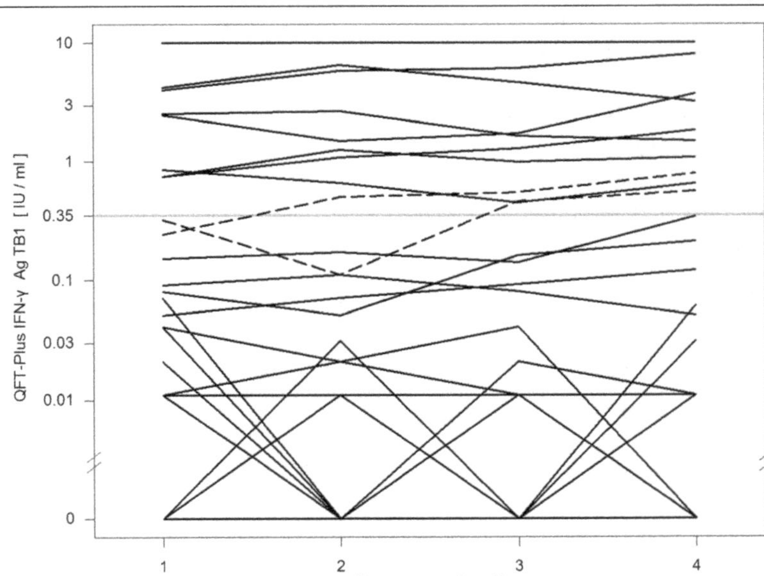

Fig. 4 QFT-Plus continuous IFN-γ courses during the four study weeks of TB Antigen Tube 1 (TB1)

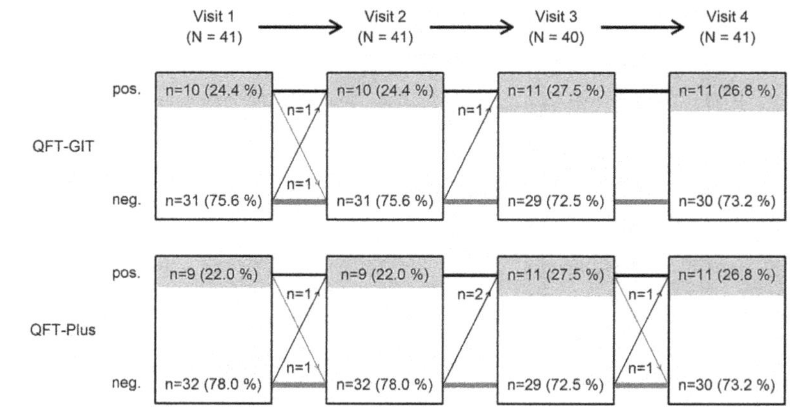

Fig. 5 Flow chart of study population and IGRA results

random fluctuation around a true mean. Each time the same subject undergoes repeated measurement, extreme observations might be followed by ones that are closer to the subject's true mean. This could lead to natural variation looking like real change in serial testing of the same subject [29]. Ringshausen et al. and Tagmouti et al. identified this phenomenon as an additional source of test variability in serial IGRA testing [8, 17], especially when IGRA positive subjects are longitudinal followed.

As all variations took place within a narrow range close to the manufacturers' cutoff, the use of a borderline zone like already proposed for the QFT-GIT might as well be useful for the interpretation of changes around the cutoff in the QFT-Plus. For the QFT-GIT Ringshausen et al. in their review advocate the use of a borderline zone from 0.2–0.7 IU/ml. The authors suggest that subjects with borderline zone results and suspected infection should be retested before recommending preventive chemotherapy [9]. Using this definition for the QFT-Plus and defining a conversion as a cross passing of the borderline zone from below to above and a reversion as a cross passing from above the borderline zone to below the borderline zone, we did not observe a conversion or reversion. Applying this definition for conversions will reduce the number of preventive treatments needed when a positive QFT is observed in serial testing.

Table 3 Concordance between the two IGRAs at each study visit

Visit No.	No. of valid results	Pos. QFT-Plus *n* (%)	Pos. QFT-GIT *n* (%)	Discordant results *n* (%)	Agreement between IGRAs
1	41	9 (22.0)	10 (24.4)	3 (7.3)	92.7%
2	41	9 (22.0)	10 (24.4)	3 (7.3)	92.7%
3	40	11 (27.5)	11 (27.5)	2 (5.0)	95.0%
4	41	11 (26.8)	11 (26.8)	0 (0.0)	100%
Total	163	40 (24.5)	42 (25.8)	8 (4.9)	95.1% (κ = 0.89)

Test results of QFT-Plus for individuals were very similar, with a high ICC of 0.88.

Furthermore it is worth noticing that in four cases only the IFN-γ value of the antigen TB2 tube crossed the manufacturer's cutoff leading to conversion and reversion in those participants. The overall number of inconsistent results is too low to suggest that tube TB2 was the sole cause of the higher rate of variability. This observation seems plausible because of a further source of variation but deserves further investigation in follow-up studies.

Overall, inconsistent IGRA results of less than 7% occurred, which is less frequently than what can be found in the literature. Ringshausen et al. described reversion rates of 22.1% to 71.4% and conversion rates of 0.7% to 14.4% in their systematic review [9].

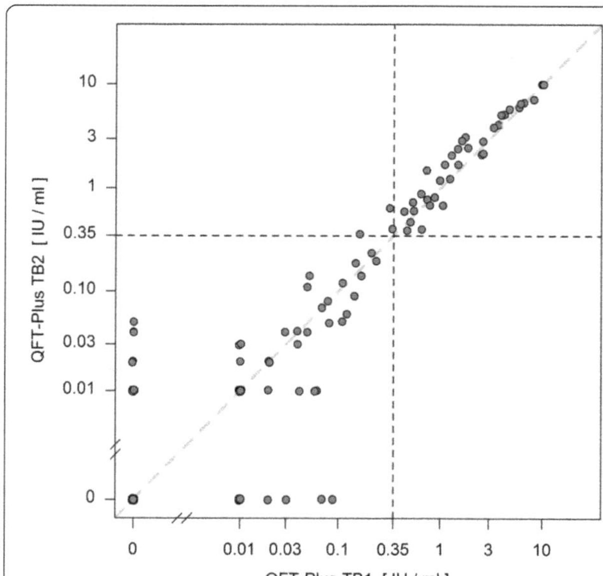

Fig. 6 Concordance between the QFT-Plus tubes TB1 and TB2

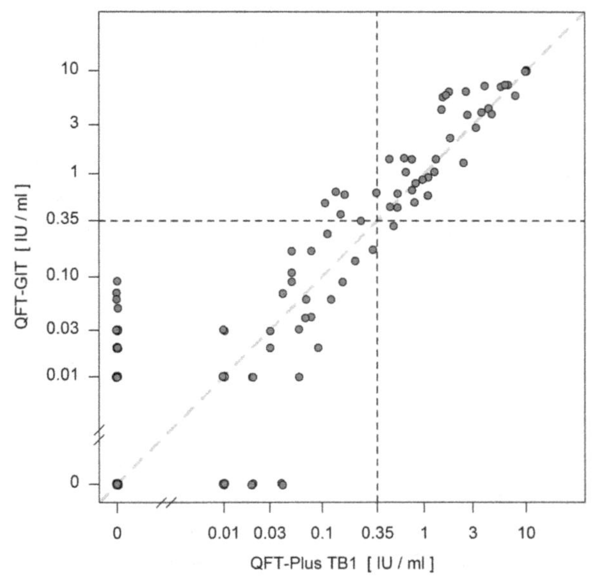

Fig. 7 Concordance between QFT-GIT and QFT-Plus tube TB1

In another systematic review Zwerling et al. found 7% to 70% of reversions and 11.6% to 21% of conversions in serial testing of healthcare workers (HCW) in high-incidence countries, and 11% to 33% of reversions and 1.8% to 14.4% of conversions in HCW serial testing in low-incidence countries [6].

As our numbers, especially occurrence of reversions, are lower, it is important to note that these studies were undertaken with data from screening of HCWs and that the interval between subsequent visits varied between the studies but were in most cases longer than our seven-day interval.

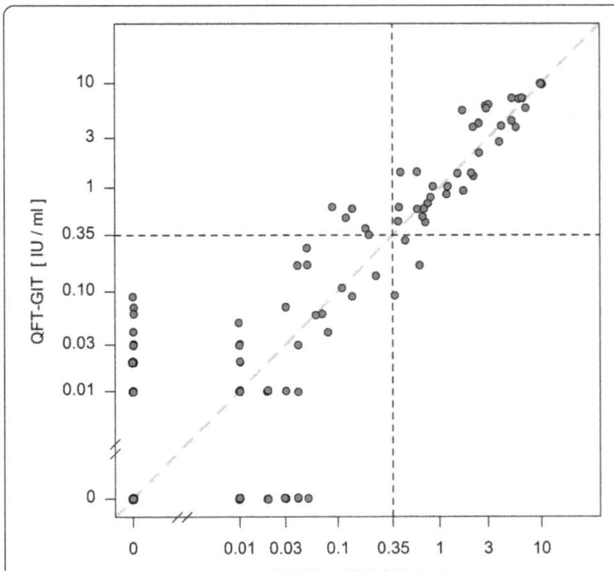

Fig. 8 Concordance between QFT-GIT and QFT-Plus tube TB2

In a study undertaken in a similar timeframe to ours, but also using HCWs as its study population and five time points, Ringshausen et al. found 28.6% of inconsistent results (inconsistency in 10 out of 35 subjects). Comparing results of subsequent visits to baseline results, they had 50% of reversions (6 out of 12 initial positive subjects) and 17.4% of conversions (4 out of 23 initial negative subjects) [17].

King et al. in their variability study on a large cohort of U.S. HCWs investigating the other commercially available IGRA, the T-SPOT.TB, showed lower conversion rates: 0.8% conversions and 17.6% reversions (or 1.6% conversions and 26.4% reversions if including borderline zone results). Their study shows a strong correlation between the risk of conversion and the reported TB incidence rates of the state in which the HCWs were located [30]. The lower conversion rates in the study by King et al. could as well be inherent to the different assay that was used. Compared to the ELISPOT based assay the ELISA based assays like QFT-GIT and QFT-Plus might show higher variability due to the limited control of the number of T-cells in the vials. This was suggested by an assay comparison concerning Cytomegalovirus (CMV) infection comparing CMV ELISPOT and CMV QuantiFERON: Saldan et al. assume interassay differences like the comparison of CMI responses in a volume of blood in QuantiFERON assays versus a given number of cells in ELISPOT assays to be a potential source of variability [31].

Systematic testing of HCWs for LTBI is a main area of use for serial IGRA testing. As stated above, most studies on IGRA variability are undertaken on HCWs with longer intervals between blood collections. New TB exposure at intervals between the study visits might cause IGRA conversion. Zwerling et al. note in their systematic review that occupational TB risk factors correlate with IGRA positivity but that it remains unclear whether occupational TB exposure is associated with IGRA conversion [6]. In the following, Zwerling et al. ran different studies to evaluate the impact of occupational TB exposure on IGRA conversion. Such an association could not be shown in Canadian HCWs [24] but was present in another study with nursing students in India [32]. In order to eliminate TB exposure as a factor of IGRA variability during our study, intervals between blood collections were short and a cohort with low probability of recent TB contact was chosen. On the other hand untargeted systematically testing of low risk groups could lead to higher false positive rates [2]. So we chose a group of participants with a higher risk than the native population in Germany (German TB incidence 6.2:100,000): students with a migration background from countries with a TB incidence of at least 10 incident cases per 100,000 per year. As a matter of fact, all participants with an initial positive IGRA come from a country with high TB incidence ≧ 125:100,000 or from a country classified as a high TB burden country by the WHO. Therefore it is likely that the positive results at baseline were 'true positive' results. This might explain the low reversion rate we observed compared to the HCW studies mentioned above. However, no gold standard for LTBI testing exists to which IGRA results can be compared. As no active TB was found in our study, it is impossible to say if positives are 'true positives' in respect of LTBI.

Yet all 11 participants with a positive baseline result in one of the two IGRAs stayed positive in at least one of the two IGRAs through all four visits. One of those 11 students was treated for active TB and had consistently positive results in both IGRAs. It was shown in other studies that IGRA positivity can persist in people formerly infected with active TB after completion of antituberculosis chemotherapy and that IGRAs therefore are not a sufficient tool for monitoring antituberculosis chemotherapy [33]. It seems plausible that the other 10 participants with positive results in both IGRAs on the final visit were indeed true positives with regard to LTBI. All conversions in those participants were stable conversions.

Even the 12th participant that only had one positive QFT-Plus result on visit 3 and later reverted was born in a high-incidence country and reported a close contact to active TB over ten years ago (contact with a relative). The positive QFT-Plus result might indeed be an immunological footprint of that former contact but because of the unstable conversion and all-negative results in the other visits this case was not classified as LTBI.

Still it is important to notice that reversion does not mean that the previous QFT was false positive as suggested by a recent study from South Africa. Andrews et al. demonstrated that the predictive value of a positive IGRA result is higher than the predictive value of a negative test result, even if the test reverts to negative at the following control. Incident tuberculosis was 8-fold higher among QFT reverters than in participants with all negative QFT results [34].

Strengths and limitations

Our study is the first study we are aware of that investigated variability of the new generation QFT-Plus in serial testing in a direct head-to-head comparison with QFT-GIT.

The number of participants tested was rather small (n = 41) but a total of 163 serial measurements were analyzed for each IGRA. These numbers align with similar studies on IGRA variability [17].

Choosing students with a migration background studying at a German university as our study subjects gave us an opportunity to evaluate the IGRAs in a cohort with higher LTBI risk than the native population in a low TB incidence setting. Therefore it is highly unlikely that our participants had new contact to active TB during the study period.

The students proved to be a reliable cohort with all of the participants attending their appointments punctually. The only missing result was caused by a blood sample that could not be analyzed. None of the participants dropped out of the study.

Letting individuals with a recent TST application (less than 3 or even 6 months prior first study visit) participate although other studies tend to exclude these individuals due to possible IGRA boosting [17, 24] might be a limitation of the study as well as a strength because we investigated all of the subjects without any censoring. Other sources also indicate no IGRA boosting following TST application. These studies advise against attributing IGRA positivity to possible boosting induced by a previous TST [8, 35].

Conclusions

Although an initial recent study certifies the new generation IGRA QFT-Plus as delivering results with good sensitivity and specificity [22], our study could not confirm improvements in the area of test variability. Inclusion of an additional test tube elucidating $CD8^+$ T-cell response can give rise to further variability. However, following our data the increase in variability was rather small due to the high agreement between QFT-GIT and QFT-Plus. Assuming that the additional tube used in the QFT-Plus will improve sensitivity, the similarity in variability suggests that QFT-Plus has the potential to be advantageous compared to its predecessor.

Abbreviations

BCG: Bacillus calmette-guérin; BGW: Institute for Statutory Accident Insurance and Prevention in the Health and Welfare Services; CI: Confidence interval; CMI: Cell-mediated immune response; CMV: Cytomegalovirus; CVcare: Center of Excellence for Health Services Research in Nursing; ECDC: European Centre for Disease Prevention and Control; ELISA: Enzyme-linked immunosorbent assay; FDA: U.S. Food and Drug Administration; GPR: Principles of Prevention and Rehabilitation Department; HCW: Healthcare worker; ICC: Intraclass correlation coefficient; IFN-γ: Interferon-gamma; IGRA: Interferon-gamma release assay; LTBI: Latent tuberculosis infection; NTM: Nontuberculous mycobacteria; QFT-GIT: QuantiFERON-TB Gold In-Tube; QFT-Plus: QuantiFERON-TB Plus; SD: Standard deviation; TB: Tuberculosis; TST: Tuberculin skin test; UKE: University Medical Center Hamburg-Eppendorf; WHO: World Health Organization

Acknowledgments

We thank all of the students who participated in our study, attending their appointments punctually and reliably despite exams, internships or even personal tragedies and agreeing to anonymous analysis of their data. Furthermore we thank M. Hentschke and I. Büchner-Horstmann and all medical technicians of Dr. Fenner & Colleagues Laboratory for their dedicated work and E. Muth, O. Kleinmüller and P. Koch of the Center of Excellence for Health Services Research in Nursing (CVcare) for contributing analysis tools and helping with literature.

Funding
No special funds were received for this study. However, the Institute for Health Services Research in Dermatology and Nursing of the University Medical Centre Hamburg-Eppendorf (UKE) receives an unrestricted fund from the Institution for Statutory Accident Insurance and Prevention in the Health and Welfare services (BGW) on an annual basis to maintain the working group at the UKE. The funds are provided by a non-profit organization that is part of the social security system in Germany. The funder had no role in study design, data collection and analysis, decision to publish, or preparation of the manuscript.

Authors' contributions
Conceived and designed the experiments: JK, ENGM, AS, JFK, AN. Performed the experiments: JK, ENGM. Analyzed the data: JK, JFK, ENGM, AS, AN. Created figures and tables: JFK, JK, ENGM. Wrote the paper: JK, JFK, ENGM, AS, AN. All authors read and approved the final manuscript.

Competing interests
The authors declare that they have no competing interests.

Author details
[1]University Medical Center Hamburg-Eppendorf (UKE), Center of Excellence for Health Services Research in Nursing (CVcare), Hamburg, Germany. [2]Institute for Statutory Accident Insurance and Prevention in the Health and Welfare Services (BGW), Principles of Prevention and Rehabilitation Department (GPR), Hamburg, Germany.

References
1. U.S. Food and Drug Administration CfDaRH. QuantiFERON® -TB - P010033. Rockville; 2016. Approval letter. http://www.accessdata.fda.gov/cdrh_docs/pdf//p010033a.pdf. Accessed 16 Jun 2016.
2. Nienhaus A, Ringshausen FC, Costa JT, Schablon A, Tripodi D. IFN-gamma release assay versus tuberculin skin test for monitoring TB infection in healthcare workers. Expert Rev Anti Infect Ther. 2013;11:37–48.
3. Pai M, Zwerling A, Menzies D. Systematic review: T-cell-based assays for the diagnosis of latent tuberculosis infection: an update. Ann Intern Med. 2008; 149:177–84.
4. Diel R, Loddenkemper R, Nienhaus A. Evidence-Based Comparison of Commercial Interferon-gamma Release Assays for Detecting Active TB. Chest. 2010;137:952–68.
5. Sester M, Sotgiu G, Lange C, Giehl C, Girardi E, Migliori GB, Bossink A, Dheda K, Diel R, Dominguez J, et al. Interferon-gamma release assays for the diagnosis of active tuberculosis: a systematic review and meta-analysis. Eur RespirJ. 2011;37:100–11.
6. Zwerling A, van den Hof S, Scholten J, Cobelens F, Menzies D, Pai M. Interferon-gamma release assays for tuberculosis screening of healthcare workers: a systematic review. Thorax. 2012;67:62–70.
7. Pai M. Serial Testing With TB Interferon-gamma Release Assays Toward a Nuanced Understanding. Chest. 2012;142:1366–8.
8. Tagmouti S, Slater M, Benedetti A, Kik SV, Banaei N, Cattamanchi A, Metcalfe J, Dowdy D, van Zyl SR, Dendukuri N, et al. Reproducibility of interferon gamma (IFN-gamma) release Assays. A systematic review. Ann Am Thorac Soc. 2014;11:1267–76.
9. Ringshausen FC, Schablon A, Nienhaus A. Interferon-gamma release assays for the tuberculosis serial testing of health care workers: a systematic review. J Occup Med Toxicol. 2012;7.
10. Schablon A, Harling M, Diel R, Ringshausen FC, Torres Costa J, Nienhaus A. Serial testing with an interferon-γ release assay in German healthcare workers. GMS Krankenhhyg Interdiszip. 2010;5:Doc 05.
11. Perry S, Sanchez L, Yang SF, Agarwal Z, Hurst P, Parsonnet J. Reproducibility of QuantiFERON-TB gold in-tube assay. Clin Vaccine Immunol. 2008;15:425–32.
12. Pai M, Kunimoto D, Jamieson F, Menzies D. Diagnosis of latent tuberculosis infection. Can Respir J. 2013;20:23a–34a.
13. Mazurek GH, Jereb J, Vernon A, LoBue P, Goldberg S, Castro K, IGRA Expert Committee, Centers for Disease Control and Prevention. Updated guidelines for using Interferon Gamma Release Assays to detect Mycobacterium tuberculosis infection - United States. MMWR Recomm Rep. 2010;59:1–2.
14. European Centre for Disease Prevention and Control. Use of interferon-gamma release assays in support of TB diagnosis. Stockholm: ECDC; 2011:3–38.
15. Pai M, Elwood K. Interferon-gamma release assays for screening of health care workers in low tuberculosis incidence settings: dynamic patterns and interpretational challenges. Can Respir J. 2012;19:81–3.
16. Schablon A, Nienhaus A, Ringshausen FC, Preisser AM, Peters C. Occupational screening for tuberculosis and the use of a borderline zone for interpretation of the IGRA in German healthcare workers. PLoS One. 2014;9, e115322.
17. Ringshausen FC, Nienhaus A, Costa JT, Knoop H, Schlosser S, Schultze-Werninghaus G, Rohde G. Within-Subject Variability of Mycobacterium tuberculosis-Specific Gamma Interferon Responses in German Health Care Workers. Clin Vaccine Immunol. 2011;18:1176–82.
18. Thanassi W, Noda A, Hernandez B, Newell J, Terpeluk P, Marder D, Yesavage JA. Delineating a Retesting Zone Using Receiver Operating Characteristic Analysis on Serial QuantiFERON Tuberculosis Test Results in US Healthcare Workers. Pulm Med. 2012;2012:291294.
19. Thanassi W, Noda A, Hernandez B, Friedman L, Dorman S, Yesavage J. Negative Tuberculin Skin Test and Prediction of Reversion of QuantiFERON Interferon Gamma Release Assay in US Healthcare Workers. Infect Control Hosp Epidemiol. 2016;37(4):478–82.
20. Ringshausen FC, Nienhaus A, Schablon A, Schlosser S, Schultze-Werninghaus G, Rohde G. Predictors of persistently positive Mycobacterium-tuberculosis-specific interferon-gamma responses in the serial testing of health care workers. BMC Infect Dis. 2010;10:220.
21. Qiagen. QIAGEN launches QuantiFERON®-TB Gold Plus – a new generation of the most accurate test for detecting tuberculosis infections 2015, press release 7 Jan 2015. https://www.qiagen.com/de/about-us/press-releases/pressreleaseview?ID={C861949E-DF50-475B-8148-B4C70034C49E}&lang=en. Accessed 16 Jun 2016.
22. Barcellini L, Borroni E, Brown J, Brunetti E, Codecasa L, Cugnata F, Dal Monte P, Di Serio C, Goletti D, Lombardi G, et al. First independent evaluation of QuantiFERON-TB Plus performance. Eur Respir J. 2016;47:1587–90.
23. WHO World Health Oraganization. Global Health Observatory data repository. Incidence Data by country (2007 - present) http://apps.who.int/gho/data/node.main.1320?lang=en (2016). Accessed 16 Jun 2016.
24. Zwerling A, Benedetti A, Cojocariu M, McIntosh F, Pietrangelo F, Behr MA, Schwartzman K, Menzies D, Pai M. Repeat IGRA Testing in Canadian Health Workers: Conversions or Unexplained Variability? Plos One. 2013;8.
25. Qiagen. QuantiFERON®-TB Gold Plus (QFT®-Plus) ELISA Package Insert. http://www.quantiferon.com/irm/content/PI/QFT/PLUS/2PK-Elisa/UK.pdf (2015). Accessed 16 Jun 2016.
26. Gaur RL, Pai M, Banaei N. Impact of blood volume, tube shaking, and incubation time on reproducibility of QuantiFERON-TB gold in-tube assay. J Clin Microbiol. 2013;51:3521–6.
27. Cicchetti DV. Guidelines, Criteria, and Rules of Thumb for Evaluating Normed and Standardized Assessment Instruments in Psychology. Psychol Assess. 1994;6:284–90.
28. WHO. Global Tuberculosis Report 2015. Geneva: World Health Organization; 2015. p. 1–192.
29. Barnett AG, van der Pols JC, Dobson AJ. Regression to the mean: what it is and how to deal with it. Int J Epidemiol. 2005;34:215–20.
30. King TC, Upfal M, Gottlieb A, Adamo P, Bernacki E, Kadlecek CP, Jones JG, Humphrez-Carothers F, Rielly AF, Drewry P, Murray K, DeWitt M, Matsubara

J, O'Dea L, Balser J, Wrighton-Smith P. T-SPOT.TB Interferon-γ Release Assay Performance in Healthcare Worker Screening at Nineteen U.S. Hospitals. Am J Respir Crit Care Med. 2015;192(3):367–73.
31. Saldan A, Forner G, Mengoli C, Tinto D, Fallico L, Peracchi M, Gussetti N, Palù G, Abate D. Comparison of the Cytomegalovirus (CMV) Enzyme-Linked Immunosorbent Spot and CMV QuantiFERON Cell-Mediated Immune Assays in CMV-Seropositive and –Seronegative Pregnant and Nonpregnant Women. J Clin Microbiol. 2016;54(5):1352–6.
32. Zwerling A, Pai M, Michael JS, Christopher DJ. Serial testing using interferon-gamma release assays in nursing students in India. Eur Respir J. 2014;44:257–60.
33. Pai M, Denkinger CM, Kik SV, Rangaka MX, Zwerling A, Oxlade O, Metcalfe JZ, Cattamanchi A, Dowdy DW, Dheda K, Banaei N. Gamma Interferon Release Assays for Detection of Mycobacterium tuberculosis Infection. Clin Microbiol Rev. 2014;27:3–20.
34. Andrews JR, Hatherill M, Mahomed H, Hanekom WA, Campo M, Hawn TR, Wood R, Scriba TJ. The dynamics of QuantiFERON-TB gold in-tube conversion and reversion in a cohort of South African adolescents. Am J Respir Crit Care Med. 2015;191(5):584–91.
35. Ritz N, Yau C, Connell TG, Tebruegge M, Leslie D, Curtis N. Absence of interferon-gamma release assay conversion following tuberculin skin testing. Int J Tuberc Lung Dis. 2011;15:767–9.

10

Attitude, reporting behaviour and management practice of occupational needle stick and sharps injuries among hospital healthcare workers in Bale zone, Southeast Ethiopia

Tolesa Bekele[1*], Alem Gebremariam[2], Muhammedawel Kaso[1] and Kemal Ahmed[1]

Abstract

Background: Although the prevalence of blood borne pathogens in many developing countries is high, documentation of infections due to occupational exposure is limited. Seventy percent of the world's HIV infected population lives in Sub-Saharan Africa, but only 4 % of cases are reported from this region. Under reporting of needle stick and/or sharps injuries in healthcare facilities was common.

Methods: An institutional based cross-sectional study was conducted in December 2014 among healthcare workers in four hospitals of Bale zone, Southeast Ethiopia. A total of 362 healthcare workers were selected randomly from each of the working departments. Data were collected using self-administered questionnaire and were entered using Epi-Info version 3.5 and analysed using SPSS version 20.0. Multivariable logistic regression analysis was used to identify independent effect of each variable on the reporting behaviour of needle stick and/or sharp injury.

Results: Nearly six out of ten injuries (58.7 %) were not reported to the concerned body. The main reasons for not reporting the injuries were time constraint (35.1 %), sharps which caused injury were not used on any patient (27.0 %), the source patients did not have disease of concern (20.3 %), and lack of knowledge that it should be reported (14.9 %). Half of healthcare workers (HCWs) those who experienced injury had sought medical care next to self based action. Respondents with monthly salary of 450 to 1000 Ethiopian Birr (1 US Dollar = 22.00 Ethiopian Birr) were about six times more likely to report occupational needle stick and/or sharps injury (NSSI) than HCWs with salary of 2001 to 8379 birr (AOR = 5.73). However, HCWs who had no knowledge about probability of infection transmission through NSSI and not taking any self based measures after occurrence of injury were 45 % (AOR = 0.55) and 93 % (AOR = 0.07) less likely to report occupational injury than their counterparts, respectively.

Conclusions: Occupational needle stick and/or sharps injuries are common among HCWs at the study area. Even though majority of respondents were concerned about the risk of NSSI exposure, most respondents did not report it to the concerned body. Therefore, provision of on job training on the risk of occupational NSSI exposure may strengthen HCWs to practice timely reporting and its management in case of occupational injury exposure.

Keywords: Reporting behavior, Injury, Healthcare workers, Bale zone, Oromia, Ethiopia

* Correspondence: tolesa2003@yahoo.com
[1]Department of Public Health, College of Medicine and Health Sciences, Madda Walabu University, Oromia, Ethiopia
Full list of author information is available at the end of the article

Background

World Health Organization (WHO) in 2007 endorsed the Global Plan of Action on Workers' Health from 2008 to 2017 to provide political framework for development of policies, infrastructure, technologies and partnerships for achieving basic level of health protection in all workplaces throughout the world. The Global Plan of Action addresses all aspects of workers' health, including primary prevention of occupational hazards, protection and promotion of health at work, employment conditions and improving the response of health systems to workers' health. In such a way it links occupational health to public health [1].

While as many as twenty blood borne pathogens can be transmitted through accidental needle and/or sharps injury, the potentially life threatening are Human Immunodeficiency Virus (HIV), hepatitis B virus (HBV) and hepatitis C virus (HCV) [2]. Needle stick and sharps injury (NSSI) is an injury with needles, scalpel blade, catheter stylet or other pointed objects which were used for any invasive procedure with a patient and contaminated with blood or body fluids. Sharps injuries are hidden problem; after it happens most of workers forget and get on with their work. Neither the magnitude of the risk of needle stick and sharps injury nor the practices associated with it has been well understood among HCWs [3].

A number of policy strategies are available for avoiding disease burden associated with NSSI, including vaccination against HBV, post exposure prophylaxes (PEP) for HBV, HCV and HIV, reducing the number of injections and invasive procedures where appropriate, using safer devices and properly disposing of needles and other sharps. Despite the presence of many opportunities to reduce the disease burden, the full impact of NSSI is not yet recognized [4]. Most of people at risk for occupational exposures are in developing countries where there is paucity of reporting standard protocols. In addition, poor knowledge and practices related to the risk and hazard of sharps injuries substantially contribute to the probability of the injuries [5].

Although the prevalence of blood borne pathogens in many developing countries is high, documentation of infections caused by occupational exposure in these countries is scarce. Seventy percent of the world's HIV infected population lives in Sub-Saharan Africa but only 4 % of worldwide cases of occupational HIV infection are reported from this region [6]. Underreporting of sharps injuries by employees is documented in different literatures. The magnitude of underreporting ranges from 22 to 99 % [7]. There are many reasons why healthcare workers do not report sharp injuries. They may perceive that the injuries or the source patients are low risk, they may fear the diseases to which they have potentially been exposed, they may have concerns about job security or the extra paperwork and time involved in follow-up. In addition, they may lack information and training about appropriate reporting procedures or the reporting procedures themselves may be inadequate [8, 9].

Ethiopian healthcare facilities do not have adequate reporting system. This is why most of incidents are not reported and inadequately treated. Tangible evidence on the reporting system and its management in healthcare facilities is very limited and varies from setting to setting. There are few studies conducted on occupational NSSI exposure. However, the reason why HCWs do not report incidents of sharp injuries was not yet well addressed. To the best of our knowledge, there is no any available data reported before about occupational NSSI reporting behaviour and its management among HCWs from the study area.

Methods

The study was carried out in December 2014 at four hospitals namely Ginnir, Robe, Delo mena and Goba. The four hospitals are found in Bale Zone, Oromia Regional State, at Southeast of Ethiopia. By the year 2014, these four hospitals were offering different types of healthcare services for the surrounding community. Hospital based cross-sectional study design was employed. All healthcare workers working in the four hospitals who have direct contact with patients or equipments used on patients were involved in the study. These were doctors, anaesthetists, health officers, nurses, midwives, laboratory personnel, laundry workers and waste handlers. All individuals out of work during data collection due to annual leave and those who could not respond to the questions due to illness were excluded from the study.

The sample size was determined using single population proportion formula with the following assumptions: the proportion of HCWs who experienced needles stick and/or sharp injury in the previous 12 months was 31.0 % [10], 1.96 values of 95 % confidence interval, 5 % margin of error and 10 % non-response rate. The total sample size became 362.

All hospitals in Bale zone were included in the study. Before selection of study participants, first we obtained the list of workers and categorized them into their specific working department. Then proportionate allocation to size was used for each department to share the total sample size. Study participants who fulfil the inclusion criteria were selected by simple random sampling technique using the list of workers taken from each working department.

Questionnaire was developed by referring published literatures [10–13]. The questionnaire was first written in English and then translated to Afan Oromo and Amharic (local languages) by experts in both languages and then retranslated to English to check for consistency. Eight data collection facilitators (BSc nurses) were assigned to the four hospitals (two per hospital). Pre-testing was done on 5 % of the same source population other than the sampled population in Goba and Robe hospitals. Based on the pre-test result, necessary correction was made for the questionnaire. Data were collected using self-administered questionnaire.

The questionnaire included background information, attitude about risk of NSSI, its management and reporting behaviour of the respondents. Finally, the questionnaire was administered by data collection facilitators who were trained for 1 day ahead of data collection. Supervision during data collection was done by investigators to see how the data collection facilitators were handling data collection process. Each filled questionnaire was checked for its completeness and consistency on daily basis.

The collected data were checked for completeness and consistency by the principal investigators before data entry for analysis. Prior to data entry, each questionnaire was given a unique code by principal investigator. The principal investigator prepared template and entered data using Epi Info version 3.5 and 20 % of the data were double entered in computer software. Data cleaning were done to check missing values and inconsistencies by running frequencies for each variable. Cleaned data were exported from Epi Info to Statistical Program for Social Sciences (SPSS) version 20.0 for analysis. Frequency distribution and percentage were used to present the results of uni-variate analysis. Logistic regression model was used to identify the independent effect of each predictor variable on the dependent variable. Those variables which were significant on bi-variate analysis (P-value < 0.05) were entered to multivariable logistic regression analysis. The association between the reporting behaviour of NSSI and independent variables was determined using odds ratio (OR) with 95 % confidence interval (CI). The level of significance was taken at $\alpha = 0.05$.

Ethical clearance was obtained from the Ethical and Review Committee of Madda Walabu University, College of Medicine and Health Sciences. An official permission was communicated through formal letter from Madda Walabu University Research and Community Service Directorate Office to the respective hospital. Written consent was secured from each participant. Participants were told that the information provided was confidential and that their identities were not revealed in association with the information they provided.

Results

Socio-demographic characteristics of participants

From a total of 362 HCWs working in four hospitals, 340 fully responded the questionnaire, giving a response rate of 93.9 %. The mean age of the respondents were 28.3 (SD = ± 7.7) years. More than eight out of ten (82.1 %) of the respondents were found in the age group of 18 to 32 years. Majority of the participants were Orthodox Christian (62.1 %) by religion and were Oromo (79.1 %) by Ethnicity. Nearly half of the respondents (49.7 %) were nurses by profession (Table 1).

Attitude about risk of needle stick and sharp injury

Almost all of the respondents 334 (98.2 %) knew about the risk of NSSI exposure. Among the HCWs who knew

Table 1 Socio-demographic characteristics of hospital healthcare workers in Bale zone, December, 2014 ($n = 340$)

Socio- demographic characteristics	Frequency (n)	Percentage (%)
Participants' working hospital		
Ginir	90	26.5
Goba	115	33.8
Delo mena	70	20.6
Bale Robe	65	19.1
Sex of respondents		
Male	153	45.0
Female	187	55.0
Age group of participants		
18–32	279	82.1
33–47	44	12.9
48–62	17	5.0
Marital status		
Ever married	191	56.2
Never married	149	43.8
Religion		
Orthodox	211	62.1
Muslim	67	19.7
Protestant	58	17.0
Wakefata	4	1.2
Ethnicity		
Oromo	269	79.1
Amhara	59	17.3
Gurage	6	1.8
Tigrie	3	0.9
Others (Harari, Somali and Wolayita)	3	0.9
Educational level		
Grade(5–12th)	55	16.2
College diploma and above	285	83.8
Monthly salary		
450–1000	77	22.7
1001–2000	60	17.6
2001–8379	203	59.7

about the risk, 273 (81.3 %), 46 (13.7 %) and 17 (5.1 %) rated as high, moderate and low risk, respectively. More than eight out of ten 283 (83.2 %) respondents perceived that NSSI is avoidable. The main perceived prevention methods of NSSI were proper disposal of the used needles (35.7 %), careful collection of needles and/or sharps (25.1 %) and adherence to universal precautions (21.2 %). Significant proportion (16.2 %) of respondents also perceived that personal protective equipment and other methods such as not recapping needle and sterilizing before disposal (1.8 %) as a method of prevention. Nearly all respondents 338 (99.4 %) knew that diseases can be transmitted through NSSI exposure. Respondents were asked about type of diseases which can be transmitted due to occupational NSSI exposure. Almost eight out of ten (81.1 %) HCWs reported at least three diseases including HIV, HBV and HCV. Only ten respondents reported that malaria can be transmitted through occupational NSSI.

Respondents were asked about what contributed to NSSI in their respective hospital. Thirty one percent of the participants reported that lack of personal protective equipment in the working place could put HCWs at increased risk of injury. Similarly, excess workload (28.5 %), improper disposing of needles into safety box after use (22.9 %), and other such as over crowed in working department, waste handling and lack of hand washing facility in the working unit account for 17.6 % of injuries. Most of the respondents (95.6 %) reported that safety box was available in their working department. Whereas 148 (43.5 %) of the respondents reported that there was no occupational NSSI reporting protocol in their working department. Only 20 % of HCWs received their vaccination after starting their career at the hospital. From a total of the respondents, 119 (35.0 %) got tested for HIV, HBV and HCV at the time of the study. Of those who got tested, nearly half (54.9 %) of the respondents had been tested for at least one of the three diseases (HIV, HBV and HCV).

NSSI management and reporting behaviour of the respondents

Of those HCWs experienced NSSI, majority 107 (84.9 %) of them took self based measures. The most common self based actions taken were washing the injured body part with soap and water (53.3 %), washed with iodine or alcohol solution (42.1 %), and HIV testing (40.2 %). However, 19 (15.1 %) of HCWs did not take any action for their injury. Nearly six out of ten (58.7 %) respondents did not report the accident of their injury to concerned body. The main reasons for not reporting the injury were: time constraints (35.1 %), sharps caused injury were not used on any patient (27.0 %), it was used on patient but the patient did not have disease of concern (20.3 %) and lack of knowledge that it should be reported (14.9 %).

Half of the HCWs who experienced injury had sought medical care next to self based action. Of those who sought medical care, 39.7 % took post exposure prophylaxes such as antiretroviral agents (zidovudine) and tetanus anti-toxoid (TAT). Among the NSSI events reported to infection prevention department, 94.2 % were reported immediately after the injury (Table 2).

Factors associated with reporting behaviour of needle stick and/or sharp injury

On bi-variate analysis respondents from Goba hospital were four times more likely to report occupational NSSI compared to respondents from other hospitals in the study area. But this becomes not significant after controlling other variables in the multivariable analysis (Table 3). Respondents with educational status (5–12th grade), presence of occupational injury reporting protocol and safety guideline in working department were the predictors of reporting the NSSI events compared to their counterparts. But these were also not significant on multivariable analysis. Respondents with monthly salary of 450 to 1000 Ethiopian Birr (1 US Dollar = 22.00 Ethiopian Birr) were about six times more likely to report occupational NSSI than HCWs with salary of 2001 to 8379 birr (AOR = 5.73, 95 % CI: 1.71, 19.23). However, HCWs who did not know that diseases can be transmitted through needle stick and/or sharp injury and who did not take self based measures after occurrence of injury were 45 and 93 % less likely to report occupational injury than their counterparts (AOR = 0.55, 95 % CI: 0.47, 0.68) and (AOR = 0.07, 95 % CI: 0.01, 0.63), respectively (Table 3).

Discussion

Nearly four out of five respondents in this study rated the level of risk of infection after exposure to NSSI is as high risk. This result is much higher than the study done in Royal College of nursing in London in which 15 % of the respondents perceived that the level of risk of contracting a blood borne that disease from their last injury is as high risk [14]. Almost all respondents (99.4 %) knew diseases can be transmitted through NSSI. This finding is comparable with the study done in Felege Hiwot Referral hospital in Bahir Dar (98.5 %) [10]. It is also indicated in other study that most of HCWs know the possibility that NSSI could lead to the contracting of diseases such as HIV, hepatitis B and C [15].

The current study found that two fifth of the respondents reported that there was no reporting protocol for NSSI in their respective working department. In similar way the study done in two hospitals of Tanzania reported that more than half of the observed hospital

Table 2 Management and reporting behaviour of NSSI among hospital healthcare workers, Bale zone, December, 2014

Variables	Frequency (n)	Percentage (%)
Ever experienced NSSI at work ($n = 340$)		
Yes	126	37.1
No	214	62.9
Self management taken after injury ($n = 126$)		
Yes	107	84.9
No	19	15.1
Type of action taken after injury[a]		
Washed with soap and water	57	53.3
Washed with iodine or alcohol	45	42.1
Get tested for HIV	43	40.2
Take post exposure prophylaxis (PEP)	25	23.4
Take tetanus anti-toxoid (TAT)	31	29.0
Squeezing to extract more blood	10	8.5
Applying pressure to stop bleeding	18	16.8
Ever reported NSSI to concerned body ($n = 126$)		
Yes	52	41.3
No	74	58.7
Time of injury reported ($n = 52$)		
Immediately after injury	49	94.2
Late before going off work place	2	3.8
After two days of injury	1	1.9
Reasons for not reported injury[a]		
Being too busy at the time of injury	26	35.1
Sharps caused injury never used on patient	20	27.0
Used on patient but was not disease of concern	15	20.3
They did not know as they should report	11	14.9
They did not know how to report	7	9.5
Their colleagues told them not to worry	1	1.4
Sought medical care after injury ($n = 126$)		
Yes	63	50.0
No	63	50.0
Treatment given ($n = 63$)		
Tested for different diseases	15	23.8
Pre-test counselling	4	6.3
Post-test counselling	19	30.2
PEP was given and follow-up started	25	39.7

[a]Each of the percentages does not add up to 100 % because respondents could choose several responses which could be more than one

Table 3 Multivariable analyses of factors associated with NSSI reporting behaviour among hospital healthcare workers in Bale zone, December, 2014

Variables	Reporting of NSSIs exposure	
	Crude OR (95 % CI)	Adjusted OR (95 % CI)
Working hospital		
Ginir	1.63 (0.52, 510)	1.04 (0.27, 4.05)
Goba	4.1 (1.37, 12.30)*	2.08 (0.46, 9.44)
Delo mena	1.62 (0.44, 5.95)	0.48 (0.08, 2.90)
Bale Robe	Ref	Ref
Educational level		
Grade(5-12th)	2.95 (1.07, 8.11)*	7.54 (0.46, 12.56)
College diploma and above	Ref	Ref
Monthly income		
450–1000	3.05 (1.17,7.98)*	5.73 (1.71, 19.23)*
1001–2000	1.68 (0.68, 4.15)	2.67 (0.88, 8.10)
2001–8379	Ref	Ref
Diseases can be transmitted by NSSI		
Yes	Ref	Ref
Do not know	0.70 (0.31, 0.89)*	0.55 (0.47, 0.68)*
Self management taken after injury		
Yes	Ref	Ref
No	0.06 (0.01, 0.47)*	0.07 (0.01,0.63)*
Presence of protocol for reporting		
Yes	2.62 (1.26, 5.46)*	2.17 (0.74, 6.34)
No	Ref	Ref
Safety guidelines available		
Yes	2.87 (1.34, 6.15)*	2.39 (0.95, 6.07)
No	Ref	Ref

*Significant at $P < 0.05$, *Ref* Reference

departments did not have guidelines for prevention and management of occupational exposure to HIV infections [16]. Lack of reporting protocol supplies may seriously hampers reporting effort and puts both patients and HCWs at increased risk of infection. Current study showed that there was low HBV vaccination coverage (20.3 %) in the study area. This result is much lower compared to study done in Pakistan where 86.3 % of HCWs received their vaccination after starting their job at the hospital [17]. It is recommended that the need for immunization against HBV in the start of career in healthcare settings [4] but no such policy is implemented in Ethiopian healthcare facilities and specifically at the study area.

In this study it was revealed that half of the injured workers did not seek medical care after they sustained NSSI. This is inconsistent with the study done in

Mongolian public hospitals in which out of the respondents who reported at least one NSSI in the previous 3 months, 35.9 % answered as they did not seek medical assistance after the occurrence of an injury [12]. This may imply that a system should be introduced in healthcare facilities to ensure that all healthcare workers should be pre-informed where to seek medical treatment after the occurrence of NSSI.

Nearly 60 % of the respondents did not report the injury to the concerned body. The main reasons stated for not reporting were time constraint, needles or sharps caused injury were not used on patients and low perceived risk of diseases transmission due to injury. This result is almost in agreement with Ahmadabad (64 %) [18], and in Alexandria (74.7 %) [19]. But it is higher as compared to the report from Felege Hiwot Referral hospital in Bahir Dar, Ethiopia (46.1 %). The reason for not reporting the occurrence of injury was; the victims perceived that the patient had low probability of being HIV positive especially when the disease status of the patient is unknown [10]. Barriers that hinder reporting of injuries should be appropriately identified in order to provide counselling and treatment for HCWs after exposure to the event.

Respondents who had lower monthly salary were six times more likely to report occupational NSSI. The possible justification might be those HCWs with lower income may seek help from employer to get medical expenses. In addition, those workers with high income may not report to employer to seek money for treatment since they can afford expenses by themselves. Healthcare workers who did not know probability of diseases transmission through NSSI had 45 % lower odds of reporting their injury. Similarly, those who did not take self based measures after occurrence of injury were 93 % less likely to report occupational injury to the concerned body. This may suggest that providing on job training for HCWs on the importance of reporting after injury could improve the victim's medical seeking behavior.

In interpreting the findings of this study, taking the limitations into consideration is important. Since the study was based on self-reported data in assessing reporting behaviour and management of occupational NSSI exposure; a common threat to the validity of the self-report that can lead to information bias is social desirability and recall bias. In addition, cross-sectional study by its nature cannot establish temporal cause and effect relationships.

Conclusions

Based on the findings of the study it is concluded that HCWs working in the four hospitals of Bale zone are at increased risk of blood borne pathogens infection due to NSSI. Knowledge of the risk of blood borne pathogens transmission due to occupational exposure and whom to contact in the event of NSSI exposure seems to affect practices of HCWs in relation to its management and timely reporting. Therefore, more rigorous control measures and occupational injury prevention and its management programs need to be implemented by national and institutions. In addition, monitoring and control of health of healthcare workers in order to promote decent and safe work throughout the health facilities is important. Furthermore, regular reporting, provision of hepatitis B immunoglobulin (HBIG) for victims and evaluation of occupational NSSI exposures need to be introduced in the study area.

Competing interests

The authors declare that they have no competing interests.

Authors' contributions

TB and AG carried out the conception and designing of the study, data collection, performed statistical analysis and wrote the manuscript. MK and KA participated in designing the study, data collection, reviewing and editing the final draft of the manuscript. All authors read and approved the final manuscript.

Authors' information

TB (MPH), MK (MPH) and KA (MPH are lecturers at Madda Walabu University, College of Medicine and Health Sciences. AG (MPH in Epidemiology), lecturer at Adigrat University, College of Medicine and Health Sciences.

Acknowledgements

We would like to acknowledge Madda Walabu University, College of Medicine and Health Sciences for giving us this important opportunity. Our acknowledgement also goes to our friends who give us comments on the proposal structure and arrangement. Finally, we would like to acknowledge Bale zone health office, respective hospital administrators, our data collection facilitators and study subjects.

Author details

[1]Department of Public Health, College of Medicine and Health Sciences, Madda Walabu University, Oromia, Ethiopia. [2]Department of Public Health, College of Medicine and Health Sciences, Adigrat University, Adigrat, Tigray, Ethiopia.

References

1. World Health Organization. The Global Occupational Health Network: GOHNET Newsletter. 2007; Issue No 14.
2. De Laune S. Risk reduction through testing, screening, and infection control precautions with special emphasis on needle stick injuries. Infect Control Hosp Epidemiol. 1990;11:563–5.
3. Stewardson DA. Occupational exposures occurring among dental assistants in a UK dental school. Prim Dent Care. 2003;10:23–6.
4. Rapiti E, Prüss ÜA, Hutin Y. Sharps injuries: assessing the burden of disease from sharps injuries to health-care workers at national and local levels. Geneva: WHO Environmental Burden of Disease Series; 2005. Issue No 11.
5. Sagoe MC, Pearson RD, Perry J, Jagger J. Risks to health care workers in developing countries. New England J Med. 2001;345:538–41.
6. Ippolito G, Puro V, Heptonstall J, Jagger J, De-Carli G, Petrosillo N. Occupational human immunodeficiency virus infection in health care workers: worldwide cases. Clin Infect Dis. 1999;28:365–83.
7. Nagao M, Iinuma Y, Igawa J, Matsumura Y, Shirano M, Matsushima A, et al. Accidental exposures to blood and body fluid in the operation room and the issue of underreporting. American Journal of Infection Control. 2009;37:541–544.

8. Haiduven DJ, Simpkins SM, Phillips ES, Stevens DA. A survey of percutaneous/ mucocutaneous injury reporting in a public teaching hospital. Journal of Hosp Infect. 1999;41:151–4.
9. Massachusetts. Department of Public Health Occupational Health Surveillance Program. Sharps Injuries among Hospital Workers in Massachusetts,(Unpublished document); 2010.
10. Lulie W, Emebet A, Medihanit T, Hanna F, Dereje B, Muluken A. Factors associated with needle stick and sharp injuries, among healthcare workers in Felege Hiwot Referral Hospital, Bahir Dar, Northwest Ethiopia. Int J Infect Control. 2013;9:1996–9783.
11. Ali G, Abasalt B, Pegah L, Amin A. Risk factors of needlestick and sharps injuries among healthcare workers. International Journal of Hospital Research. 2013;2:31–8.
12. Kakizaki M, Ikeda N, Ali M, Enkhtuya B, Tsolmon M, Shibya K, et al. Needle stick and sharps injuries among health care workers at public tertiary hospitals in an urban community in Mongolia. BMC Research Notes. 2011;4:184.
13. Reda AA, Fisseha S, Mengistie B, Vandeweerd JM. Standard precautions: occupational exposure and behavior of health care workers in Ethiopia. PLoS One. 2010;5:12. doi:10.1371/journal.pone.0014420.
14. Jane B, Geoff P. Needle sick injury in Royal College of Nursing in London. London, UK. Employment Research Ltd; 2008.
15. Sumathi M, Prashant KS, Jain RK, Meenakshi M, Manju B. Needle stick injuries among health care workers in a tertiary care hospital of India. Indian J Med Res. 2010;131:405–10.
16. Mashoto OK, Mubyazi MG, Hussein ME, Mohamed H, Malebo MH. Estimated risk of HIV acquisition and practice for preventing occupational exposure: a study of healthcare workers at Tumbi and Dodoma Hospitals, Tanzania. BMC Health Serv Res. 2013;13:369.
17. Attaullah S, Khan S, Ayaz S, Khan NS, Mullah N, Ali I, et al. Prevalence of HBV and HBV vaccination coverage in health care workers of tertiary hospitals of Peshawar, Pakistan. Virol J. 2011;8:275.
18. Goswami M, Patel P, Nayak S, Mehta HK, Shah R, Devmurari D, et al. Needle stick and sharp instruments injuries among health care providers at cardiology institute, Ahmedabad. National Journal of Community Medicine. 2010;1:114–7.
19. Hanafi M, Mohamed AM, Kassem MS, Shawki M. Needle stick injuries among health care workers of University of Alexandria hospitals. East Mediterr Health J. 2011;17:26–35.

11

Tobacco smoke particles and indoor air quality (ToPIQ-II) – a modified study protocol and first results

Alexander Gerber*, Alexander V Hofen-Hohloch, Johannes Schulze and David A Groneberg

Abstract

Background: Environmental tobacco smoke (ETS)-associated particulate matter (PM) has to be seen as an independent health hazard and needs to be discussed separately from the already well-known toxic and carcinogenic compounds contained in cigarette smoke. We believe that brand-specific amounts of PM are of public interest and should be investigated.

Methods: An automatic environmental tobacco smoke emitter was developed and placed into a glass-chamber to generate cigarette smoke as reliably as possible. Cigarettes were smoked automatically according to a standardized protocol. Mean concentrations (C_{mean}) and area under the curve (AUC) of PM2.5 released by the brands P&S, Virginia (without filter) and the 3R4F standard research cigarette of the University of Kentucky, USA, were measured and compared with each other.

Results: C_{mean} PM2.5 of 3R4F reference was 1,725 μg/m^3, for P&S: 1,982 μg/m^3 and for Virginia without filter: 1,525 μg/m^3. AUC PM2.5 for 3R4F reference was: 527,644 μg/m^{3}xsec, for P&S: 606,171 μg/m^{3}xsec, and for Virginia without filter: 464,788 μg/m^{3}xsec.

Conclusions: Our modified ToPIQ-II study protocol shows significant brand-specific differences in the amounts of PM2.5 released by cigarettes into the environment, when compared to 3R4F reference cigarettes. We believe that information about PM-release of all relevant brands in relation to reference cigarettes should be published. In the light of PM as an independent risk factor for morbidity and mortality, this may serve as a basis for further epidemiologic investigations.

Keywords: Particulate matter, Cigarettes, Automatic environmental tobacco smoke emitter

Introduction

Health effects of air pollution have been the subject of scientific research for decades, and airborne particulate matter (PM) is one important aspect of air pollution and generally considered a great health hazard [1].

PM is the term for a mixture of microscopic solid and liquid matter suspended in the air. It is attributable to both natural sources — such as volcanoes, dust storms or fires —, and to human activities (anthropogenic PM), such as the burning or fossil fuels, traffic, industrial processes or tobacco smoke. Composition, size and shape of PM depend on its source. PM can be made up of hundreds of different chemicals. The United States Environmental Protection Agency (EPA) has defined, categorized and regulated inhalable PM (particles up to 10 micrometers) since 1987 in the National Air Quality-Standard for Particulate Matter (PM-Standard) [2]. Two groups of inhalable particles are distinguished: "Inhalable coarse particles" with aerodynamic diameters larger than 2,5 μm but smaller than 10 μm, and "fine particles" with aerodynamic diameters of 2.5 μm and less. All inhalable particles smaller than 10 μm are categorized as PM10, while inhalable particles smaller than 2.5 μm are categorized as PM2.5. Their potential to cause harm depends on size, shape and solubility. The smaller the particles are, the deeper they can be inhaled. Coarse particles generally pass

* Correspondence: gerber@med.uni-frankfurt.de
Institute of Occupational, Social and Environmental Medicine, Goethe-University, Theodor-Stern-Kai 7, Haus 9b, 60590 Frankfurt am Main, Germany

nose and throat and enter into the lungs. Fine particles tend to penetrate into the gas exchange regions of the lung and some may even enter into the bloodstream [3]. Surface area and solubility limit the extent of absorption of gasses and vapors. Depending on their origin, fine particles may serve as carriers for carcinogens like benzopyrenes, by absorbing them on their surface. Both long-term and short-term exposure to inhalable PM are associated with increased cardiovascular-, pulmonary- and neurological morbidity and mortality as well as with premature delivery, birth defects and premature death [4-10].

According to the "Global Burden of Disease study", exposure to air pollution and particulate matter ranks as one of the top ten risk factors for health globally [11]. WHO recommended critical values for PM concentration in public environments are exceeded regularly [12]. While indoor particulate matter air pollution by solid fuel use for cooking is a major problem in developing countries and according to the WHO, 4.3 million people a year die from the exposure to household air pollution [13], second-hand smoke exposure is a leading contributor to the disease burden in high-income countries [14]. Apart from many toxic substances contained in ETS, epidemiological data suggests particulate matter itself to be a harmful component of ETS and demonstrates its association with many detrimental effects on human health, such as increased morbidity and mortality [5-7,15].

Therefore, not only information about nicotine and tar yield of a cigarette are of interest for the consumer. Also, information about the amount of PM emitted by a cigarette should be published, as PM seems to be an independent risk factor.

Several studies have shown a high brand loyalty, predominantly among older smokers in high-income-countries [16,17]. These smokers are likely to expose their personal environment to ETS of one brand for years or even decades. We believe that the consumer and the public have the right to be informed about brand-specific PM-amounts. In order to supply information about brand-specific PM release in relation to a 3R4F standard research cigarette, the ToPIQ-II study protocol was developed to automatically smoke cigarettes and to measure PM amounts as standardized, reliable and repeatable as possible.

Aims

The aim of the ToPIQ-II study is to measure brand-specific amounts of PM- release of different tobacco products in a standardized way and reliably and repeatable as possible. In contrast to the original ToPIQ study protocol [18], an electric and programmable smoking machine (automatic environmental tobacco smoke emitter) is used this time to generate environmental tobacco smoke.

Methods

Tobacco products

Both analyzed brands (P&S and Players Virginia No. 6) are produced by Reemtsma Cigarettenfabriken GmbH, a 100% daughter company of the Imperial tobacco group. Tar and nicotine yield of Virginia without filter adds up to 10 mg and 0,8 mg. P&S cigarettes contain the same tar and nicotine yield (10 mg, 0,8 mg). The 3R4F reference cigarette has an average tar yield of 9.5 mg and a nicotine yield of 0.73 mg per cigarette.

Automatic environmental tobacco smoke emitter (AETSE)

An automatic environmental tobacco smoke emitter was developed and constructed by Schimpf-Ing, Trondheim Norway. The AETSE consists of a 200 ml glass syringe, a stepper motor, a microcontroller, aluminium profiles and mechanical parts such as hoses and valves (Figure 1). The stepper motor imitates puffing by pulling and pushing the syringe plunger, thus sucking the mainstream smoke (MS) into the syringe and exhaling it into the chamber. Igniting and extinguishing is carried out via two rubber gloves embedded into the glass wall,

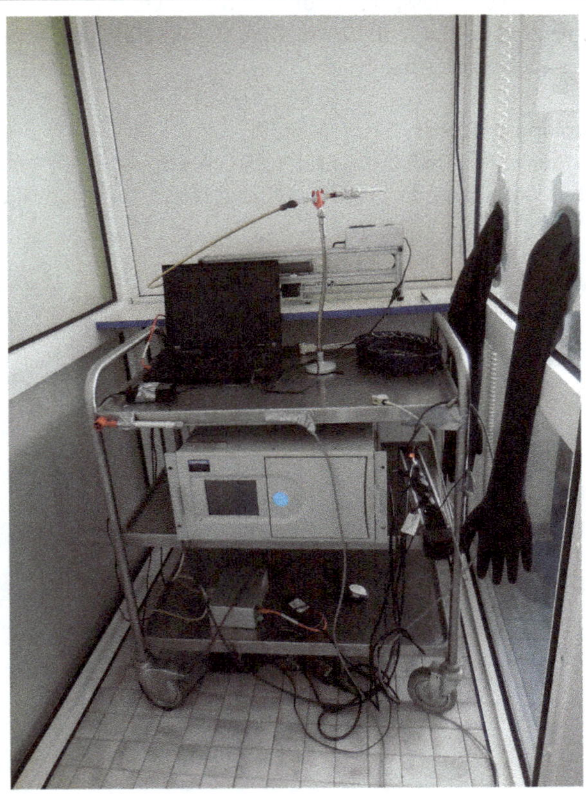

Figure 1 Automatic environmental tobacco smoke emitter: the AETSE consists of a glass syringe with a plunger, a stepper motor to pull and push the plunger, a microcontroller that drives the motor and aluminium parts. Two rubber gloves are embedded into the glass panel to operate the system.

providing an isolated access to the chamber (Figure 1). Between puffs the smouldering cigarette continuously emits sidestream smoke (SS), which, together with the MS, forms environmental tobacco smoke (ETS). Frequency and tidal volume of the smoking machine were set according to a self-developed smoking protocol. The AETSE is placed inside a 2.88 m^3 glass chamber in order to protect the researcher from exposure to ETS. To quantify the concentrations of particulate matter (PM2.5), an aerosol spectrometer was used (Model 11.09, Grimm Co., Ainring, Germany). The PM2.5 concentration was measured with a time resolution of 6 seconds. According to the EPA categorization from 1997, measurement of PM2.5 includes fine particles with an aerodynamic diameter of 2.5 μm or smaller. Using a special weighting function for PM measurement, particles are counted in different weightings depending on their aerodynamic diameter (particles < 0,5 μm: 100%, particles = 2.5 μm: 50%, particles > 3,5 μm: 0%). All measurements were conducted in air-conditioned laboratory rooms at temperatures of 22,7 ± 1,9°C and a humidity of 29% ± 5%. Since the chamber was placed inside our laboratory rooms, measurement procedures were not influenced by biases due to daily variations of PM environmental concentrations. Nevertheless, background PM concentrations were controlled permanently by reading the baseline before and after each measuring cycle.

Smoking protocol

To generate environmental tobacco smoke from cigarettes in a standardized way, cigarettes were smoked according to a self-developed smoking protocol. It consists of 10 identical puffs of 3 seconds duration each. Every puff has a volume of 40 ml and is followed by 27 seconds of smouldering until the next puff is being started.

We first measured baseline values of particulate matter for 10 minutes. Then smoking started with an initial double-puff while igniting the cigarette manually with a cigarette lighter using the rubber gloves embedded into the glass wall. After 5 minutes, the cigarette was extinguished manually in a water bowl and baseline reading continued for 10 minutes after extinguishing each cigarette. Each measuring cycle finished with dust extraction by means of a high performance industrial suction, installed in the backboard and roof of the chamber.

Data processing and analysis

The timespan between ignition and extinction of each smoking cycle (Figure 2) was analyzed and the area under the curve (AUC) of PM2.5 (AUC-PM2.5) and mean concentrations of PM2.5 (PM2.5) were calculated (Figure 3) (Graph Pad Prism 5.03). Results for the ETS exposure parameters C_{mean} (Figure 4) and AUC (Figure 5) from 40 3R4F reference cigarettes, 19 P&S cigarettes and 19 Virginia (without filter) cigarettes were tested for significant differences between the cigarette types. The one-sample t-test was used to compare each tobacco product with the reference cigarette and Bonferroni's correction was used to counteract the problem of multiple comparisons. Significance was assumed when $p < 0,05$. To ensure that equal amounts of reference cigarettes and brand

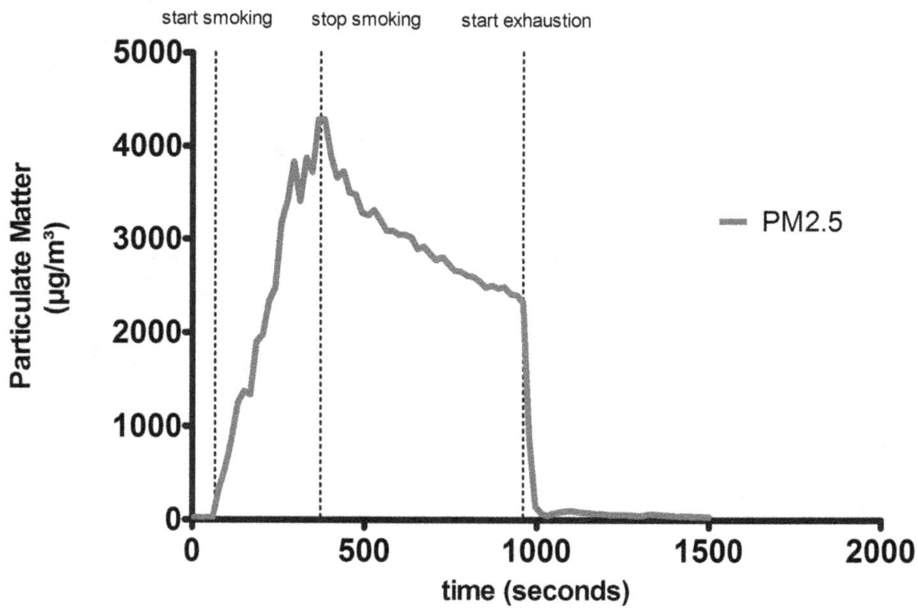

Figure 2 The measuring cycle: complete measuring cycle illustrated exemplarily.

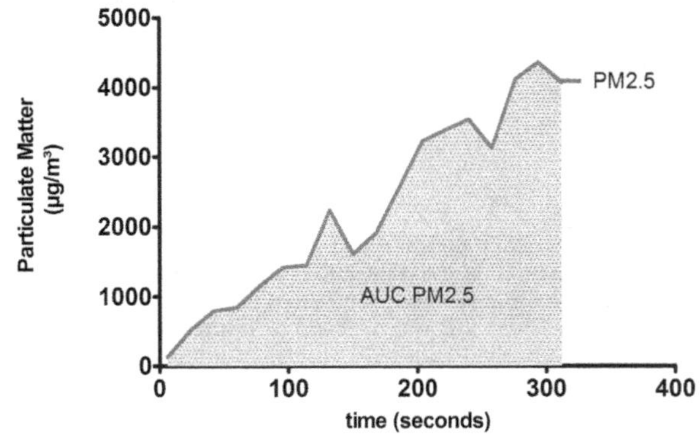

Figure 3 **Measurement of AUC: the interval from ignition to extinction (five minutes) was evaluated.**

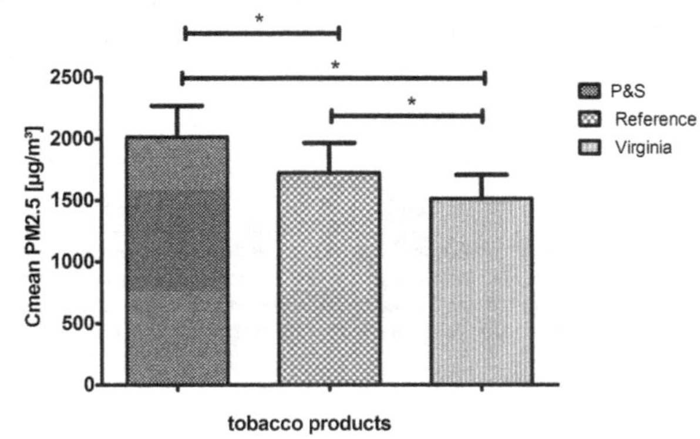

Figure 5 **Comparison of 3R4, P&S and Players Virginia No. 6.** Significance was assumed, when p< 0,05 (* means significant): PM2.5 AUC are compared.

cigarettes being smoked for our test, we smoked two packets of 3R4F and one packet of each brand cigarette. A Gaussian distribution of individual parameters was found for all tested brands.

Results

We found significant differences between the tested brands for C_{mean} PM2.5 and AUC PM2.5, respectively (Figures 4 and 5, Table 1).

Discussion

To our knowledge, assessments of fine particulate matter between cigarette brands, as issued in our current ToPIQ-II study, have not been carried out so far. In some studies ETS-associated PM was measured. In those studies, however, PM-amounts were not compared between brands and occasionally, human smokers were made to sit in test chambers in order to produce the needed environmental tobacco smoke [19-21]. While human smokers guarantee a realistic ETS-generation, it endangers the health of the test-smokers. In our ToPIQ-II study protocol, an AETSE is used to ensure that no humans be exposed to health-hazarding ETS. Besides the unrealistic simplification of human smoking behavior, another methodological weak point of using an AETSE to generate environmental tobacco smoke is the composition of mainstream smoke exhaled by a smoking machine compared to mainstream smoke exhaled by a real smoker. In our study we assessed ETS, which consists to about 85% of sidestream smoke, released directly into the chamber by the burning cigarette and to about 15% of mainstream smoke, exhaled by the AETSE. Real smokers retain approximately 30-66% of the particulate phase contained in the MS, when puffing a cigarette, and the amount of particulate absorption by the smoker's respiratory tract is related to size and solubility of the substance [22]. Sahu et al. compared the particle size distribution of MS and exhaled MS to predict the likelihood of deposition in the human respiratory tract. They found a ratio of the calculated deposition fraction of 0,613 for MS and 0,471 for exhaled MS [23]. The particulate phase of exhaled cigarette smoke showed a growth factor of 1.5 ± 0,3 due to coagulation and hygroscopic growth of smoke particles in the respiratory system. The AETSE most likely does not alter MS during ventilation to a comparable degree. One may ask why we did not use an internationally accepted smoking regime (e.g. the ISO machine smoking regime or the Canadian Intense). As mentioned above, our experiments were not intended to provide absolute PM data for defined situations, but rather to enable a comparison of different brands and tobacco products. We cannot compare our findings in a 2.88 m^3 chamber with the findings of other groups, and our own health ethics don't allow us to imitate real-life smoking conditions. Therefore, and considering that there is no really approved standardized and non-controversial method — as

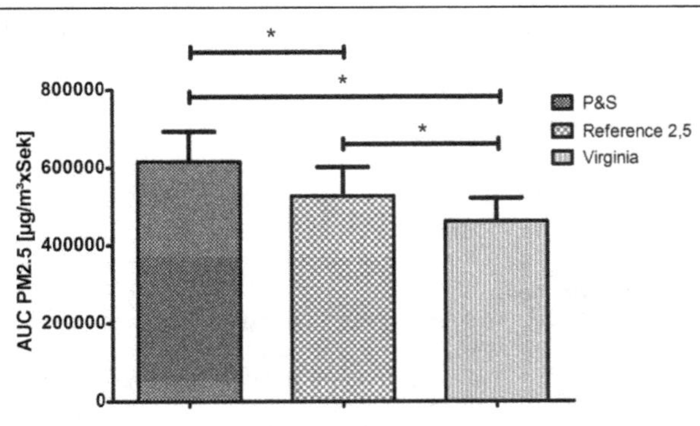

Figure 4 **Comparison of 3R4F, P&S and Players Virginia No. 6.** Significance was assumed, when p< 0,05 (* means significant): PM2.5 Mean concentrations are compared.

Table 1 Shows average PM2.5 mean concentrations, average AUC PM 2.5 and tar- yield for 3R4F reference cigarettes, P&S cigarettes and Virginia cigarettes without filter

Tobacco product	C_{mean}PM2.5 (µg/m^3)	AUC PM2.5 (µg/m^3 × sec)	Combustion time (seconds)	Tar yield per cigarette (mg)
3R4F reference	1,725 ± 244	527,644 ± 74,812	300	9,5
P&S	1,982 ± 252	606,171 ± 77,311	300	10
Virginia	1,525 ± 193	464,788 ± 59,417	300	10

PM concentrations of the P&S brand cigarette exceeded the reference cigarette values significantly ($p < 0{,}05$) (Figures 4 and 5). For all parameters and brands, individual values were statistically distributed according to a Gaussian distribution. Surprisingly, PM values of Virginia without filter were significantly lower than the corresponding values of 3R4F research cigarettes and P&S cigarettes ($p < 0{,}05$). This means that the mere existence of cigarette filters might have less influence on PM release than other aspects of cigarette designs, such as tobacco mixture, cellulose content and other additives that influence burning-characteristics.

above mentioned protocols have been heavily criticized [24]—, we find it legitimate to use a self-developed protocol to smoke cigarettes in a standardized way according to our requirements. Despite the large brand-specific differences in ETS formation, heterogeneity between individual packs of the same brand was low. Normally, a power analysis is performed in advance to determine sample size needed to prove significance. Contrary to this usual procedure, we decided not to do so, since this being a pilot study and we could not predict the differences between the groups to be expected. However, the null hypothesis can be rejected and thus, the sample size must have been sufficient. A Gaussian distribution of individual results and a standard deviation of <15% for all brands supports our believe that our protocol, when used for experimental purposes as in our setup, is practicable and liable. A potential disadvantage of our approach is that our presently used AETSE, performing a standardized smoking protocol, is not able to adapt automatically to a possible heterogeneity of flow resistance between the different tobacco products, as human smokers would do by increasing suction power, puff volume of puff frequency to achieve the usual dosage. As cigarettes are filled with machine-cut tobacco and cellulose as binder and stabilizing components, flow resistance can vary considerably between brands and even between cigarettes of the same brand, as we found out. Using the AETSE, a large flow resistance would lead to smaller C_{mean} PM and a longer smoke duration. Comparing fix 300 seconds time intervals may lead to differently-advanced smoked cigarettes, and C_{mean} and AUC could not be compared seriously. Under real-life conditions, smokers usually smoke their cigarettes or cigarillos until they are finished. They do not adhere to an exact time interval. As P&S and Players Virginia No. 6 cigarettes show similar flow resistances and were in average equally-advanced burned down after 300 sec., we considered a fixed time interval reasonable for our present study. For future cases with great differences in flow resistance, however, as it is occasionally seen when comparing cigarettes and low-priced cigarillos, we plan to compare fixed lengths of the tobacco products [25].

Currently, reproducible data of brand-specific PM release of tobacco products under real-life conditions are not available to consumers. We do consider them to be of general public interest.

As mentioned in the introduction, exposure to particulate matter has to be seen as an independent risk factor for morbidity and mortality. Several studies have linked the rate of hospital admissions due to cardiovascular or pulmonary reasons to the levels of short-term high impact exposure to PM [26-28]. It has been shown that long-term exposure to PM correlates with cardiovascular and respiratory morbidity and mortality [29-31]. Pope et al. have assessed the relationship between long-term exposure to fine particulate air pollution and all-cause, lung cancer, and cardiopulmonary mortality. They demonstrated statistically that PM2.5 pollution was associated with all-cause, lung cancer, and cardiopulmonary mortality and that an increase of about 10 µg/m^3 PM2.5 was associated with approximately 4%, 6%, and 8% increased risk of all-cause, cardiopulmonary, and lung cancer mortality, respectively [32].

In the light of this, it appears to be even more necessary to assess PM2.5 data in relation to reference cigarettes for all known brands as a basis for later examinations and comparisons.

Despite several limitations in this study due to the chosen experimental method, it is still reasonable to draw insightful conclusions regarding brand-specific amounts of ETS-associated PM, and further investigations of all relevant brands should be performed.

Competing interests

The authors declare that they have no competing interests.

Authors' contributions

AG, JS and DAG have made substantial contributions to the conception and design of the study, acquisition of the data and have been involved in drafting and revising the manuscript. A v. H-H conducted the measuring of the cigarettes. All authors have read and approved the final manuscript.

Acknowledgement

We thank G. Volante for expert help.

References

1. Brunekreef B, Holgate ST. Air pollution and health. Lancet. 2002;360:1233–42.
2. Particulate Matter. (PM) http://www.epa.gov/pm/.
3. Siponen T, Yli-Tuomi T, Aurela M, Dufva H, Hillamo R, Hirvonen MR, et al. Source-specific fine particulate air pollution and systemic inflammation in ischaemic heart disease patients. Occup Environ Med. 2014.
4. Repace JL, Lowrey AH. Indoor air pollution, tobacco smoke, and public health. Science (New York, NY). 1980;208:464–72.
5. Atkinson RW, Anderson HR, Sunyer J, Ayres J, Baccini M, Vonk JM, et al. Acute effects of particulate air pollution on respiratory admissions: results from APHEA 2 project. Air Pollution and Health: a European Approach. Am J Respir Crit Care Med. 2001;164:1860–6.
6. Bell ML, Ebisu K, Peng RD, Walker J, Samet JM, Zeger SL, et al. Seasonal and regional short-term effects of fine particles on hospital admissions in 202 US counties, 1999–2005. Am J Epidemiol. 2008;168:1301–10.
7. Brook RD, Rajagopalan S, Pope 3rd CA, Brook JR, Bhatnagar A, Diez-Roux AV, et al. Particulate matter air pollution and cardiovascular disease: An update to the scientific statement from the American Heart Association. Circulation. 2010;121:2331–78.
8. Turner MC, Krewski D, Pope 3rd CA, Chen Y, Gapstur SM, Thun MJ. Long-term ambient fine particulate matter air pollution and lung cancer in a large cohort of never-smokers. Am J Respir Crit Care Med. 2011;184:1374–81.
9. Beelen R, Raaschou-Nielsen O, Stafoggia M, Andersen ZJ, Weinmayr G, Hoffmann B, et al. Effects of long-term exposure to air pollution on natural-cause mortality: an analysis of 22 European cohorts within the multicentre ESCAPE project. Lancet. 2014;383:785–95.
10. Qiu J, He X, Cui H, Zhang C, Zhang H, Dang Y, et al. Passive smoking and preterm birth in urban China. Am J Epidemiol. 2014;180:94–102.
11. Lozano R, Naghavi M, Foreman K, Lim S, Shibuya K, Aboyans V, et al. Global and regional mortality from 235 causes of death for 20 age groups in 1990 and 2010: a systematic analysis for the Global Burden of Disease Study 2010. Lancet. 2012;380:2095–128.
12. Gerber A, Bohn J, Groneberg DA, Schulze J, Bundschuh M. Airborne particulate matter in public transport: a field study at major intersection points in Frankfurt am Main (Germany). J Occup Med Toxicol. 2014;9:13.
13. Household (Indoor) Air Pollution. http://www.who.int/indoorair/en/.
14. Arku RE, Adamkiewicz G, Vallarino J, Spengler JD, Levy DE. Seasonal variability in environmental tobacco smoke exposure in public housing developments. Indoor air 2014.
15. Sunyer J, Basagana X. Particles, and not gases, are associated with the risk of death in patients with chronic obstructive pulmonary disease. Int J Epidemiol. 2001;30:1138–40.
16. Cowie GA, Swift E, Borland R, Chaloupka FJ, Fong GT. Cigarette brand loyalty in Australia: findings from the ITC Four Country Survey. Tob Control. 2014;23 Suppl 1:i73–9.
17. Chen CM, Chang KL, Lin L, Lee JL. Brand switching or reduced consumption? A study of how cigarette taxes affect tobacco consumption. J Health Econ. 2014;15:991–8.
18. Mueller D, Uibel S, Braun M, Klingelhoefer D, Takemura M, Groneberg DA. Tobacco smoke particles and indoor air quality (ToPIQ) - the protocol of a new study. J Occup Med Toxicol. 2011;6:35.
19. Leaderer BP, Hammond SK. Evaluation of vapor-phase nicotine and respirable suspended particle mass as markers for environmental tobacco-smoke. Environ Sci Technol. 1991;25:770–7.
20. Martin P, Heavner DL, Nelson PR, Maiolo KC, Risner CH, Simmons PS, et al. Environmental tobacco smoke (ETS): A market cigarette study. Environ Int. 1997;23:75–90.
21. Nelson PR, Conrad FW, Kelly SP, Maiolo KC, Richardson JD, Ogden MW. Composition of environmental tobacco smoke (ETS) from international cigarettes and determination of ETS-RSP: Particulate marker ratios. Environ Int. 1997;23:47–52.
22. Moldoveanu SC, St Charles FK. Differences in the Chemical Composition of the Particulate Phase of Inhaled and Exhaled Cigarette Mainstream Smoke. Contributions Tobacco Res. 2007;22:290–302.
23. Sahu SK, Tiwari M, Bhangare RC, Pandit GG. Particle Size Distribution of Mainstream and Exhaled Cigarette Smoke and Predictive Deposition in Human Respiratory Tract. Aerosol Air Qual Res. 2013;13:324–32.
24. Hammond D, Wiebel F, Kozlowski LT, Borland R, Cummings KM, O'Connor RJ, et al. Revising the machine smoking regime for cigarette emissions: implications for tobacco control policy. Tob Control. 2007;16:8–14.
25. Gerber A, Bigelow A, Schulze M, Groneberg DA. Brand cigarillos - a cheap and less harmful alternative to cigarettes? Particulate matter emissions suggest otherwise. Int J Environ Res Public Health. 2015;12:428–38.
26. Almeida SM, Silva AV, Sarmento S. Effects of exposure to particles and ozone on hospital admissions for cardiorespiratory diseases in SetuBal, Portugal. J Toxicol Environ Health A. 2014;77:837–48.
27. Milojevic A, Wilkinson P, Armstrong B, Bhaskaran K, Smeeth L, Hajat S. Short-term effects of air pollution on a range of cardiovascular events in England and Wales: case-crossover analysis of the MINAP database, hospital admissions and mortality. Heart (British Cardiac Society). 2014;100:1093–8.
28. Wang Y, Eliot MN, Wellenius GA. Short-term changes in ambient particulate matter and risk of stroke: a systematic review and meta-analysis. J Am Heart Assoc. 2014;3.
29. Jakubiak-Lasocka J, Lasocki J, Badyda AJ. The influence of particulate matter on respiratory morbidity and mortality in children and infants. Adv Exp Med Biol. 2014.
30. Xie W, Li G, Zhao D, Xie X, Wei Z, Wang W, et al. Relationship between fine particulate air pollution and ischaemic heart disease morbidity and mortality. Heart. 2015;101:257–63.
31. Lu F, Xu D, Cheng Y, Dong S, Guo C, Jiang X, et al. Systematic review and meta-analysis of the adverse health effects of ambient PM and PM pollution in the Chinese population. Environ Res. 2015;136C:196–204.
32. Pope 3rd CA, Burnett RT, Thun MJ, Calle EE, Krewski D, Ito K, et al. Lung cancer, cardiopulmonary mortality, and long-term exposure to fine particulate air pollution. JAMA. 2002;287:1132–41.

12

Usage of gloves for hair shampooing in German hairdressing salons

Madeleine Dulon[1*], Björn Kähler[1], Sandra Kirvel[2], Günter Schlanstedt[2] and Albert Nienhaus[3]

Abstract

Background: Occupational skin disease caused by wet work is particularly common in employees in hairdressing salons. The objective of this paper was to determine the frequency of glove use for hair shampooing.

Methods: Data on the usage of gloves for hair shampooing were collected by covert observations in four cross-sectional surveys of newly opened hairdressing salons located in Cologne. Measurements were conducted between 2009 and 2012. A team of five trained observers were involved in the measurements. As a second assessment method, salon owners of other newly opened salons from five districts of Germany were interviewed by telephone at three of the four measurement points. Trend analysis was performed with the Mantel-Haenszel test for trends and simple linear regression. Differences in proportions of glove use between the two assessment methods were compared by chi-squared tests.

Results: In total, 435 hair shampoos were observed and 630 salon owners interviewed. Gloves were worn in 14 % of the observed hair shampoos. Proportions of glove use differed significantly according to assessment measurement. Proportions of glove use assessed by covert observation increased from 10.5 % to 18.5 % ($p_{trend} = 0.044$) whereas the proportions obtained by telephone interview decreased over the study period from 84 % to 76 % ($p_{trend} = 0.037$). No trend was found for the intensity of glove use ($p_{trend} = 0.2C4$).

Conclusions: Gloves were worn in less than 20 % of hair shampoos. This rate is much lower than values reported from other written or verbal surveys. Future measures for skin protection in hairdressing sa ons should take this into account.

Keywords: Hairdressers, Wet work, Skin disease, Occupational disease, Prevention

Background

Occupational hand eczema is one of the most prevalent occupational diseases (OD) in Europe [1]. The complications and consequences of occupational hand eczema include chronic severe eczema, prolonged sick leave, unemployment, and impaired quality of life [2]. In Germany, claims of occupational skin disease (OD No. 5101) accounted for around 34 % of all workers' compensation claims in 2013 [3]. Around 4.5 % of all claims of occupational skin disease (OSD) were notified by hairdressers (Berufsgenossenschaft für Gesundheitsdienst und Wohlfahrtspflege, Statistical Department 2014, personal communication). However, more than 14.2 % of the recognised cases with OSD concerned hairdressers. Hairdressers have an increased risk of developing skin disease, as they are exposed to several hair dressing chemicals, such as perming agents, hair dyes and bleaches and work with irritants such as shampoos and water [4–6]. The duration of wet work in the hairdresser trade - measured by direct observation – ranges between 2 and 4 h per day [7, 8].

Preventive programs for employees in hairdressing salons were first introduced in Germany in 1992 and there has been a downward trend in suspected and recognised cases of OSD in hairdressers over the last 15 years (see also in Additional file 1). This seems to reflect improvements in working conditions in hairdressing salons, due to

* Correspondence: madeleine.dulon@bgw-online.de
[1]Department of Occupational Health Research, German Social Accident Insurance Institution for the Health and Welfare Services, Pappelallee 33/35/37, 22089 Hamburg, Germany

both new legislation [9, 10] and the introduction of measures for secondary and tertiary individual prevention [11]. Although the annual numbers of skin disease claims reported by hairdressers have decreased over the last decade, the annual incidence of new reports is still high - with approximately 4.0 to 5.0 cases per 1,000 full time employees (Berufsgenossenschaft für Gesundheitsdienst und Wohlfahrtspflege, Statistical Department 2014, personal communication). The annual workers' compensation-related costs in Germany for medical treatment, professional rehabilitation and pensions for hairdressers with an OD No. 5101 were approximately 12 million Euro in 2000, but continuously decreased until 2007. Since 2007, the annual costs have stagnated at just under 8 million Euro (see Additional file 1). In this context, a campaign to prevent hand eczema in hairdressers was started in 2009 by the workers' compensation board responsible for hairdressers in Germany - the Social Accident Insurance Institution for the Health and Welfare Services (Berufsgenossenschaft für Gesundheitsdienst und Wohlfahrtspflege, BGW).

The prevention campaign for the hairdressing craft

The campaign *Live your dream* was directed towards employees in hairdressing salons. The campaign was designed to increase skin protection measures among hairdressers and ultimately reduce disability and workers' compensation-related costs. The objective was to persuade employees in hairdressing salons to wear gloves for wet work. If gloves were worn more often for shampooing hair, this should lead to a reduction in the daily exposure to wet work and should correspond to increased skin protection.

The campaign's claim was "with glamour, style and beautiful hands". All the media and products used in the campaign were specifically designed to be appropriate to the target group. This was particularly the case for the central product in the campaign, the champagne coloured disposable nitrile glove, which was intended to be regarded as smart and trendy by the hairdressers and to encourage them to wear gloves for shampooing hair. Communication focussed on advertisements in the printed media, together with the Internet platform "Lebe deinen Traum" (*Live your dream*) and the social networks Facebook and Twitter. The Facebook page offered various links to skin protection measures by the BGW. An average of two contributions per day was posted in Facebook. The posts dealt with campaign topics, but also contained infotainment or referred to offers such as the Monday discount for ordering gloves. During the campaign, an online shop was operated, which sold skin care products including the campaign gloves.

The aim of our study was to quantify how often gloves were used by hairdressers for shampooing hair.

Methods

Study Design

Glove usage in the salons was assessed by two disparate methods - covert observations of hair shampoos and telephone interviews of salon owners. Cross-sectional surveys were conducted in hairdressing salons annually in August between 2010 and 2012 (Survey 2, 3 and 4). A baseline survey was administered prior to the start of the campaign in August 2009 (Survey 1).

Participants and data collection

The data base consisted of German hairdressing salons which had been registered between January 2008 and June 2012 as newly opened salons in the address database of the workers' compensation board (BGW). The inclusion criteria were that the salon had opened in the 12 months before the corresponding survey and was registered in one of the five district administrations of the BGW chosen as study regions (Munich, Dresden, Cologne, Magdeburg and Hamburg). In total, 10,264 newly opened salons were identified during the study period. Lists of salons were generated for each survey, consecutively numbered and transmitted to a research institute in the social sciences, that had been commissioned to perform the observations and to a market research institute, that had been commissioned to perform the telephone interviews. Random samples were drawn by the commissioned institutes, using random numbers generated by a random number generator. In order to compensate for drop-outs, the sample contained twice as many salons as the target number of observations, or five-fold the number of interviews. If no observation was possible in the salon or an interview was refused, this was replaced by the next entry in the list of random numbers.

Covert observation

The observation of shampooing was based on the methods of participant and non-participant observation [12]. In the participating variant, the researcher became part of the situation being studied, e.g. had his or her hair shampooed; in the non-participating variant, the researcher attempted to observe whether the hairdressers wore gloves for shampooing the hair of other customers. The observations were covert. The salon owner was not informed about the observation, in order to avoid the effect of social desirability. The trained observer team consisted of four females and one male person. The participating and non-participating observations were performed in a standard manner (including for example making an appointment or leafing through hairdressing magazines). Each observation was documented retrospectively with the help of a structured observation form. The documentation form contains information on the date and time of the observation, as well as the number and gender of the customers and employees, the number of observed hair shampoos and whether these were performed in gloves. The endpoint of the analysis was, whether gloves were used for shampooing during the observation, with the options yes and no. The distinction between the participating and non-participating variants was dispensed with. If no shampooing had been performed within a limited time frame of 20 min, the observation was coded as unsuccessful.

A pre-test was performed in 10 salons - five each from an urban area and a rural area of Cologne. It became apparent that too much time was needed for observations in rural areas - long drives, few customers or long waiting times for non-participating observations. For this reason, a sample of salons located in the greater Cologne area was selected. The address database for observations included a total of 3,019 salons. A random sample of 749 salons was visited to conduct the observation of shampoos (32 % out of 2,339 salons with verified addresses; 241 in survey 1, 163 in survey 2, 88 in survey 3 and 257 in survey 4). Routes were arranged for the observation team along the addresses in the random sample. Observation was successful in every second salon (385 out of 749).

Telephone survey

Telephone interviews were restricted to the owners, as they bear the responsibility for implementing the health and safety regulations in their salons. A computer-assisted telephone interview questionnaire was used. The questionnaire comprised two main topics; the first topic contained questions on implementation of skin protection measures in the salon, glove use during daily work (including hair shampooing) and reasons for non-use of gloves for hair shampooing. The second topic contained questions on the perception of the campaign and the use of the campaign materials; these results will be reported elsewhere [13]. Glove use was assessed with two questions: The first question was "Are gloves used for shampooing in your salon?" with the options yes and no; the second question was "How often do the employees in your salon use gloves for shampooing?" with the options never, rarely, frequently and always.

Data collection by telephone interview was limited to surveys 1, 2 and 4. The address database for the telephone surveys included a total of 7,578 salons. A random sample of 2,958 salons with verified phone numbers was used. Contact by telephone interview was made with 1,820 salons (433 from survey 1, 575 from survey 2, and 812 from survey 4).

Compliance with the rules on data protection was confirmed by the data protection manager of the BGW.

Statistical analysis

Data analysis was based on the number of hair shampoos that had been observed and — in the case of the telephone survey — on the number of salon owners who had agreed to participate in the interview. Data from each survey were used as cross-sectional samples. The Mantel-Haenszel test for trend and linear regression were used for the analysis of trends in the proportion of glove use across the study period. Differences in proportions between the two assessment measurements were compared by the Chi-square test. A p value of less than 0.05 was considered as statistically significant. The statistical analyses were performed using IBM SPSS version 20 and MedCalc software.

Results

A total of 435 hair shampoos were observed and a total of 630 salon owners (35 %) agreed to be interviewed. Gloves were worn in 14.0 % of the observed hair shampoos (Table 1). The proportion of glove use increased from 10.5 % in survey 1 to 18.5 % in survey 4, with a mean increase of 2.7 percentage points per year ($p_{trend} = 0.044$). According to the interviews, protective gloves were available in the salons of nearly all interviewed salons owners (Table 1). However, gloves were used for shampooing in only 80.3 % of the salons using protective gloves generally. The proportion of glove use decreased from 84.4 % to 76.2 % over the study period with a mean decrease of 2.6 percentage points per year ($p_{trend} = 0.037$).

Rates for the intensity of glove use showed that gloves were worn in 39 % of hair shampoos always (Table 2). The figure is similarly high for frequent use of glove. In around 25 % of shampoos gloves were worn only rarely or never. Rates for the intensity of glove use did not change statistically significantly across the three surveys ($p_{trend} = 0.204$).

The rates of glove use provided by the salon owners were much higher for all surveys than the rates determined by observation - by a factor of about 6 (Table 1). However, if the comparison is restricted to hairdressers who always use gloves for shampooing (39 %, Table 2), this gap is narrowed to a factor of 3.

Discussion

The campaign *Live your dream* was developed to make hairdressers more aware of the issue of skin protection. The principle objective of the campaign was to reduce the high exposure to wet work by increasing the use of gloves for shampooing hair. The campaign focused on enhancing the attractiveness of glove use for hairdressers so that this desirable procedure became routine for them.

There is currently no gold standard for assessing wet work that is stressful for the skin during the working

Table 1 Proportions of glove use for hair shampooing in hairdressing salons; separated by methods of assessment

		Observation of shampoos			Telephone interview of salon owners				Comparison of proportion for glove use for hair shampooing	
		Number of salons	Glove Usage		Glove Usage					
					Generally		For shampoos			
Survey	Data collection	N	N	%[a]	N	%[a]	N	%[b]	χ^2	P
1	August 2009	172	18	10.5	218	99.1	184	84.4	207.564	<.001
2	August 2010	69	9	13.0	199	99.5	159	79.9	95.068	<.001
3	August 2011	75	12	16.0	-	-	-	-	-	-
4	August 2012	119	22	18.5	198	94.3	151	76.2	97.763	<.001
Total		435	61	14.0	615	98.0	494	80.3	446.824	<.001

[a]Relative to number of salons (observed/interviewed)
[b]Relative to number of salons using gloves generally

day [8]. In epidemiological studies, video cameras or hand-held computers are often used to record occupational exposure. However, neither of these can be used without the knowledge of the observed employees and it is conceivable that they may change their behaviour.

According to the assessment method of covert observation, the overall rate of glove use for hair shampoos is around 14 %. To our knowledge, this is the first study to apply the method of covert observations in hairdressing salons in order to assess the usage of gloves for hair shampooing. Therefore no directly comparable figures exist. Rates of glove use for shampooing published by other studies vary between 6 % and 76 % [14–18]. Our rate of 14 % lies at the lower end of this broad range. One explanation for the discrepancy may be that the published figures for glove use were predominantly collected by questioning hairdressers. The rates of glove usage provided by the salon owners fit well with the range of the published data. The high rates suggest that the answers were influenced by the social desirability of the responses, as the salon owners were aware that the survey had been commissioned by the workers' compensation company that is responsible for hairdressers. This may indicate that cognitive dissonance is given, that the salon owners possessed the requisite knowledge, but that they often failed to implement it. There is no conclusive explanation for the decrease in glove use over time assessed by interview.

Table 2 Intensity of use of gloves when shampooing hair according to telephone survey (N = 603)

	Always		Frequently		Rarely/never	
Survey	N	%	N	%	N	%
1	87	40.6	86	40.2	41	19.2
2	71	36.4	72	36.9	52	26.7
4	77	39.7	63	32.5	54	27.8
Total	235	39.0	221	36.6	147	24.4

As shown by the observations, there was a positive trend for glove use for shampooing across the four surveys. Although measurement points cover the duration of the prevention campaign, it is unclear whether this improvement was caused by the campaign's activities.

Strength and limitations

The method of covert observation has been applied for the first time to a large group of hairdressing salons, in order to assess the frequency of glove use. The method of covert observation gives the opportunity to document workplace behaviour in hairdressing salons without the employees being aware and acting in the sense of social desirability. On the other hand, the observations were very tedious, with respect to both time and costs. The limitation to one observation per salon can lead to bias.

The present study design cannot be used for an evaluation of the effectiveness of the prevention campaign *Live your dream*, as no control group was included and no cohort of salons with repeated pre-/post measurements beyond the end of the campaign was provided. As it is not known whether the hairdressers in the campaign salons had changed their intentions and accepted glove wearing for shampooing as their new behaviour, no association can be established between the campaign's activities and proportions of glove usage assessed by our study.

Conclusions

The rate of glove use for hair shampoos is less than 20 % and is thus considerably lower than reported in earlier studies based on data provided by questionnaire-based surveys.

Competing interests

There is no perceived conflict of interest.

Authors' contributions

MD participated in the design of the study and drafted the manuscript. BK conceived the campaign and participated in the design of the study. SK participated in the acquisition of data and has been involved in drafting the manuscript. GS participated in the design of the study, performed the statistical analysis and was involved in drafting the manuscript. AN has been involved in revising the manuscript critically for important content. All authors read and approved the final manuscript.

Acknowledgements
We wish to thank the staff member of the Forschungsgruppe g/d/p for performing the computer assisted telephone interviewing and the research assistants of the Gesellschaft für Forschung und Beratung im Gesundheits- und Sozialbereich (FOGS) for carrying out observations in hairdressing salons.

Financial support
All costs associated with this campaign were funded by the German Social Accident Insurance Institution for the Health and Welfare Services. The Research group g/d/p and the FOGS Institute were commissioned by the BGW to carry out the projects related to the evaluation. The CVcare is supported by an unrestricted fund of the BGW. The funder of the campaign had no role in the analysis, decision to publish, or preparation of the manuscript.

Author details
[1]Department of Occupational Health Research, German Social Accident Insurance Institution for the Health and Welfare Services, Pappelallee 33/35/37, 22089 Hamburg, Germany. [2]Society for Research and Consulting in the Health and Welfare Sector, Prälat-Otto-Müller-Platz 2, 50670 Cologne, Germany. [3]Institute for Health Services Research in Dermatology and Nursing (IVDP; CVcare), University Medical Centre Hamburg-Eppendorf, Martinistrasse 52, 20246 Hamburg, Germany.

References

1. Diepgen TL. Occupational skin-disease data in Europe. Int Arch Occup Environ Health. 2003;76:331–8.
2. Meding B, Wrangsjo K, Jarvholm B. Fifteen-year follow-up of hand eczema: persistence and consequences. Br J Dermatol. 2005;152:975–80.
3. Lipka B, Scherer K. Deutsche Gesetzliche Unfallversicherung - Die Kennziffern des Jahresberichts 2013 [German Statutory Accident Insurance - the Parameters of the 2013 Annual Report]. DGUV Forum. 2014;9:29–41.
4. Dickel H, Kuss O, Schmidt A, Kretz J, Diepgen TL. Importance of irritant contact dermatitis in occupational skin disease. Am J Clin Dermatol. 2002;3:283–9.
5. Diepgen TL. Occupational skin diseases. J Dtsch Dermatol Ges. 2012;10:297–313.
6. Khumalo NP, Jessop S, Ehrlich R. Prevalence of cutaneous adverse effects of hairdressing: a systematic review. Arch Dermatol. 2006;142:377–83.
7. Anveden I, Liden C, Alderling M, Meding B. Self-reported skin exposure–validation of questions by observation. Contact Derm. 2006;55:186–91.
8. Kralj N, Oertel C, Doench NM, Nuebling M, Pohrt U, Hofmann F. Duration of wet work in hairdressers. Int Arch Occup Environ Health. 2011;84:29–34.
9. Ausschuss für Gefahrstoffe. Technische Regeln für Gefahrstoffe - Gefährdung der Haut durch Arbeiten im feuchten Milieu (Feuchtarbeit) (TRGS 531) [Technical Rules for Hazardous Substances - Risk to the Skin from Working in a Moist Environment (Wet Work) (TRGS 531). BArbBl. 1996;9:65-67.
10. Ausschuss für Gefahrstoffe. Technische Regeln für Gefahrstoffe - Friseurhandwerk (TRGS 530) [Technical Rules for Working with Hazardous Substances in Hairdressing (TRGS 530). Gemeinsames Ministerialblatt. 2007;58:497–514.
11. Dickel H, Kuss O, Schmidt A, Diepgen TL. Impact of preventive strategies on trend of occupational skin disease in hairdressers: population based register study. BMJ. 2002;324:1422–3.
12. Diekmann A. Empirische Sozialforschung, Grundlagen, Methoden, Anwendungen. Reinbek: Rowohlt Taschenbuch Verlag; 2002.
13. Gruber J, Hirschberger A. Facebook motiviert Friseure zum Hautschutz. Social Media in der Prävention. [Facebook motivate hairdresser for skin protection. Social media in the prevention]. DGUV Forum. 2012;10:22–3.
14. Dulon M, Kähler B, Kirvel S, Schlanstedt G, Schoening S. Neues Ansprachekonzept zur Primärprävention beruflicher Hauterkrankungen für die Friseurbranche [A new approach for primary prevention of occupational skin disease in hairdressers]. Arbeitsmed Sozialmed Umweltmed. 2011;46:618–23.
15. Ling TC, Coulson IH. What do trainee hairdressers know about hand dermatitis? Contact Derm. 2002;47:227–31.
16. Nienhaus A, Rojahn K, Skudlik C, Wulfhorst B, Dulon M, Brandenburg S. Sekundäre Individualprävention bei FriseurInnen mit arbeitsbedingten Hauterkrankungen [Secondary individual prevention and rehabiltation in female hairdressers suffering from skin diseases]. Gesundheitswesen. 2004;66:759–64.
17. Nixon R, Roberts H, Frowen K, Sim M. Knowledge of skin hazards and the use of gloves by Australian hairdressing students and practising hairdressers. Contact Derm. 2006;54:112–6.
18. Schlesinger T, Revermann K, Schwanitz HJ. Dermatosen bei Auszubildenden des Friseurhandwerks in Niedersachsen - Ein Vergleich zwischen 1989, 1994 und 1999 [Dermatoses in Trainee Hairdressers - a comparison between 1989, 1994 and 1999]. Dermatologie in Beruf und Umwelt. 2001;49:185–92.

Health of the corporate worker: health risk assessment among staff of a corporate organization in Ghana

Henry Aidoo[1], Akye Essuman[2], Phyllis Aidoo[1], Anita O. Yawson[3] and Alfred E. Yawson[4*]

Abstract

Introduction: Health promotion at the workplace and for workers is important to promote workers' health, improve working environments and work practices. The goal of this analysis was to provide an example of health risk assessment conducted in a large media organization in Ghana for its workers and to identify correlates of health risks identified among different categories of workers.

Methods: This was a cross sectional study of the health risk of staff in a large corporate media organization in Accra, Ghana, conducted in 2012. In all 161 members of staff were screened and records included in the analysis. An abstraction form was used to collect data on age and sex of staff, staff category, self-reported health risk, history of chronic disease and self-rated health status. Measurements included weight, height, Body Mass Index, fasting blood sugar, total cholesterol/ HDL cholesterol and blood pressure. Data were entered into SPSS version 21, and analyzed by simple frequencies, proportions and ratios. Measured health indices were analyzed by mean ± standard deviation. Significant association between categorical outcome measures were determined with chi-square test at the 95 % confidence level.

Results: The sex characteristics of the workers indicated more males than females, male: female sex ratio of 2.3: 1. Close to half of the workers 66 (41.0 %) self-reported history of chronic disease and 40 (24.8 %) self-rated their overall state of health as poor. In all, 31.7 % of workers self-reported hypertension, while measured blood pressure indicated 60.2 % prevalence of diastolic blood pressure. Prevalence of obesity was 63.8 %; 49.1 % of staff had above normal total cholesterol levels and 12.4 % had blood glucose indicative of diabetes. Senior and management staff had relatively higher prevalence of obesity, high blood pressure, above normal cholesterol and fasting blood sugar levels.

Conclusion: More staff were unaware of their individual health risks and the health risks were higher among senior staff and management members. Adoption of regular health educational and health promotion activities as well as health surveillance procedures is essential to improve health of workers and promote positive social climate at the work place.

Keywords: Health promotion, Corporate worker, Risk assessment, Ghana, Low income setting

* Correspondence: aeyawson@yahoo.com
[4]Department of Community Health, School of Public Health, College of Health Sciences, University of Ghana, Room 46, P. O. Box 4236, Korle-Bu, Accra, Ghana
Full list of author information is available at the end of the article

Introduction

Health promotion at the workplace and for workers is important. It includes promoting healthy lifestyles, the maintenance and promotion of workers' health and working capacity, improvement of working environments and work practices [1, 2]. This is to ensure they are conducive to safety and health, as well as the development of work organization and working cultures in a direction that supports health and safety at work, promotes a positive social climate, which may enhance the productivity of the enterprise [1–3].

Companies governed by a collective bargaining agreement have a responsibility for staff to undergo routine medical screening. These medical screening done as part of health surveillance in the workplace aims to identify health risks and improve worker productivity [3]. Health surveillance procedures are usually established in the workplace to contribute to the prevention of work related ill health and to promote general health, i.e. the physical, mental and social well-being of employees [1, 3]. Health surveillance at the workplace may be established to identify work-related effects or non-work related effects of risks that workers are exposed to. Pre-employment, fitness-for-work, occupational risk, and periodic medical examinations are all well recognized health surveillance procedures [2, 3].

Workers are expose to numerous risk such as air pollution and contamination from workplace activities, handling and dismantling of e-waste, ingestion and inhalation of poisonous chemicals, gases, heavy metals or semivolatile organic compounds [4–6]. In recent years there has been a steady growth of work related psychosocial stressor characterized by strenuous work arrangements and increased job instability, which holds particularly true for the media industry [7]. These hazardous exposures and stressors have implications on the health and wellbeing of workers; periodic medical examinations and work place assessments are imperative.

However clear objectives for carrying out these medical examinations, the basis for any sound workplace programme are often absent [8]. Organizational health should be viewed as one link in the chain of organizational effectiveness. A company can be healthy for itself by growing and being efficient, healthy for its employees by offering a healthy work environment and meeting their growth needs. In addition, the company may be healthy for its customers by offering good products and services, and healthy for the community by exhibiting concern not only for its viability but also for the environment [9].

One way of making these workplace screening programmes meaningful, is to organize a health risk assessment (HRA) for staff at the workplace [10]. This is a systematic approach to collecting information from individuals that identifies risk factors, provides individualized feedback, and links the person with intervention to promote health, sustain function and/or prevent disease [10]. A typical HRA instrument obtains information on demographic characteristics (e.g. sex, age), lifestyle (e.g. smoking, exercise, alcohol consumption, diet), personal medical history, and family medical history. In some cases, physiological data (e.g., height, weight, blood pressure, cholesterol levels) are also obtained [1, 10, 11].

There have been suggestions for employers to contain health expenditures of their workers through demand management programs at the workplace [12]. These programs are designed to reduce utilization by focusing on disease prevention, work site health promotion, wellness programs, and access management. Work site health promotion is a comprehensive approach to improving health through awareness creation, health education, behavioral change, and organizational health initiatives [12].

It is critical to explain the benefits of the health risk assessment to workers, usually the health professional asks asymptomatic individuals to participate in some diagnostic or investigative procedure which may or may not seem directly beneficial to him or her. Lifestyle health risk assessments aim to identify those lifestyles which contribute to ill health and which can be modified to result in the prevention of illness, promote the health of the individual worker and garner economic benefit to the company and country [1, 2, 13]. These workplace assessments may not be done regularly by employers especially in low income setting where national incomes are low and capacity to increase labour cost are limited [14, 15].

The goal of this analysis was to provide an example of health risk assessment conducted in a large media organization in Ghana for its workers and to identify correlates of health risks among different categories of workers. A large media organization was selected to provide a baseline assessment to promote this healthful activity among employers and corporate enterprises in Ghana and other low income settings.

Methods

This was a cross sectional study of the health risk of staff in a large corporate media organization in Accra, Ghana, conducted in May-June 2012.

Site of study

This large corporate media organization has over 400 employees. The staff are categorized into three, Management staff, Senior staff and Junior staff. The company also has temporary staff who are outsourced from employment agencies. The institution has an offsite clinic with one permanent Senior Medical Officer (an occupational health practitioner), two Nursing Officers, two pharmacy staff and three support staff. The clinic renders out-patient curative services and attends to between 30 and 40 clients daily from 8:00 am to 5:00 pm. Medical emergencies and severe disease conditions are referred to other hospitals in Accra. Periodic health assessments are conducted by members of the health team for all categories of staff in the organization. This analysis is one such assessment conducted in 2012.

Study population

The subjects for this analysis were categorized into three, management staff, senior staff and junior staff. Management staff include the Managing director, directors of various departments and managers of various units who are mainly engaged in administrative and supervisory duties. Senior staff include technical and administrative staff who are mainly involved in technical services associated with the electronic and print media. Junior staff are mainly support staff to the technical officers, messengers and hospitality staff who engage in housekeeping, carting, transportation and sale of media products.

Sampling methods

All members of staff who provided consent and were available were screened and records were included in the analysis. Members of all the three categories of staff, management staff, senior staff and junior staff were involved.

Data collection

An Abstraction form was used to collect data on the personal characteristics of staff, such as; age and sex of staff and description of staff category (i.e. Junior staff, Senior staff, Management staff) and the departments of each staff in the organization. Data on self-reported health risk (tobacco use); self-reported history of chronic disease (hypertension) and self-rated health status (as good or poor) were collected. Self reported data was compared to the clinical records for accuracy.

Measurements

Data were collected on weight in kg, height in cm, Body Mass Index (BMI) in Kg/m^2, fasting blood sugar (FBS) in mmol/L, total cholesterol and HDL cholesterol in mmol/L and blood pressure in mmHg. In this analysis, normal ranges for measured health indices were: Fasting Blood Sugar 4.1–5.9 mmol/L; Total Cholesterol <5.2 mmol/L; HDL Cholesterol <1.0 mmol/L as Low, >1.55 mmol/L as High. BMI ranges, <18.5 as underweight, 18.5–24.9 as normal weight, 25–29.9 as overweight and ≥ 30 as obesity.

Data handling

All data were treated with a high level of confidentiality. Unique identifiers and codes were employed to depersonify the participants and were used for computer-based data entry. In all cases, abstraction forms and documentations were kept securely locked. Computerized records of the survey were kept in locked files. These documents were accessible to the occupational physician only.

Data analysis

Data from the abstraction form were entered into Statistical Package for the Social Sciences (SPSS) version 21, and analyzed. Age and sex characteristics of staff, history of chronic disease and use of tobacco were analyzed by simple frequencies, proportions, ratios and presented as tables. Measurements of health indices were analyzed by mean ± standard deviation. Outcome measures were disaggregated by staff category (MS, SS and JS). The current analysis did not assess health risk by sex of the corporate worker. Significant association between categorical outcome measures were determined with chi-square test at the 95 % confidence level.

Ethical issues

Clearance was obtained from Management and Occupational Health Unit of the corporate media organization. No reference has been made to identify or link the organization to this analysis.

Results

In all, there were 161 workers involved in the health risk assessment, constituting 40.3 % of the entire staff population of the organization. There were more males (112) than females (49), giving a male: female sex ratio of 2.3: 1.

Table 1 Age and sex characteristics of staff and categories of staff involved in health assessment of the organization, Accra, Ghana

Age group	Sex of staff		Total
	Male	Female	
21- 30 years	7 (6.3)	11 (22.4)	18 (11.2)
31-40 years	22 (19.6)	11 (22.4)	33 (20.5)
41-50 years	40 (35.7)	12 (24.5)	52 (32.3)
51-60 years	43 (38.4)	15 (30.6)	58 (36.0)
Total	112 (100)	49 (100)	161 (100)
Number and staff categories involved in health risk assessment			
Staff categories	Frequency	Percent	Cumulative percent
Junior staff	37	23	23
Senior staff	90	55.9	78.9
Management staff	34	21.1	100.0
Total	161	100.0	

As shown in Table 1, the overall mean and standard deviation of the age of staff was 45.1 ± 9.6 years, it was 46.4 ± 8.8 years among males, and 42.2 ± 10.7 years in females. Senior staff were in the majority, 90 (55.9 %), and management staff were the least, 34 (21.1 %).

Among all staff, 66 (41 %) reported presence of a chronic disease condition, this report was significantly higher in senior staff (42.2 %) compared to management staff and junior staff (p-value = 0.001) as shown in Table 2. In all, only 10 of the 161 staff members reported ever using tobacco (i.e. Self-reported prevalence of tobacco use among staff was 6.2 %). More than a third of all senior staff (35.6 %) and management staff (35.3 %) self-reported the presence of hypertension. Close to a quarter 40 (24.8 %) of all staff self-rated their current health status as poor.

Overall mean ± standard deviation (SD) of BMI of staff was 27.0 ± 5.1, and was highest among management members (28.3 ± 6.6), as shown in Table 3. Overall fasting blood sugar was 4.9 ± 1.6 mmol/L and was within normal for all categories of staff. Mean total cholesterol level of all three staff categories indicated a value above the normal range expected for the age of staff members. Interestingly, the mean total cholesterol level was 5.2 mmol/L for each staff category. Mean systolic blood pressure (SBP) and mean diastolic blood pressure (DBP) were 127.8 ± 16.4 mmHg and 86.3 ± 11.6 mmHg respectively.

Table 2 Self-reported medical history and self-rated health status of staff in the organization, Accra, Ghana

Staff category	Personal medical history			
	Yes (%)	No (%)	Total (%)	*P*-value
Self-reported Chronic disease				
Junior staff	14 (37.8)	23 (62.2)	37 (100)	0.001
Senior staff	38 (42.2)	52 (57.8)	90 (100)	
Management staff	14 (41.2)	20 (58.8)	34 (100)	
Total	66 (41.0)	95 (59.0)	161 (100)	
Self-reported tobacco use				
Junior staff	5 (13.5)	32 (86.5)	37 (100)	
Senior staff	4 (4.4)	86 (95.6)	90 (100)	
Management staff	1 (3.0)	33 (97.0)	34 (100)	
Total	10 (6.2)	151 (93.8)	161 (100)	
Self-reported hypertension				
Junior staff	7 (18.9)	30 (81.1)	37 (100)	0.230
Senior staff	32 (35.6)	58 (64.4)	90 (100)	
Management staff	12 (35.3)	22 (64.7)	34 (100)	
Total	51 (31.7)	110 (68.3)	161 (100)	
Self-rated current health status				
	Good (%)	Poor (%)	Total (%)	*P*-value
Junior staff	28 (75.7)	9 (24.3)	37 (100)	0.592
Senior staff	66 (73.3)	24 (26.7)	90 (100)	
Management staff	27 (79.4)	7 (20.6)	34 (100)	
Total	121 (75.2)	40 (24.8)	161 (100)	

Further assessment of health risk factors among staff in Table 4 shows that, more than half of all staff (63.8 %) were obese, and almost half (49.1 %) had above normal total cholesterol levels. Diastolic blood pressure (≥90 mmHg) was above normal for 60.2 % of all staff and 20 (12.2 %) of all staff had blood glucose indicative of diabetes.

Over 70 % of senior staff and management members were either overweight or obese, and close to a third had systolic blood pressure ≥ 140 mmHg. More than half of senior staff had above normal total cholesterol levels and above normal diastolic blood pressure.

Discussion

This health risk assessment of staff in a large corporate media organization in Accra, Ghana provides an example of the conduct of a healthful corporate activity by employers to ensure health and safety at the work place and enhance productivity [1–3]. In all 40 % of total staff population were involved in the assessment. It was voluntary, some workers refused consent to participate and others were unwilling for the blood samples to be taken, while others were absent on official assignments (i.e. 239; 60 %). The sex characteristics of the workers indicate more males than females with a male: female sex ratio of 2.3: 1 which is not surprising as men dominate in most corporate organizations and institutions in Ghana [16]. The current analysis however, did not assess health risk by sex of the corporate worker; and does not speak to sex differences in occupational risk of the corporate worker; this was not an objective of the study.

It is essential that employers especially in low income settings identify health risk assessment in the workplace as a cost saving measure to improve productivity. It may increase labour cost but the benefits garnered from productive workforce may be greater [13]. Early detection of risk provides opportunity to implement measures to prevent development of health complication and loss of productivity [1, 6, 7]. In this review close to half of the workers self-reported history of a chronic disease and almost a quarter self-rated their overall state of health as poor. Demand management programmes at the workplace designed to focus on disease prevention and health promotion including work site health promotion, wellness programmes, and improved access to health care services are important. Comprehensive health-promoting activities such as creating awareness, health education, behavioral change communication, and organizational health initiatives to engender increased physical activity is imperative [7, 12].

One critical observation from this assessment was that 66 (41 %) of staff self-reported history of chronic disease and 51 (32 %) self-reported hypertension, however measured blood pressure indicated the overall prevalence of diastolic

Table 3 Measured Health indices of staff per staff category in the Corporate Organization, Accra, Ghana

Staff category		Measured Health indices							
		Weight in kg	Height in cm	Body mass index of staff	Fasting blood sugar mmol/L	Total cholesterol mmol/L	HDL cholesterol mmol/L	Systolic blood pressure mmHg	Diastolic blood pressure mmHg
Junior staff $N = 37$	Mean ± SD	71.3 ± 12.4	169.6 ± 8.6	24.7 ± 3.7	4.6 ± 0.8	5.2 ± 1.3	1.2 ± 0.2	126.6 ± 13.5	88.6 ± 10.4
Senior staff $N = 90$	Mean ± SD	76.5 ± 14.5	166.8 ± 7.0	27.5 ± 4.9	5.0 ± 1.9	5.2 ± 0.8	1.2 ± 0.2	128.1 ± 17.2	85.3 ± 12.3
Management staff $N = 34$	Mean ± SD	82.2 ± 19.6	170.2 ± 5.4	28.3 ± 6.6	4.8 ± 1.1	5.2 ± 1.0	1.3 ± 0.6	128.7 ± 18.2	86.8 ± 10.3
Total $N = 161$	Mean ± SD	76.4 ± 15.7	168.2 ± 7.3	27.0 ± 5.1	4.9 ± 1.6	5.2 ± 1.0	1.2 ± 0.3	127.8 ± 16.4	86.3 ± 11.6

Normal range for Fasting Blood Sugar 4.1-5.9 mmol/L; Total Cholesterol < 5.2 mmol/L; HDL Cholesterol <1.0 mmol/L Low, >1.55 mmol/L High. BMI ranges: < 18.5 is underweight, 18.5-24.9 is normal weight, 25–29.9 is overweight and ≥ 30 is obesity

blood pressure to be 60 % . The health implication is that more staff are unaware of being hypertensive. This finding conforms to that of the World Health Organization's Study on Global AGEing and Adult Health (SAGE Wave 1), nationwide survey among older person 50 years and above in Ghana, which showed that the prevalence of self-reported hypertension was 14 %, while the prevalence of measured systolic and/or diastolic hypertension was 51 %. It indicated further that among the hypertensive, the percentage of persons whose treatment is effective was very low (4 %), and that most older adults who are hypertensive are not on treatment (83 %) [17]. The major point being made by this comparison of the results is that health risks are not always identified by individuals and that self-reported ill-health tends to underestimate the prevalence of measured disease [18, 19].

Apart from high blood pressure, other health risks were identified in the workers. More than half of all staff (64 %) were obese, and almost half (49 %) had above normal total cholesterol levels and 12 % had blood glucose indicative of diabetes. This indicates the burden of risk in this corporate worker group which otherwise would have gone undetected. In this relatively younger and working population, health risk assessment in the work place provides a great opportunity to identify health risk and link persons at risk to health care. The adoption of regular educational sessions with appropriately selected health topics addressed by experts, departmental health education sessions, health and safety meetings, training of first aid personnel and peer educators are measures that could improve health of workers and promote positive social climate at the work place [1, 10]. In addition, aerobic sessions at the workplace, biannual corporate games consisting of inter-departmental games and inter-organization games may be useful measures to promote health at the workplace.

Health risks varied across the different categories of health workers. Senior staff and management members had relatively higher prevalence of being overweight or obese, high systolic and/or diastolic blood pressure, above normal total cholesterol levels and above normal fasting blood sugar. This observation may be associated with the work practices and habits of these senior level staff whose duties are more sedentary and tend to be physically inactive. They may be more exposed to attending meetings and conferences, these make it more difficult for one to maintain the usual dietary habits and practices. Health surveillance at the workplace is essential to identify work-related effects or non-work related effects of risks that workers are exposed to. Pre-employment, fitness-for-work, occupational risk, and periodic medical examinations are all well recognized health surveillance procedures [1–3].

For the employer in low income setting, the margin to increase labour cost is limited and poses a real challenge [14, 15] and any activity- no matter how useful- may be looked at primarily from the cost it imposes on the organization. In settings where enforcement of law on corporate responsibility are not stringent, some employers may ignore work place health assessment and other recognized health surveillance procedures.

Table 4 High risk groups among each staff category in the Corporate Organization, Accra, Ghana

Staff category	Overweight/obesity BMI > 29.9	Fasting blood sugar > 5.9 mmol/L	Total cholesterol ≥ 5.2 mmol/L	Systolic blood pressure ≥ 140 mmHg	Diastolic blood pressure ≥ 90 mmHg
	n (%)	*n* (%)	*n* (%)	*n* (%)	*n* (%)
Junior staff $N = 37$	16 (43.2)	3 (8.1)	17 (45.9)	6 (16.2)	25 (67.6)
Senior staff $N = 90$	63 (70)	13 (14.4)	47 (52.2)	29 (32.2)	50 (55.6)
Management staff $N = 34$	24 (70.6)	4 (11.8)	15 (44.1)	10 (29.4)	22 (64.7)
Total $N = 161$	103 (63.8)	20 (12.4)	79 (49.1)	45 (28)	97 (60.2)

Limitations

The under- or over-estimation of chronic disease/risk through self-report is of great concern for epidemiological studies and surveys [18]. This health risk assessment relied on individual submissions and the self-report of health conditions, (such as hypertension), is likely to result in underestimation of prevalence rates compared to measured rates [19]. In addition, this paper presented only cross sectional observations. We believe the paper would have been much stronger if an intervention expected to improve the quality of the workers' health had been instituted and assessed to determine the effect. The analysis however, provides useful baseline information on health risks among workers for corporate organizations in Ghana to promote health among workers and the work place.

Conclusion

The assessment reveals that more staff have high health risks they are not aware of and that health risks varied across the different categories of health workers. Health risks are higher among senior staff and management members. Adoption of regular health educational and health promotion activities as well as health surveillance procedures to identify risk among all category of workers are essential to improve health of workers and promote positive social climate at the work place.

Competing interests

The authors declare that they have no competing interests. The views expressed in this paper are those of the authors. No official endorsement by any corporate organization in Ghana is intended or should be inferred.

Authors' contributions

HA and AEY developed the concept, AEY analyzed the survey data. HA and AEY, contributed to the writing of the first draft manuscript. AE, PA, AOY contributed and reviewed various sections of the manuscript. All the authors reviewed the final version of the manuscript before submission. All authors read and approved the final manuscript.

Authors information

H Aidoo is an Occupational Health Practitioner.
A Essuman is a Consultant Family Health Physician and University Lecturer.
P Aidoo is a Senior Critical Care Nursing Officer.
AO Yawson is a Senior Critical Care Nursing Officer.
AE Yawson is a Consultant Public Health Physician and University Lecturer.

Acknowledgement

We are thankful to all the workers and health personnel of this large corporate media organization in Ghana who undertook this health risk assessment, especially the two special ladies who assisted in the data collection. We are grateful to the management of the organization for their support and willingness to share the information with the corporate world.

Author details

[1]125 Row House, Michener Park, Edmonton, AB T6H, 4M4, Canada. [2]Family Medicine Unit, Department of Community Health, School of Public Health, College of Health Sciences, University of Ghana, Korle-Bu, Accra, Ghana. [3]Department of Anaesthesia, Korle-Bu Teaching Hospital, Korle-Bu, Accra, Ghana. [4]Department of Community Health, School of Public Health, College of Health Sciences, University of Ghana, Room 46, P. O. Box 4236, Korle-Bu, Accra, Ghana.

References

1. Burton J. WHO Healthy Workplace. Framework and model: background and supporting literature and practices. Geneva: World Health Organization, Switzerland; 2010. p. 47–55.
2. Naumanen P, Liesivuori J. Populations at risk across the lifespan: population studies. Workplace health promotion activities of Finnish occupational health nurses. Public Health Nurs. 2009;26 Suppl 3:218–28.
3. International Labour Organization. Global strategy on occupational health for all. Recommendation of the second meeting of the WHO Collaborating Centres in Occupational Health. Switzerland, Geneva: World Health Organization; 1995.
4. He ZG, Li GY, Chen JY, Huang Y, An TC, Zhang CS. Pollution characteristics and health risk assessment of volatile organic compounds emitted from different plastic solid waste recycling workshops. Environ Int. 2015;77:85–94. doi:10.1016/j.envint.2015.01.004.
5. An TC, Huang Y, Li GY, Chen JY, Zhang CS. Pollution profiles and health risk assessment of VOCs emitted during e-waste dismantling processes associated with different dismantling methods. Environ Int. 2014;73:186–94.
6. McCarthy MC, O'Brien TE, Charrier JG, Hafner HR. Characterization of the chronic risk and hazard of hazardous air pollutants in the United States using ambient monitoring data. Environ Health Perspect. 2009;117:790–6.
7. Ertel M, Pech E, Ullsperger P, Von Dem Knesebeck O, Siegrist J. Adverse psychosocial working conditions and subjective health in freelance media workers. Work & Stress: An International Journal of Work, Health & Organisation. 2005;19 Suppl 3:293–9. doi:10.1080/02678370500307289.
8. Bell JG, Bishop C, Gann M, Gilbert MJ, Howe W, et al. A systematic approach to health surveillance in the workplace. Occup Med. 1995;45 Suppl 6:305–10.
9. Shoaf C, Genaidy A, Karwowski W, Huang SH. Improving performance and quality of working life: a model for organisational health assessment in emerging enterprises. Hum Factors Ergon Manuf. 2004;14 Suppl 1:81–95.
10. Anderson D, Staufacker M. The impact of worksite-based health risk appraisal on health-related outcomes: a review of the literature. Am J Health Promot. 1996;10 Suppl 6:499–508.
11. World Health Organization. Global strategy on occupational health for all: The way to health at work. Recommendation of the second meeting of the WHO Collaborating Centres in Occupational Health, October 11–14, 1994, Beijing, China. Retrieved October10, 2014 from: http://www.who.int/occupational_health/publications/globstrategy/en/index.html.
12. Fronstin P. Health promotion and disease prevention: a look at demand management programs. EBRI Issue Brief. 1996;177:1–14.
13. Phillips JF. Using an ounce of prevention: does it reduce health care expenditures and reap pounds of profits? A study of the financial impact of wellness and health risk screening programs. J Health Care Finance. 2009;36 Suppl 2:1–12.
14. Carrin G, James C. Reaching universal coverage via social health insurance: key design features in the transition period. Geneva: World Health Organization, Switzerland; 2004. p. 5–13.
15. Carrin G. Social health insurance in developing countries: a continuing challenge". Int Soc Secur Rev. 2002;55 Suppl 2:57–69.
16. Yawson AE, Malm KL, Adu AA, Wontumi G, Biritwum RB. Patterns of health service utilization at a medical school clinic in Ghana. Ghana Med J 2012;46 Suppl 3:128–35.
17. Department of Community Health, University of Ghana Medical School. Ghana national report on world health organization's study on global AGEing and adult health (SAGE) in Ghana, wave 1. Switzerland, Geneva: World Health Organization; 2014.
18. Vellakkal S, Subramanian SV, Millett C, Basu S, Stuckler D, Ebrahim S. Socioeconomic inequalities in non-communicable diseases prevalence in India: disparities between self-reported diagnoses and standardized measures. PLoS One. 2013;8:e68219.
19. Andresen E, Malmstrom TK, Miller DK, Miller JP, Wolinsky FD. Retest reliability of self-reported function, self-care and disease history. Med Care. 2005;43 Suppl 1:93–7.

14

Standardized assessment of psychosocial factors and their influence on medically confirmed health outcomes in workers

Susel Rosário[1*], João A. Fonseca[1,2,3], Albert Nienhaus[1,4,5] and José Torres da Costa[1,6]

Abstract

Previous studies of psychosocial work factors have indicated their importance for workers' health. However, to what extent health problems can be attributed to the nature of the work environment or other psychosocial factors is not clear. No previous systematic review has used inclusion criteria based on specific medical evaluation of work-related health outcomes and the use of validated instruments for the assessment of the psychosocial (work) environment.

The aim of this systematic review is to summarize the evidence assessing the relationship between the psychosocial work environment and workers' health based on studies that used standardized and validated instruments to assess the psychosocial work environment and that focused on medically confirmed health outcomes. A systematic review of the literature was carried out by searching the databases PubMed, B-ON, Science Direct, Psycarticles, Psychology and Behavioral Sciences Collection and the search engine (Google Scholar) using appropriate words for studies published from 2004 to 2014. This review follows the recommendations of the Statement for Reporting Systematic Reviews (PRISMA). Studies were included in the review if data on psychosocial validated assessment method(s) for the study population and specific medical evaluation of health-related work outcome(s) were presented.

In total, the search strategy yielded 10,623 references, of which 10 studies (seven prospective cohort and three cross-sectional) met the inclusion criteria. Most studies (7/10) observed an adverse effect of poor psychosocial work factors on workers' health: 3 on sickness absence, 4 on cardiovascular diseases. The other 3 studies reported detrimental effects on sleep and on disease-associated biomarkers. A more consistent effect was observed in studies of higher methodological quality that used a prospective design jointly with the use of validated instruments for the assessment of the psychosocial (work) environment and clinical evaluation.

More prospective studies are needed to assess the evidence of work-related psychosocial factors on workers´ health.

Keywords: Psychosocial work environment, Psychosocial factors, Risk assessment, Workers' health, Occupational health

* Correspondence: skrosario@gmail.com
[1]Faculty of Engineering of the University of Porto, Porto, Portugal
Full list of author information is available at the end of the article

Background

The significant changes occurring in the world of work over the last several decades have been associated with profound effects on the health and well-being of workers. The European Union (EU) countries are facing escalating health care costs and costs linked to absenteeism, presenteeism and employee turnover, these being determinant factors and considered as issues of great concern to many employers and providers of health care services [1]. According to the Statistical Office of the European Union (EUROSTAT), public health care costs in EU-27 countries amount to an average of 8.3 % of annual gross domestic product each year [1]. In accordance with the Community Strategy Health and Safety at Work of the European Agency for Safety and Health, prevention and health promotion at work should be regarded as one of the priorities [2]. Employers are recognizing the competitive advantage that a healthy workplace can provide to them, as the development and maintenance of a healthy working environment and workforce has clear benefits for organizations and employees [3].

International Labour Organization defines psychosocial risk factors as the interactions among job content, work organisation and management, and other environmental and organisational conditions, on the one hand, and the employees' competencies and needs on the other that prove to have a hazardous influence over employees' health through their perceptions and experience [4].

Currently, psychosocial risks are recognized as one of the biggest challenges for occupational health and safety, as they are able to cause serious deterioration in workers' physical and mental health, leading to significant consequences for organizations and society [5–9]. These risks are considered to be a growing threat to the health of employed people, especially so in association with factors such as globalization, the free market economy, new information technologies, the economic crisis and subsequent recession [5, 8–11], which present challenges to better identifying the fit between the workplace conditions and labor force characteristics that might impact health [12].

According to the Framework Directive (89/391/EEC) [13] employers have a legal responsibility to ensure the safety and health of workers in every aspect related to work, and this includes psychosocial risks in the workplace [14]. Although the implementation of these provisions varies from one country to another, the Framework specifies that these risks must be identified, assessed, prevented and managed [15–17]. One of the most important aspects to consider is that risk assessment at work requires the use of valid and reliable methods in order to identify the risk factors in organizations [15, 17, 18]. So occupational safety and health legislation confers a central place in risk assessment to preventive approaches [9], which should be considered a priority in organizations [16, 19, 20].

In recent decades, a growing body of research developed through multiple theorectical frameworks (e.g., Job Demand-Control Model; Effort-Reward Imbalance Model; Model of Work, Copenhagen Psychosocial Model; Family and Inter-role Conflict) and innumerable measures for assessing the work environment (e.g., Job Content Questionnaire; Effort-Reward Imbalance; Copenhagen Psychosocial Questionnaire; Copenhagen Burnout Inventory, Work-Family Conflict Scale and Family-Work Scale, Family Supportive Supervisors' Behaviors and Family, Pressure Management Indicator, Job Diagnostic Survey, among others) have investigated the influence of working conditions on health, and of psychosocial hazards at work on adverse health outcomes.

According to the recent publication of the Eurofound & EU-OSHA (2014) [5] it is important to note that establishing the link between working conditions associated with psychosocial risks related to the health of workers is a very complex relationship, considering that there are many factors that influence health such as: *(a) personal behaviour, lifestyle and living conditions, institutional and economic context and genetic make-up of workers; (b) workplace exposure to different risks that themselves differ in the way they affect health; (c) exposure to others' risks affecting health indirectly; (d) some health problems are caused by a combination of factors, rather than exposure to a single physical or psychosocial factor; (e) the effect of exposure to risk factors is likely to differ depending on a wide number of individual worker characteristics; (f) the extent to which negative direct or indirect effects of work on health affect the capacity of people to engage in paid work and their general quality of work and life depends on the extent to which these effects can be mitigated or remedied.*

Considering the major progress that has been made in this subject by national and European governments and world bodies, this is a challenging and active area of research due to the current dynamic environment of workplaces and the need to cross multiple domains (psychology, sociology, occupational safety and health, epidemiology, medicine and other areas of knowledge). Although the study results are not fully consistent, professionals have lacked the strength to evaluate the associations fully, because the causal associations are still poorly understood. The recently published Second European Survey of Enterprises on New and Emerging Risks (ESENER-2) (2015) [9] reported the use of health and safety services where occupational doctors (68 %), health and safety generalists (63 %) and experts in accident prevention (52 %) were the professionals most often used, while as regards psychosocial risks the use of a psychologist was reported by only 16 % of establishments in the

EU-28. The results may indicate that EU-28 workplaces are experiencing a changing paradigm in organizations as regards the importance placed on psychosocial risk management, as they are starting to show efforts to integrate psychology experts (16 %) in the Occupational Safety and Health Services.

A critical limitation of the current research at a methodological level involves the scarcity of studies which present two main aspects: the use of validated instruments to assess psychosocial factors for the study population in conjunction with specific medical evaluation of related work health outcomes in order to ascertain the link between work-related psychosocial factors and workers´ health. Accordingly, the organizational and occupational health psychosocial literature has emphasized the importance of increased utilization of objective measures of health [21, 22] to accurately examine the complex interrelationships between work, the physical and mental health of workers and the health of organizations.

To our knowledge, no previous systematic review is available that has studied the link between work-related psychosocial factors on workers´ health using high-quality data based on validated assessment method(s) for the study population and clinical evaluation of health-related work outcome(s). This paper reviews the existing high-quality evidence for the influence of work-related psychosocial factors on workers´ health.

Materials and methods

Electronic searches were performed in the following database sources: PuBmed, B-ON (Elsevier, Springer, Taylor & Francis, Wiley, CINAHL, Emerald), Science Direct, Psycarticles, Psychology and Behavioral Sciences Collection and GOOGLE (http://scholar.google.com) for the period from 2004 to June 2014. This is because the role of psychosocial factors has been documented to change over time and this review aimed to reflect the current situation.

The search strategy consisted of a combination of three search strings: terms related to psychosocial work factors; terms related to risk assessment (according to the European Union Occupational Health and Safety Legislation Directive 89/391/EEC, it involves the use of psychosocial validated intruments for measuring psychosocial work factors and validated protocols for medical evaluation) and terms related to workers´ physical and mental health outcomes (Additional file 1). The references of the articles found were screened for additional relevant studies.

The publications had to be available in peer-reviewed journals. Original studies in English, French, Portuguese and Spanish were eligible for the review.

We followed a standard protocol for this review according to the validated PRISMA guidelines and recommendations for systematic reviews [23]. (The PRISMA checklist is given in Additional file 2).

Study selection was conducted based on the inclusion criteria: (i) participants are adult workers; (ii) exposure to one or more psychosocial work characteristics/factors measured [24]; (iii) workers´ physical and mental health outcomes as reflected through psychosocial validated instruments for the study population and through evidence of specific medical evaluation(s) of health-related work outcomes or evidence of registered data on sickness absence (not due to accidents) and (iv) design was either cross-sectional or prospective study.

Opinion articles, abstracts, book chapters and reviews were excluded.

Actually, the use of register-based data of sickness absence as an objective assessment is increasingly considered a reliable measure of health [25]. Moreover, longitudinal studies have demonstrated that the psychosocial work environment can be found to be a key element for the prediction of rates of sickness absence [26].

The psychosocial work factors considered eligible in this review are based on two categories: context at work (organizational culture and function; role in the organization; career development, decision latitude/control; interpersonal relationships at work; home-work interface) and content of work (work environment and work equipment; task design and job content; workload/pace of work; work schedule) [24].

The screening of articles was carried out in two phases. In the first phase, articles were screened on the basis of title and abstract. The abstracts of all the selected titles were sorted for a more detailed information. Two independent reviewers (S.R and J.T.C) read the abstracts and categorized them as relevant, not relevant and possibly relevant. In the second phase, the full-text articles were assessed for eligibility. Two reviewers (S.R and J.T.C) independently applied inclusion and exclusion criteria to potentially eligible papers and both reviewers then independently extracted data from the original articles. Any disagreement were independently checked by the second reviewer (J.A.F) and consensus reached.

Data were extracted for the following study characteristics: study design; country; setting/workplace; professional activity studied; sample size; age range of participants; participation rate at baseline (all designs), participation rate at the moment of follow-up (cohort design); confounders measured; psychosocial work factors; validated psychosocial work factors assessment instruments(s) for the study population, and specific medical evaluation(s) of health-related work outcomes or evidence of registered data on sickness absence (validated and confirmed with the company registered sickness absence).

As a criterion of quality of the articles included in the review as regards participation rate and attrition rate, we used a specific methodological quality assessment based on Nieuwenhuijsen et al. [27]. According to the specific criteria, the participation rate at baseline of the population study should be at least 50 % and the participation rate at the moment of follow-up between 60 and 80 %.

The association of work-related psychosocial factors on workers health (based on validated assessment method(s) for the study population and clinical evaluation of health-related work outcomes) was examined for the effects measures (differences in means, correlation coefficients, beta coefficient, rate ratios (RR), odds ratios (OR), hazard ratios (HR), risk ratios (*P*-value or 95 % confidence interval (95 % CI) and were presented for each study if available. Results were synthesized according to study design (cross-sectional, prospective cohort), validated psychosocial work factors assessment instruments for the study population (questionnaires, scales) and outcome(s) (diseases, sickness absence).

Ethical approval was not required, as the study was a systematic review based on published data.

Results

The literature search yielded a total of 10,623 references. After removing the 140 duplicates, 10,483 records were screened on the basis of titles and abstracts. Of these, 170 were selected as potentially relevant. From these, 160 full text articles were excluded because they: (i) did not use psychosocial validated instruments for the study population ($N = 98$), (ii) did not present evidence of specific medical evaluation of health-related work outcomes ($N = 41$), or (iii) did no use psychosocial validated instruments for the study population and did not present evidence of specific medical evaluation of health-related work outcomes ($N = 21$). A total of 10 studies fulfilled the inclusion criteria [28–37]. The results of the search in the different databases and the selection process are reported in Fig. 1.

The characteristics and findings of the ten original studies included in this review are presented in Tables 1 and 2.

Of the 10 included studies, 5 originated in Europe, 2 were performed in Asia and 2 were performed in North America. The 10 studies were published between 2006 and 2014; 7 were prospective cohort and 3 cross-sectional. A variety of population were studied, including

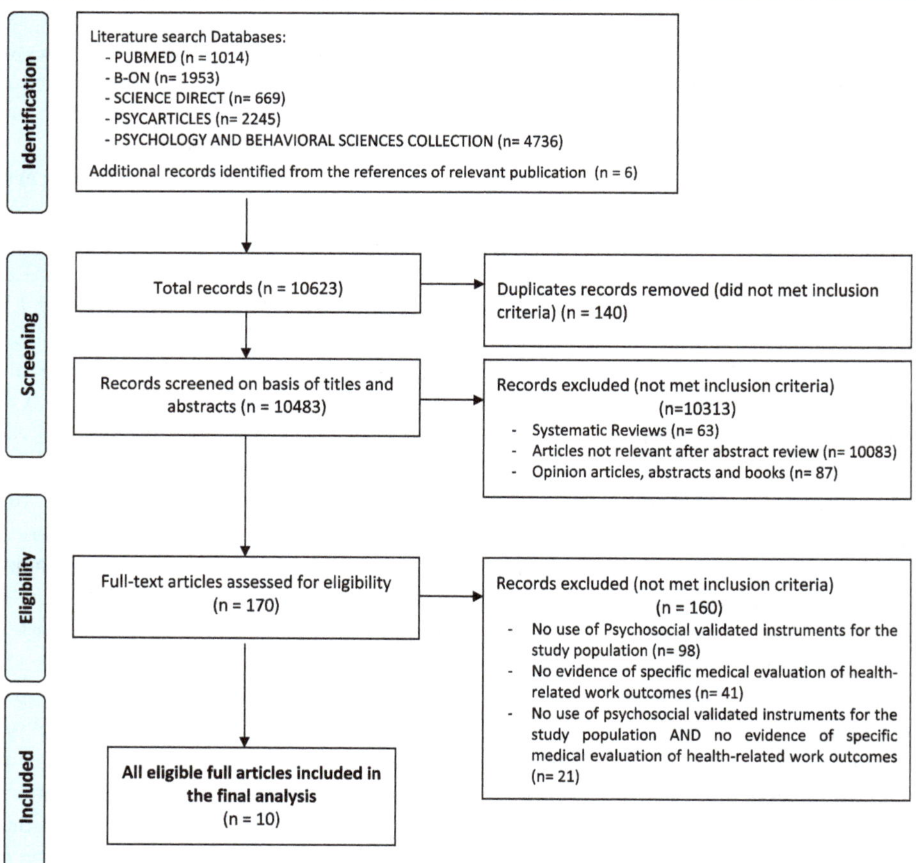

Fig. 1 Flow of information through the different phases of the systematic review

Table 1 Descriptive data for the studies included

Author, Year, Country, Reference	Setting/Workplace	Study Design	Study sample (N)	Age range of participants (years)	Participation rate baseline (%)	Participation rate follow-up (%)
Rugulies et al. 2007 Denmark [28]	5 different organizations in the human service sector	Prospective Cohort	Human service professionals (890)	43.9 years (SD 8.8)	1999–2000 80 %	2002–03 83.0 %
Borritz et al. 2010 Denmark [29]	7 different organizations within the human service sector	Prospective Cohort	All occupational groups (1734)	44.5 years (SD 10.2)	1999–2000 80 %	2005 68.0 %
Nyberg et al. 2009 Sweden [30]	20 Occupational Health Units	Prospective Cohort	White collar occupations (3122)	19–70 years	1992–1995 76 %	2003 ———
Tsutsumi et al. 2009 Japan [31]	Employees engaged in non-industrial occupations	Prospective Cohort	All occupationally non-industrial groups (6553)	18–65 years	1992–1995 65.4 %	2003 ———
Guimont et al. 2006 Canada [32]	22 Public Organizations	Prospective Cohort	Full range of white collar occupations (6719)	18–65 years	1991–1993 75 %	1999–2003 89 %
Sabbath et al. 2011 France [33]	French Gas and Electricity Company (EDP-GDF)	Prospective Cohort	Employees of EDP-GDF) (13179)	40–50 years (male) 35–50 years (female)	1995–1998 75 %	1999–2003 75 %
Aboa-Éboulé et al. 2011 Canada [34]	Workers who returned to work after a myocardial infarction	Prospective Cohort	89 % full-time workers11 % non full-time workers (738)	49.9 (SD 6.3)	1995–1997 82 %	1998–2000 80 % 2003–2005 78 %
Bellingrath et al. 2010 Germany [35]	Schools	Cross-Sectional	School teachers (55)	50.0 years (SD 8.47)	na[a]	na
Su-Shan Tsai et al. 2014 China [36]	Taiwanese Transportation Company	Cross-Sectional	Male long-haul bus drivers (825)	42.0 years (SD 0.25)	na	na
Crain et al. 2014 USA [37]	Information Technology Firm	Cross-Sectional	Information technology employees (623)	46 years (SD 8.38)	na	na

[a]na – not applicable

human service professionals, general working population, school teachers, long haul bus drivers, information technology employees).

The follow-up durations of the prospective studies ranged from 18 months to 11 years.

According to the specific criteria of the methodological quality assessment based on Nieuwenhuijsen et al. [27], 7 prospective cohort studies reported a high participation rate at baseline (≥50 %). Of the 7 prospective studies, 4 presented a participation rate at follow-up between 60 and 80 % and 2 did not present information. (We tried to obtain the missing data by sending an email to the two authors, but unfortunately did not receive a response) (Table 1).

All the studies used at least one psychosocial validated instrument for the study population and reported health-related work outcomes (Table 2). Considering the psychosocial validated instruments for the study population presented in this review, four studies used a Job Content Questionnaire (JCB), two studies used the Copenhagen Psychosocial Questionnaire (COPSOQ) and Copenhagen Burnout Inventory (CBI), one study used ERI, one study included both JCQ and ERI and one study used the Stress Profile. There were 4 studies on the demand-control support model [30–34, 36], 2 studies on the effort-reward imbalance model [34, 35], 1 study considered both models JCQ and ERI [34] and 2 studies on "theory-based without being based on one specific theory" [38] as the COPSOQ is covering a broad range of aspect of currently leading concepts and theories [such as: the Job Characteristics model; the Michigan organizational stress model; the Demand-control-(support) model; the sociotechnical approach; the action-theoretical approach; the Effort-reward-imbalance model and the Vitamin model] [28, 29].

The medical evaluation of health was based on: biochemistry indices [30, 35, 36], self-reported sickness absence from work (validated and confirmed with the company registered sickness absence), use of national database, and certified and diagnosed by a physician, hospital records [28, 29, 33], medical history [30, 31], body mass index (BMI) [30, 32, 33], blood pressure [30, 32, 34, 36] and actigraphic measurement of sleep quality and quantity [37].

All the studies included in this review controlled for at least one potential confounder. Potential confounders were sociodemographic (age, gender, marital status, ethnicity, number of children, children below the age of 7), socioeconomic (educational attainment, income, profession); biological factors (body-mass index, waist circumference, family history of health problems, cholesterol, hypertension, diabetes mellitus); lifestyle factors/personal habits (smoking status, alcohol or caffeine consumption, physical activity, weekly leisure time); work organization

Table 2 Descriptive data of the ten manuscripts. Confounders measured, validated assessment method(s), medical evaluation of health-related work outcomes, and health-related work outcomes measures are included

Author, Year, Country, Reference	Confounders measured	Psychosocial validated assessment method(s)	Medical evaluation of health-related work outcomes	Health-related work Outcome(s)
Rugulies *et al.* 2007 Denmark [28]	Age, gender, type of organization, family status, children below the age of 7 living with the respondent, smoking, alcohol consumption, weekly leisure time physical activity, body-mass index and socio-economic status.	Copenhagen Burnout Inventory (CBI); Copenhagen Psychosocial Questionnaire I (COPSOQ I)	Self-reported sickness absence days (validated/confirmed with company records).	A wide range of psychosocial work characteristics (exposure to violence and threats,high emotional demands, high requirement to hide emotions, low influence at work, low meaning of work, low quality of management and role conflicts showed an increased number of sickness absence days at follow-up.
Borritz *et al.* 2010 Denmark [29]	Gender, age, socioeconomic status, family status, health-related lifestyle, prevalence of self-reported disease.	Copenhagen Burnout Inventory (CBI);Copenhagen Psychosocial Questionnaire II (COPSOQ II)	Long-term sickness absence register, database of Danish social transfer payment (˃ 2 weeks, with medical certification) during 18 months of follow-up.	Poor level of specific psychosocial work characteristics predicted increased risk of long-term sickness absence during follow-up.
Nyberg *et al.* 2009 Sweden [30]	Education, social class, supervisory status, income from work, perceived physical load at work, physical exercise, smoking status.	The Stress Profile	Systolic and diastolic blood pressure (mm Hg) measured twice; height, weight and waist measured to determine body mass index (BMI Kg/m^2) and waist circumference (cm). Blood samples (cholesterol, HDL, triglycerides, fibrinogen and diabetes. Records of hospital admissions and death during follow-up obtained.	Better leadership was associated with lower ischaemic heart disease (IHD). There is a prospective, dose-response relationship between specific managerial behaviors and ischaemic heart disease among employees.
Tsutsumi *et al.* 2009 Japan [31]	Demographic characteristics (age, educational attainment, smoking status, alcohol consumption, physical activity index, body mass index, hypertension, diabetes mellitus, hypercholesterolemia.	Job Content Questionnaire (JCQ)	Current health status through direct interview, via telephone or letter annually to determine the participants´ current health status .In case of an incident medical records were reviewed and exams made.	Occupational stress related to job strain was associated with the incidence of strokes among Japanese men.
Guimont *et al.* 2006 Canada [32]	Demographic Characteristics (age, marital status, education, number of children living with the worker) risk factors for hypertension and cardiovascular disease (smoking, low level of physical activity, high cholesterol, diabetes), family history of cardiovascular diseases or hypertension, characteristics of work and social life.	Job Content Questionnaire (JCQ)	At worksite, trained nurses measured blood pressure, weight, height and waist circumference using validated protocols.	Cumulative exposure to job strain resulted in a significant increase in systolic blood pressure among male white-collar workers, especially those with low levels of social support at work.
Sabbath *et al.* 2011 France [33]	Age, marital status, alcohol consumption, current smoker, social ties and occupational grade.	Job Content Questionnaire (JCQ)Berkman´s Questionnaire on Social Networks and Social Suppot	EDP-GDFs records for sickness absence from work certified and diagnosed by a physician. Body weight (BMI).	High work-family demands predict long-term all causes of sickness absence across a socio-economically diverse occupational cohort.
Aboa-Éboulé *et al.*2011 Canada [34]	Age, marital status, education, alcohol consumption, physical activity.	Effort-Reward-Imbalance (ERI)	Medical information about acute MI and medical history were documented during hospitalization at baseline. Hospital summary database for Quebec residents (MED-ECHO) and Canadian Mortality Data Base.	High ERI and low reward were associated with recurrent coronary heart disease. The effects were more pronounced among women.

Table 2 Descriptive data of the ten manuscripts. Confounders measured, validated assessment method(s), medical evaluation of health-related work outcomes, and health-related work outcomes measures are included *(Continued)*

Bellingrath *et al.* 2010 Germany [35]	Sex, age, years of employment, type of school, health status and health behavior.	Trier Social Stress Test (TSST)Effort-Reward-Imbalance (ERI)Hospital Anxiety and Depression Scale-Depression (HADS-D)	Lymphocyte subset counts and lymphocyte production of tumor-necrosis-factor (TNF)-α, interferon (IFN)-ϒ, interleukin (IL)-2, -4, -6 and -10 were measured before and after the challenge.	In teachers with high levels of ERI and OC was found significantly lower natural killer cell numbers before as well as after the stressor which might be indicative of a dampened innate immune defence.
Su-Shan *et al.* 2014 China [36]	Demographic data (age, marital status, ethnicity, educational levels, height, weight, body mass index) Lifestyle and personal habits (smoking, alcohol drinking, coffee drinking, betel nut chewing, level of physical activity), work conditions.	Job Content Questionnaire (JCQ)	Biochemistry indices (blood lipids, blood sugar, blood pressure) assessed in the annual health examination.	The risk of inflammatory disease markers in a group of young drivers subject to high strain.
Crain *et al.* 2014 USA [37]	Race, gender, number of children and work schedule.	Work-family conflict; Family-suportive supervisor behaviors short form (FSSB-SF)	Actigraphic measurements of sleep quality and quantity.	The combination of predictors (work-to-family confict; family-to-work conflict, family-suportive supervisor behaviors-short form) was significantly related to both objective and self-report measures of sleep quantity and quality.

factors (number of hours worked per week, shift schedule, frequency of unexpected schedule changes); clinical prognostic factors (prior comorbid conditions, number of in-hospital events during the first myocardial infarction, number of recommended medications); and other factors (personality profile, social support at work, work schedule, number of hours worked per week, shift schedule, frequency of unexpected schedule changes).

The overall aim of this review was to investigate the methodological quality of evidence between work-related psychosocial factors on workers′ health through data on validated assessment method(s) for the study population and specific medical evaluation of health-related work outcome(s) within the last 10 years. Most studies (7/10) observed an adverse effect of poor psychosocial work factors on workers' health: 3 on sickness absence [28, 29, 33], 4 on cardiovascular diseases [30–32, 34]. The 3 other studies reported detrimental effects on sleep and on disease-associated biomarkers [35–37]. The results were summarised qualitatively and the findings for health-related work outcomes of the studies included in the systematic review are presented in Additional file 3.

In a prospective study, Rugulies et al. assessed whether human services employees exposed to 16 different psychosocial work characteristics (contact with clients more than half the time, violence and threats from clients during the last 12 months, job involves controlling clients, emotional demands, demands for hiding emotions, quantitative demands, high work pace, influence at work, meaning of work, possibilities for development, quality of management, predictability, role clarity, role conflicts, high support from colleagues, high support from supervisors) had an increased number of sickness absence days [28]. Employee outcomes were 16 psychosocial work characteristics assessed at baseline and analysed their association with number of sickness absence days at follow-up for 3-years. A wide range of psychosocial work characteristics (exposure to violence and threats, high emotional demands, high requirement to hide emotions, low influence at work, low meaning of work, low quality of management and role conflicts) were found to be significantly related to an increase in the number of days' sickness absence at follow-up, after adjustment for confounders.

Employees who scored in the most adverse quartile of the psychosocial work environment index reported an 71 % increase [Rate Ratio (RR 1.71, 95 % CI: 1.32–2.21)] in sickness absence days. In addition, there was a clear trend that a worsening in the psychosocial work environment index predicted increases in sickness absence. Compared to employees with the most favourable psychosocial work environment (upper quartile of index), employees in the three next quartiles had 19 % ($p = .21$), 39 % ($p = .01$) and 71 % ($p = .001$, lowest quartile) more sickness absence days after adjustment for all potential confounders and for exposure to violence and threats. The analysis of etiologic fraction, found that if all study participants had been exposed to the most favourable quartile of the psychosocial work environment index, sickness absence days would have been reduced by 24 %.

Also, the elimination of exposure to violence and threats would have reduced sickness absence days by

10 %. Interestingly, in the etiologic fraction analysis, that improving the psychosocial work environment index and eliminating exposure to violence and threats would have prevented 32 % of all sickness absence days in the study population.

An additional finding was the mediating effect of work-related burnout that was recognized as a strong predictor for sickness absence when adjusted for all potential confounders and for the 16 psychosocial characteristics predicting a 28 % (RR 1.18 CI 95 %: 1.06–1.13, $p = 0.03$) more sickness absence days at follow-up.

In a prospective study, an extension of the previous study, Borritz et al. examined if burnout and psychosocial factors (emotional demands, role conflicts, role clarity, predictability and quality of leadership) predicted long-term sickness absence (>2 weeks, medically certified) at work unit level [29]. Employees outcomes were obtained through the assessment of psychosocial factors and burnout as predictors of long-term sickness absence for more than 18 months based on data from a national absence register (Database of national register of social transfer payments which contained weekly information on granted sickness absence compensation for all residents in Denmark). Poor level of specific psychosocial work characteristics aggregated at work unit level was prospectively associated with increased risk of long-term sickness absence. This study offer us two main findings: First, it found that role conflicts, the fourths (25 %) of the work unit corresponding poorest level had a double increase of future sickness absence (RR 2.18; CI 95 % 1.42–2.94), but poor levels of emotional demands, role clarity and quality of leadership too were associated with increase of sickness absence during the follow-up; Second it found that burnout was associated with more than a double increase of long-term sickness absence during the following $1^{1/2}$ years (RR 2.93; CI 95 % 1.89–3.96) regarding high level of work burnout and a double increase regarding personal burnout (RR 2.30; CI 95 % 1.58–3.02) after adjusting for confounders. In this sense, reported findings showed that a poor level of specific psychosocial work characteristics was a predictor for an increased risk of long-term sickness absence.

In a prospective study, Sabbath et al. assessed whether high work-family demands were a long-term predictor of all causes of sickness absence across a socio-economically diverse occupational cohort [33]. Employee outcomes were the three dimensions of work stress measured (decision latitude, psychological demands and social support of Job Content Questionnaire) associated with the records for sickness absence from work certified and diagnosed by a physician based on the 13179 GAZEL cohort participants of the French gas and electricity company. Employees with the highest work-family demands had a rate ratio of sickness absence of 1.78 (CI 95 % 1.47–2.14) compared with low-demand workers. To note that this association was independent of occupational grade and did not vary with gender. Also, the results were not attributable solely to psychiatric sickness absences as other categories of absences were significantly elevated among those with the highest work-family demands. These categories can be divided into systemic illnesses (circulatory and gastrointestinal disease) vs. work-related accidents and orthopaedic problems. To conclude, high work-family demands at baseline predict long-term all-cause of sickness absence across a socio-economically diverse occupational cohort.

In a study of Nyberg et al. [30] it was examined the association between employees´ perceptions of managerial behaviours and objectively measured incident ischaemic heart disease (IHD) in a prospective research design, while adjusting for conventional cardiovascular risk factors. In this prospective cohort study, baseline screening was carried out in 1992–1995 based on 3122 swedish male employees, being that a total of 74 incident IHD events occurred during the mean follow-up period of 9.7 years. As Nyberg et al. found, better leadership was associated with lower ischaemic heart disease (IHD). Thus, the inverse association was stronger the longer the participant had worked in the same workplace (age-adjusted hazard ratio) 0.76 (95 % CI 0.61–0.96) for employment for 1 year, 0.77 (95 % CI 0.61–0.97) for employment for 2 years, 0.69 (95 % CI 0.54–0.88) for employment for 3 years, and 0.61 (95 % CI 0.47–0.84) for 4 years (a robust association was identified to adjustments for education, social class, income, supervisory status, perceived physical load at work, smoking, physical exercise, BMI, blood pressure, lipids, fibrinogen, and diabetes). The dose-response association between perceived leadership behaviours and IHD among employees was demonstrated.

In the prospective study, Tsutsumi et al. [31] sought to estimate the risk of stroke onset associated with job strain in a Japanese working population. Employees outcomes were obtained through the assessment of occupational stress (Job demand-control questionnaire) and physical examination findings (routine mass screening examinations for cardiovascular diseases are held in Japan in accordance with legal requirements). It was found that a more than 2-fold increase in the risk of total stroke among with job strain (combination of high job demand and low job control) (hazard ratio, 2.73; 95 % CI 1.17–6.38) compared with counterpart men with low strain (combination of low job demand and high job control) after adjustment for age, educational attainment, occupation, smoking status, alcohol consumption, physical activity and study area. It was also found that additional adjustments for biologic risk factors attenuated the hazard ratio, but there continued to be statistical significance (hazard ratio 2.53, 95 % CI 1.08–5.94). To note, that in women no statistically significant differences were found for any stroke incidence among the job characteristics categories. The occupational stress related to job strain was significantly associated with the incidence of strokes among Japanese men.

In a prospective study, Guimont et al. assessed whether cumulative exposure to job strain increases blood pressure [32]. At baseline and follow-up, 8395 white-collar workers completed the Job Content Questionnaire and also completed questionnaire focusing on demographic characteristics, risk factor for hypertension and cardiovascular disease, family history of cardiovascular disease or hypertension and characteristics of work and social life. Moreover, at the worksite, trained nurses measured blood pressure, weight, height, and waist circumference using validated protocols. Compared with men who had never been exposed, men with cumulative exposure and those who became exposed during follow-up showed significant systolic blood pressure increments of 1.8 mmHg (95 % CI 0.1–3.5) and 1.5 mmHg (95 % CI 0.2–2.8) respectively and relative risks of blood pressure increases in the highest quintile group of 1.33 (95 % CI 1.01–1.76) and 1.40 (95 % CI 1.14–1.73). Moreover, it was found that the effect magnitudes were smaller among women and also that the effects tended to be more pronounced among men and women with low levels of social support at work.

Aboa-Éboulé et al. [34] examined prospectively the association between the effort-reward imbalance (ERI) at work and its components (effort and reward) increase in the risk of recurrent coronary heart disease (CHD) events in a 4 years of follow-up among post-myocardial infarction (post-MI) workers. Employees outcomes were measured by ERI scale and through composite of fatal CHD, nonfatal MI and unstable angina. Moreover, CHD risk factors were documented in medical files and by interview. It was found that high ERI and low reward were associated with recurrent CHD (adjusted hazard ratios, HRs = 1.75, 95 % CI: 0.99–3.08) and HR = 1.77, 95 % CI = 1.16–2.71). The authors demonstrated that there was a gender interaction showing stronger effects among women (adjusted HRs for high ERI and low reward: HR = 3.95. 95 % CI = 0.93–16.79 and HR = 9.53, 95 % CI = 1.15–78.68). In conclusion, post-MI workers holding jobs that involved ERI or low reward had increased risk of recurrent CHD.

Bellingrath et al. [35] investigated the immune response to acute stress in healthy subjects with potentially high levels of chronic work stress in order to explore whether alterations in immune regulation after an accute stressor could provide explanations for the observed links between ill-health and the ERI/OC model before actual disease manifestation. Employee outcomes were measured according to Siegrist´s effort-reward-imbalance (ERI) and Overcommitment (OC) in 62 employed school teachers which participated in a laboratory stress study. The immune regulation was assessed before and after confrontation with the acute psychosocial laboratory stressor. High levels of ERI and OC were associated with lower natural killer cell numbers (F1,49 = 7.34, $p = 0.01$, $\eta 2 = 0.13$; main effect ERI: F1,49 = 4.36, $p = 0.04$, $\eta 2 = 0.08$) whereas high levels of OC were related to a lower increase in T-helper cells after stress (F1,45 = 1.55, $p = 0.22$; main effect OC: F1.49 = 5.51, $p = 0.02$, $\eta 2 = 0.10$). Furthermore, subjects with higher ERI showed significant associations with an overall increase in post-inflammatory activity, with higher TNF – α production and elevated pre-stress IL-6 production.

The cross-sectional study of Su-Shan Tsai et al. [36] assessed the association between job strain and inflammation markers and aimed to examine factors contributing to high strain. The two measures used for employee outcomes were obtained through Job content questionnaire and the analysis of plasma high sensitivity C-reactive protein (hs-CRP) and Homocysteine as inflammation markers. The significantly increased risk of high strain on high hs-CRP was found among drivers younger than 35 years old (OR = 2.71), but not in drivers groups age 35 to 49 and older than 50. It was found a significant relationship between the risk of inflammatory disease markers and high strain in a group of young drivers.

Crain et al. [37] examined the relationships between work-family conflict (WTFC/FTWC), family-supportive supervisor behaviors (FSSB) and sleep quality and quantity, in a sample of 623 information technology workers through validated wrist actigraphy methods and also through a questionnaire.

The combination of predictors (work-family conflict; family-to-work conflict, family-supportive supervisor behavior-short form) was significantly related to both objective and self-reported measures of sleep quantity and quality (ΔF is significant for the block predictors (i.e., WTFC, FTWC, FSSB) with the two self-reported sleep quality measures, sleep insufficiency (ΔR2 = .08, ΔF =19.22, $p < .001$) and insomnia symptoms (ΔR2 = .03, ΔF = 7.09, $p < .001$), but not actigraphic WASO (ΔR2 = .00, ΔF = .81, $p < .49$). WTFC was significantly and positively associated with sleep insufficiency, B = .24, t(623) = 5.92, $p < .001$, and insomnia symptoms, B = .13, t(621) = 3.56, $p < .001$, but not WASO, B = .33, t(622) = .44, $p = .66$). It was found that work-family constructs are associated with multiple aspects of sleep quality and quantity.

Occupational health and safety

The vision of the 2016 Management Plan of the European Agency for Safety and Health at Work [39] is defined as “To be a recognised leader promoting healthy and safe workplaces in Europe based on tripartism, participation and the development of an occupational safety and health (OSH) risk prevention culture, to ensure a smart, sustainable, productive and inclusive economy". The strategic programme and activities in the management plan reflects the importance given to the effective psychosocial risks management and to work-related diseases and disabilities (Priority Area 2) and the raising of awareness about workplace risks, namelly psychosocial risks and how to prevent them (Priority Area 4).

The Occupational Safety and Health Convention, 1981 (N° 155), Convention N°161 and the Promotional Framework for Occupational Safety and Health Convention, 2006 (N°187) provide guidance on a strategic approach to integrating prevention of occupational diseases in national OSH policies and programmes [40]. The subject of work-related mental disorders is regularly examined from the prevention view point. The regular monitoring of the working environment and health surveillance of workers enables the employers to report occupational diseases.

In order to supervise the application of European legislation at the national level, the Senior Labour Inspectors′ Committe (SLIC), set up in 1982, decided to focus its 2012 information and inspection campaign on psychosocial risks [41]. Since the occurrence of the SLIC Campaign in 2012, the Labor Inspection Entities of the European member states have played a leading role in ensuring that organizations conduct psychosocial risk assessments as required according to the OSH legislation.

Also, the International Labor Organization (ILO) published in 2010 a list with the World Health Organization (WHO) entitled International Statistical Classification of Diseases and Related Health Problems, 10th Revision (ICD-10) [42]. The new list reflects the state-of-the-art development in the identification and recognition of occupational diseases. It includes a range of internationally recognized occupational diseases, from illnesses caused by chemical, physical and biological agents to respiratory and skin diseases, musculoskeletal disorders and occupational cancer. To note that mental and behavioural disorders have been, for the first time, specifically included in the ILO list.

In 2002, at the 90th Session of the International Labour Conference, the representative from the WHO spoke "of mental health as being an important part of general health, and noted furthermore that mental and behavioural disorders had proven physiological effects. Worker experts were concerned to improve the reporting of mental and behavioural disorders, noting that present notification of even well-known diseases was often poor. Reporting would then hopefully improve prevention, which was most important" [42].

In Europe, only Denmark has registered in 2005, a mental disorder designated post-traumatic stress disorder, on its list of occupational diseases. Recently, the French Parliament voted for a first step to facilitate the recognition of burnout as occupational disease [43].

This systematic review allowed to notice that current research need to conjugate occupational health and safety, medicine and psychosocial areas of knowledge in order to achieve a more accurate information.

It is important to note, there are challenges in measuring the impact of work on health due to factors such as:

(a) Limitations in national recording and notification systems of occupational diseases make it difficult to determine a causal relationship between workplace conditions and workers' health impairments, especially in the case of diseases with long latency periods and with multifactorial causes [20];
(b) The use of cross-sectional study design rather than longitudinal study design [2];
(c) The use of self-reported assessment [2]
(d) The lack of use of medically confirmed health outcomes in workers, and
(e) The lack of use of psychosocial validated assessment method(s) for the study population, as we observed in this systematic review.

Furthermore, assessment of the work environment has depended solely on quantitative evaluation methods, whereas some authors have recommended the adoption of qualitative methods as well (eg. interviews or open, semi-structured, observation) to obtain more information so as to permit a more accurate analyses [44]. Consequently, for a real understanding of the health effects of psychosocial work factors there is a need to adopt these critical methodological aspects as they can contribute to a better understanding of how the psychosocial environment (e.g., individual characteristics, interpersonal relationships, organizational factors, community factors, public policies) can influence workers' health [12, 17, 44].

Methodological considerations

Three of the studies were based on cross-sectional data. Although this design is widely used in the research fields of psychosocial work environment, it presents a recognized major limitation, in that cross-sectional may be an appropriate method at an early stage to establish inferred relations, but is insufficient draw conclusions about causality in observed associations. It is recommended to use prospective or longitudinal research designs, allowing a time period between measurements of independent and dependent variables.

A higher proportion of prospective studies yielded adverse effects on workers' health as compared to cross-sectional studies. However, the prospective design did not lead to consistent findings in the study of psychosocial factors on workers health. More studies combining a prospective cohort design and the inclusion of objective measures both for assessing psychosocial risk and health-related work outcomes are needed to assess the role of psychosocial environment in the health-adverse effects. Furthermore, more prospective studies are needed to compare results by study design.

Future epidemiological research in this area should aim to have a more rigorous assessment of the link between work-related psychosocial factors on workers´ health to advance our understanding of the potential contribution of work-related structural conditions to workers´ health.

Relatively little attention has been given to objective and repeated measures of work-related psychosocial factors and inclusion of measures of resilience, personality characteristics of workers and life events. Information linking non-work factors to workers´ health is much scarcer and it is only now beginning to emerge. Given the range of psychosocial exposures to which workers may be exposed, any future studies that focus on psychosocial factors and workers´ health should also obtain data on relevant factors outside the work including workers´ personality style, relationship, social support system, as the broader socio-economic context within which the workplace is set, in order to yield the most unbiased estimates of work-related psychosocial factors on workers´ health.

Strengths and limitations

To the best of our knowledge, this is the first systematic review assessing the methodological quality of evidence of the influence of work-related psychosocial factors on workers´ health through data on validated assessment method(s) for the study population and specific medical evaluation of health-related work outcome(s).

The major strength of the review were the broad inclusion of these two criteria, in compliance with Occupational Safety and Health legislation (Directive 89/391/EEC) of the European Union. It can be considered a strenght because it followed the European legislation of OSH (involving the use of valid risk assessment of mental and physical health of worker). This review provides an over-arching perspective, through the inclusion of objective measures of assessment in order to provide reliable findings on how the social environment and social conditions can influence health. The inclusion only of studies published in peer-reviewed journals ensured quality of the data.

There were some limitations in this review. Firstly, it is worth mentioning that because of the use of these two inclusion criteria we could have missed potentially relevant papers in the first step of data selection, for instance one Whitehall study published in 2006 [45]. Secondly, the variable body mass index (BMI) acted not only as confounders [37] as well as a medical evaluation of health-related work outcome [32, 35] which might influence the precision and magnitude of measure of the association between work-related psychosocial factors on workers´ health.

Conclusions

The results of this systematic review suggest that the social environment (workplace, community, family, etc.) can influence health outcomes. Most studies (7/10) observed an adverse effect of poor psychosocial work factors on workers' health: 3 on sickness absence [30, 31, 35], 4 on cardiovascular diseases [32–34, 36]. The 3 other studies reported detrimental effects on sleep and on disease-associated biomarkers [37–39]. However, the weight of the results is limited as only a few studies were of high methodological quality. In fact, more consistent effects were found in studies of high methodological quality using a prospective design with validated instruments to assess psychosocial work factors and objective measures of work-related health outcomes.

Therefore, more studies are need to confirm the detrimental effects of negative psychosocial work factors on health outcomes and future studies should consider a) using a prospective design, b) using validated psychosocial risk questionnaires and objective measures of health outcomes, and c) studying the complex interrelationships between work and the physical and mental health of workers.

Competing interests

The authors declare that they have no competing interests.

Authors' contributions

SR, AN, JF, and JTC have made substantial contributions to the review. All authors read and approved the final manuscript.

Acknowledgement

The authors would also acknowledge Paul Bewicke for proof-reading our manuscript. There has been no external financial support or funding of the study.

Author details
[1]Faculty of Engineering of the University of Porto, Porto, Portugal. [2]CINTESIS - Centre for Research in Health Technologies and Information Systems and Information and Decision Sciences Department, Faculty of Medicine, University of Porto, Porto, Portugal. [3]Allergy Unit, CUF Porto Institute & Hospital, Porto, Portugal. [4]Institute for Health Service Research in Dermatology and Nursing (IVDP), Center of Excellence for Epidemiology and Health Service Research for Healthcare Professionals (CVcare), University Medical Center Hamburg-Eppendorf, Martinistraße 52, Hamburg 20246, Germany. [5]Principles of Prevention and Rehabilitation Department (GPR), Institute for Statutory Accident Insurance and Prevention in the Health and Welfare Services (BGW), Hamburg, Germany. [6]Faculty of Medicine of the University of Porto, Porto, Portugal.

References

1. EU-OSHA. Motivation for employers to carry out workplace health promotion. Luxembourg: Publications Office of the European Union; 2012. Available at: https://osha.europa.eu/en/tools-and-publications/publications/literature_reviews/motivation-for-employers-to-carry-out-workplace-health-promotion.
2. EU-OSHA. Priorities for occupational safety and health research in Europe: 2013-2020. Luxembourg: Publications Office of the European Union; 2013. Available at: https://osha.europa.eu/en/tools-and-publications/publications/reports/priorities-for-occupational-safety-and-health-research-in-europe-2013-2020.
3. EU-OSHA. Well-being at work: creating a positive work environment. Luxembourg: Publications Office of the European Union; 2013. Available at: https://osha.europa.eu/en/tools-and-publications/publications/literature_reviews/well-being-at-work-creating-a-positive-work-environment.
4. International Labour Office (ILO). Psychosocial factors at work: Recognition and control. Occupational Safety and Health (Series No 56). Geneva: International Labour Office; 1986.
5. Eurofound and EU-OSHA. Psychosocial risks in Europe: Prevalence and strategies for prevention. Luxembourg: Publications Office of the European Union; 2014. Available at: https://osha.europa.eu/en/publications/reports/psychosocial-risks-eu-prevalence-strategies-prevention/view.
6. EU-OSHA. New forms of contractual relationships and the implications for occupational safety and health. Luxembourg: Office for Official Publications of the European Communities; 2002.
7. EU-OSHA. Expert forecast on emerging psychosocial risks related to occupational safety and health. Luxembourg: Office for Official Publications of the European Communities; 2007.
8. EU-OSHA. Calculating the cost of work-related stress and psychosocial risks. Luxembourg: Publications Office of the European Union; 2014.
9. EU-OSHA. The second European Survey of Enterprises on New and Emerging Risks (ESENER-2). Luxembourg: Publications Office of the European Union; 2015. Available at: https://osha.europa.eu/en/tools-and-publications/publications/second-european-survey-enterprises-new-and-emerging-risks-esener/view.
10. European Comission. Promoting mental health in the workplace: Guidance to implementing a comprehensive approach. Luxembourg: Employment, Social Affairs & Inclusion; 2014. Available at: http://ec.europa.eu/social/main.jsp?catId=716&langId=en&moreDocuments=yes.
11. Kompier MA. New system of work organization and worker's health. Scand J Work Environ Health. 2006;32(6):421–30.
12. Berkmann L, Kawachi I, Glymour M. Social Epidemiology. New York: Oxford University Press; 2014.
13. Directive 89/391/EEC of the European Parliament and of the Council of 12 June 1989 on the Introduction of measures to encourage improvements in the safety and health of workers at work. http://eur-lex.europa.eu/legal-content/EN/TXT/?uri=celex:31989L0391.
14. European Comission. Interpretative Document of the Implementation of Council Directive 89/391/EEC in relation to Mental Health in the Workplace. Employment, Social Affairs & Inclusion. 2014.
15. European Commission. Guidance on risk assessment at work. Luxembourg: Publications Office of the European Union; 1996. Available at: https://osha.europa.eu/en/legislation/guidelines/guidance-on-risk-assessment-at-work.
16. International Labour Office. ILO Guidelines on occupational safety and health management systems. Geneva: International Labour Office; 2001.
17. PRIMA-EF. The European Framework for Psychosocial Risk Management: PRIMA-EF. Nottingham: World Health Organization; 2008.
18. Nübling M, Vomstein M, Haugh A, Nübling T, Adiwidjaja A. European-Wide Survey on Teachers Work Related Stress - Assessment, Comparison and Evaluation of the Impact of Psychosocial Hazards on Teachers at their Workplace. Brussels: European Trade Union Committee for Education; 2011.
19. International Labour Organization. SOLVE integrating health promotion into workplace OSH policies: trainer's guide. Geneva: International Labour Office; 2012.
20. International Labour Office. Emerging risks and new patterns of prevention in a changing world of work. World Day for Safety and Health at Work, 28 April 2010. Geneva: 2010. Available at: http://www.ilo.org/wcmsp5/groups/public/—ed_protect/—protrav/—safework/documents/publication/wcms_123653.pdf
21. Greenhaus J, Allen T, Spector P. Health consequences of work-family conflict: The dark side of the work-family interface. In: Perrewe P, Ganster D, editors. Research in occupational stress and well being. Greenwich: JAI Press/Elsevier; 2006. p. 61–98.
22. Hurrel L, Redline S, Simmons L. Measuring job stressors and strains: Where we have been, where we are, and where we need to go. J Occup Health Psychol. 1998;3:368–89.
23. Liberati A, Altman D, Tetzlaff J, Mulrow C, Gotzsche P, Loannicis J, et al. The PRISMA statement for reporting systematic reviews and meta-analyses of studies that evaluate health care interventions: explanation and elaboration. J Clin Epidemiol. 2009;62(10):31–4. http://www.jclinepi.com/article/S0895-4356(09)00180-2/pdf.
24. Cox T, Griffiths A, Rial-Gonzalez E. Research on work-related stress. Luxembourg: Office for Official Publications of the European Communities; 2000.
25. Vahtera J, Pentti J, Kivimäki M. Sickness absence as a predictor of mortality among male and female employees. J Epidemiol Community Health. 2004; 58(4):321–6.
26. Leka S, Jain A. Health impact of psychosocial hazard at work: an overview. Geneva: World Health Organization; 2010.
27. Nieuwenhuijsen K, Bruinvels D, Frings-Dresen M. Psychosocial work environment and stress-related disorders, a systematic review. Occup Med. 2010;60:277–86.
28. Rugulies R, Christensen K, Borritz M, Villadsen E, Bültmann U, Kristensen T. The contribution of the psychosocial work environment to sickness absence in human service workers: results of a 3 year follow-up. Work Stress. 2007; 21(4):293–311.
29. Borritz M, Christensen K, Bültmann U, Rugulies R, Lund T, Andersen I, Villadsen E, Diderichsen L. Impact of burnout and psychosocial work characteristics on future long-term sickness absence. Prospective results of the Danish PUMA study among human service workers. Am Coll Occup Environ Med. 2010; 52(10):964–70.
30. Nyberg A, Alfredsson L, Theorell T, Westerlund H, Vahtera J, Kivimäki M. Managerial leadership and ischaemic heart disease among employees: the Swedish WOLF study. Occup Environ Med. 2009;66:51–5.
31. Tsutsumi A, Kayaba K, Kario K, Ishikawa S. Prospective Study on Occupational Stress and Risk of Stroke. Arch Intern Med. 2009;169(1):56–61.
32. Guimont C, Brisson C, Dagenais G, Milot A, Vézina M, Mâsse B, Moisan J, Laflamme N, Blanchette C. Effects of job strain on blood pressure: a prospective study of male and female white-collar workers. Am J Public Health. 2006;96(8):1436–43.
33. Sabbath E, Melchior M, Goldberg M, Zins M, Berkman L. Work and family demands: predictors of all-cause sickness absence in the GAZEL cohort. Eur J Public Health. 2011;22(1):101–6.
34. Aboa-Éboule C, Brisson C, Maunsell E, Bourbonnais R, Vézina M, Milot A, Dagenais G. Effort-Reward Imbalance at Work and Recurrent Coronary Heart Disease Events: A 4-Year Prospective Study of Post-Myocardial Infarction Patients. Am Psychosom Med. 2011;73(6):436–47.
35. Bellingrath S, Rohleder N, Kudielka B. Healthy working school teachers with high effort-reward imbalance and overcommitment show increase pro-inflammatory immune activity and a dampened innate immune defence. Brain Behav Immun. 2010;24(8):1332–9.
36. Tsai SS, Lai CH, Shih TS, Lin MH, Liou SH. High Job Strain is associated with inflammatory markers of disease in young long-haul bus drivers. Am Psychol Assoc. 2014;3(19):336–47.
37. Crain T, Hammer L, Bodner T, Kossek E, Moen P, Lilienthal R. Work-family conflict, family-supportive supervisor behaviors (FSSB), and sleep outcomes. J Occup Health Psychol. 2014;19(2):155–16.

38. Kristensen T, Hannerz H, Høgh A, Borg V. The Copenhagen Psychosocial Questionnaire (COPSOQ) – a tool for the assessment and improvement of the psychosocial work environment. Scand J Work Environ Health. 2005;31:438–49.
39. EU-OSHA. The 2016 Management Plan. Luxembourg: Office for Official Publications of the European Communities; 2016.
40. International Labour Office. Prevention of occupational diseases. Geneva: International Labour Office; 2013.
41. European Forum of the insurance against accidents at work and occupational diseases. (EUROGIP). What recognition of work-related mental disorders? A study on 10 European countries. EUROGIP Study Report; 2013.
42. International Labour Office. List of Occupational Diseases (revised 2010): Identification and recognition of occupational diseases: Criteria for incorporating diseases in the ILO list of occupational diseases, Occupational Safety and Health Series, No. 74. Geneva: ILO; 2010.
43. EUROFOUND. France: first step to recognising burnout as an occupational illness. 2015. European observatory of working life. EurWORK, Available at: http://www.eurofound.europa.eu/observatories/eurwork/articles/working-conditions-quality-of-life/france-first-step-to-recognising-burnout-as-an-occupational-illness.
44. Rugulies R. Studying the effect of psychosocial work environment on risk of ill-health: towards a more comprehensive assessment of working conditions. Scand J Work Environ Health. 2012;38:187–92.
45. Kivimäki M, Ferrie J, Shipley M, Brunner E, Vahtera J, Marmot M. Work stress, weight gain and weight loss: evidence for bidirectional effects of job strain on body mass index in the Whitehall II study. Int J Obes (Lond). 2006;30:982–7.

15

A decade of an HIV workplace programme in armed conflict zones: a social responsibility response of the International Committee of the Red Cross

Stéphane Du Mortier*, Silas Mukangu, Charles Sagna, Laurent Nyffenegger and Sigiriya Aebischer Perone

Abstract

The International Committee of the Red Cross (ICRC) works in fragile States and in armed conflict zones. Some of them are affected by the HIV pandemic. Within the framework of its social responsibility programme concerning HIV affecting its staff members, the organization has implemented an HIV workplace programme since 2004.
We carried out a retrospective analysis over 10 years. Data collected were initially essentially qualitative and process-oriented, but were complemented over the years by data on annual voluntary counselling and testing (VCT) uptake and on direct annual costs covering awareness, testing and antiretroviral therapy.
The number of people covered by the programme grew from none in 2003 to 4,438 in 2015, with an increase in annual VCT uptake over the years increasing from 376 persons (14 %) in 2007 to 2,663 in 2015 (60 %).
Over the years, the services were expanded from awareness raising to bringing VCT to the workplace, as well as offering testing and health coverage of other conditions and innovative approaches to facing challenges linked to situations of violence.
Within its social responsibility framework, the ICRC has shown the importance and feasibility of a workplace HIV programme in conflict zones. A sustainable workplace programme in these conflict settings requires constant adaptation, with regular follow-up given the relatively high turnover of staff, and ensuring sustainable stocks of condoms and antiretroviral drugs.

Keywords: HIV/AIDS, Social responsibility, ICRC, Workplace programme, Conflict, Humanitarian, Fragile States

Abbreviations: AIDS, Acquired Immune Deficiency Syndrome; ART, Antiretroviral therapy; CAR, Central African Republic; CD4, Lymphocytes type CD4; GIZ, Deutsche Gesellschaft für Internationale Zusammenarbeit, German society for International Cooperation; HFP, Health Focal Point; HIV, Human Immunodeficiency Virus; HR, Human Resources; ICRC, International Committee of the Red Cross; IFRC, International Federation of Red Cross and Red Crescent Societies; ILO, International Labour Organization; KAP, Knowledge, Attitude and Practices; M&E, Monitoring & Evaluation; PE, Peer Educators; PLHIV, People Living with HIV; PMTCT, Prevention Mother to Child Transmission; STI, Sexually Transmitted Infection; UNAIDS, United Nations for AIDS; VCT, Voluntary Counselling (Confidential) Testing; VL, Viral Load; WPP, Workplace Programme.

* Correspondence: daktaristephane@gmail.com
International Committee of the Red Cross, Geneva, Switzerland

Background

The use of war as a continuation of diplomacy when pursuing interest is becoming more acceptable, as systems of states are changing. State driven, inter-communal and urban violence diffuses into society destroying social fabrics. One of the definition of fragile states is weak capacity to carry out basic state functions and weak institutions. Humanitarian actors need to be agile and provide access and basic health services in places with health system failure.

The International Committee of the Red Cross (ICRC) is an independent, neutral organization ensuring humanitarian protection and assistance to victims of armed conflict and other situations of violence. It acts in response to emergencies and at the same time promotes respect for international humanitarian law and its integration into national law. Based in Geneva, Switzerland, it has a workforce of about 12,000 people in 80 countries, of whom many are affected by the HIV pandemic.

HIV workplace programmes (WPP) have been launched as new approaches in the fight against HIV [1], since HIV primarily affects populations of working age [2] and 54 % of people living with HIV (PLHIV) worldwide do not know that they are infected [3].

Publications on HIV at the workplace began to appear from 2004, many from southern Africa [4, 5], which illustrated some specific characteristics of the epidemic including higher prevalence of HIV among short-contract workers compared to permanent employees and among people in occupations with low wages. Prevalence peaks between 30 and 39 years for men and at younger ages for women [6].

In June 2013, the International Labour Organization (ILO) launched its "VCT@work initiative". Michel Sidibé, UNAIDS Executive Director, also highlighted the importance of the fight to reach the target of 5 million workers tested at work by 2015: "*We need to tell them that HIV is no longer a death sentence. They must know their status. The days when they had to hide are over. HIV is a chronic, treatable disease, and treatments are becoming less toxic*" [7].

As response to HIV affecting its staff members, the ICRC has been implementing an HIV WPP since 2004. This article reports the successes, challenges and lessons learnt from a decade of running an HIV WPP in armed conflict zones and fragile States.

ICRC and its HIV workplace programme

In 2004, 48 % of the ICRC's operational budget was spent in Africa [8], where the highly prevalent HIV pandemic had a great impact on the ICRC's workforce and its operational capacity. In order to promote the health of its staff and in line with its organizational social responsibility, ICRC representatives benchmarked other renowned WPPs, such as those of the German Society for International Cooperation (GIZ) and the Heineken breweries, and started a pilot HIV WPP which quickly expanded in numerous countries. The implementation of an HIV WPP, as well as its benefits for staff, also had economic consequences by reducing replacement costs, retaining know-how and sending a signal to the labour market, as it is more efficient to implement an HIV WPP than to lose and have to replace deceased staff members and to be obliged to develop the capacity of newly hired staff. The ICRC staff health unit wrote the HIV WPP policy, which was validated in 2006 by the ICRC Assembly, and which is in line with the ILO code of practice on HIV/AIDS and the relevant ILO guidelines [9–11]. This policy guarantees non-discrimination, confidentiality and no link between testing, status and employment. It also respects a recent ILO recommendation of 2010 [12] and ISO 26000, concerning guidance on social responsibility [13].

The desired impact of the ICRC HIV WPP is that there will be no new HIV infections among staff. The three pillars of the programme are a supportive environment, permanent access to quality HIV testing, and proper care and treatment.

The annual objectives are: (1) to increase annually the number of staff and family members who know their HIV status, with 100 % coverage of HIV testing for all pregnant women; and (2) to guarantee that HIV-infected staff and family members have access to quality care and treatment. We illustrate, below, the difficulties of guaranteeing permanent access to preventive services (especially testing) in situations of violence and armed conflicts.

Leadership of the HIV WPP

Numerous articles document the fact that one of the key factors for a successful HIV WPP is leadership [2, 14–19] resulting from a synergy between motivated, responsible personnel at three levels: national health focal points (HFPs), regional coordinators and headquarters staff.

In each country, one HFP is responsible for implementation of the WPP and for ensuring access to health services. The HFP is bound by medical confidentiality in relation with her/his colleagues from the human resources (HR) department and has responsible for peer educators (PE) selected by employees. HFPs are trained to address stigma and discrimination, to promote HIV awareness, to refer staff to voluntary counselling and testing (VCT) and to guarantee permanent condom availability, post-exposure kits and management of medical waste. They report to line managers organized in an "HIV committee", which meets at least once a year and which includes the senior management of the delegation concerned. Its members are sensitized and important boosters of the WPP especially in addressing stigma and discrimination, providing time for HIV awareness sessions and allowing VCT at the workplace, as already documented in different contexts [19, 20].

Three regional coordinators, based in Nairobi and Dakar, provide strong leadership through annual country visits and permanent technical support. At headquarters level, the health unit is available to guarantee permanent support to the programme.

Creating a supportive environment

We regularly conducted locally adapted information and education sessions on HIV/AIDS among employees by using health professionals for question-and-answer sessions, lay counsellors from among people living with HIV (PLHIV), PE groups from local businesses, and provided health insurance awareness sessions when available (e.g. in South Africa and Kenya), and through family days, 1 December (commemorative day) events, and email sensitization/video forums.

With time, the family days were revised according to needs. Instead of a family awareness day for the whole family, they were separated into young adults' day and parents' day; both events included HIV testing for eligible persons. Awareness sessions always considered the informational needs of staff and were delivered in local languages. In some contexts, "domestic violence" or "homosexuality" came out as important topics to be addressed (e.g. in South Africa, Thailand, Kenya, Haiti), while they were absent in more religious or traditional settings (e.g. Sudan, Lao People's Democratic Republic). A culture of openness and non-discrimination was promoted. Addressing possible stigma and discrimination was a daily issue [21].

VCT and ART services

HFPs identified the best VCT and ART service providers (mainly local nongovernmental organizations or in rare cases private institutions), which were scarce in some remote settings. VCT services were outsourced to HIV prevention and treatment service providers:

- to guarantee privacy and confidentiality to the staff. The only information provided to the HFPs were anonymous data on employees and family members tested yearly and on the positives tests;
- to guarantee continuum of care and access to ART according to national protocols;
- to respect local legislation, standards, criteria and epidemiology;
- for sustainability as well as to strengthen the WPP system.

The particularities of the ICRC compared to other employers are the following:

- by its mandate, the ICRC is involved in fragile States and countries in conflict where health services are often endangered and there is reduced access to care, stocks or quality services but also by lack of update of national public health policies;
- the main ICRC activities are delivered far from capital cities, near frontlines, where there is often an extreme scarcity of health services;
- in permanent adaptation to the needs generated by the conflicts, the size of the staff fluctuates over the years;
- the ICRC always respects national health policies and norms and does not develop its own ART clinics. Employees are proposed VCT services in an existing clinic, validated by the ministry of health. This guarantees confidentiality, respect of national norms concerning CD4/viral load criteria for starting treatment, inclusion of staff in the national health system and statistics for continuum of care after possible layoffs;
- there is a common HR administrative system to all delegations of the ICRC, so similarities are found in all countries (e.g. salary classes, types of contract);
- as a humanitarian organization, the ICRC delivers high-quality services at the best prices, with no logic of competition with the other health service providers or transfer of foreign investment. Very few of the affected countries have private health insurance providers. Therefore, the ICRC insures its staff and family members itself, leading to a situation in which the employer is also the insurer.

The ICRC guarantees a continuation of health insurance coverage for one year after the end of contract for patients with chronic diseases. It is one of the responsibilities of the HFP to monitor the integration of former colleagues into functional national programmes over the years.

Method

We carried out a retrospective analysis on data available over 10 years. VCT uptake is the main indicator that has been consistent throughout the years.

Some of the data came from HIV knowledge, attitude and practice (KAP) surveys established early in the relevant countries (e.g. in 2004 in Kenya, in 2005 in Ethiopia, in 2006 in Uganda, in 2008 Democratic Republic of the Congo and Burundi, and in 2010 in Zimbabwe) using a common questionnaire and showing similar results and limitations (Table 1).

A set of outcome indicators respecting national protocols was established (e.g. number of employees attending the awareness sessions, number of PE/staff), which are the same indicators as those used by the IFRC [22].

These KAP surveys eventually increased the acceptance of the HIV WPP but didn't increase the VCT

Table 1 KAP results

- Good age representation of the ICRC staff, but lower completion rate in remote offices than in the capital city
- Good knowledge (mean score of 14.3 on a scale of 20) on HIV main modes of transmission except mother to child transmission where 40 % to 55 % of them did not know the way of preventing mother to child transmission. According to countries 3 (Kenya) to 16 % (Burundi) believed HIV is transmitted by witchcraft, and for 3 (Kenya) to 23 % (DRC) it is God's punishment.
- Misconception as "birth control pills prevent HIV transmission, or mosquito transmission" were made by respectively 17.4 and 10.7 % (North Kenya) in some remote offices.
- Employees below 25 years had a significant difference in knowledge index. There is a confirmed correlation between level of education and knowledge index.
- According to countries, between 5 to 15 % of the staff reported having a diagnosed STI in the preceding 12 months and only 40 % agreed that having many sexual partners can lead to STI while 10 (Kenya) to 21 % (DRC) declared having more than two partners in the last 6 months (singles > married, but not related to number of days out of station)
- In average 70 % were willing to go for VCT, 65 % if done at the workplace with confidentiality.
- More than 80 % who were tested shared the results with someone, but disparities were documented in Kenya between the capital and remote office were, respective, 38 to 53 % were never tested due to fear.
- While 83 to 93 % declared themselves ready to take care of a PLHIV relative, 70 (North Kenya office) to 94 % (DRC) declared that a sick relative should remain a secret.
- Up to 90 % declared themselves comfortable discussing HIV/AIDS with a counsellor, only 70 % were ready to do it with their children and 65 % with their boss. Discussion about their own status was significantly lower (from 78 % with spouse to 12 % with the boss). 75 to 80 % agreed that PLHIV have an equal chance of recruitment or promotion at the ICRC
- Staff from remote offices were significantly considering themselves at low infection risk, while they were also scoring lower in knowledge index.
- In North Kenya, up to 14 % of the men and 20 % of women described having been forced to have sex.
- While few declared regular alcohol consumption, there was a correlation between daily alcohol consumption and reporting sex with a commercial sex worker.
- Condom perception and use showed better results for 25 to 39 years old. Persons younger than 25 years scored lower due to shame and misconception. The consistency of condom use was not assessed.
- More than 95 % saw a PLHIV dying of AIDS

uptake. For example, the KAP survey in Kenya was carried out in 2004, the one in Uganda in 2006, and the one in Burundi in December 2008. Figure 1 illustrates the lack of correlation between the KAP surveys and the VCT uptake.

After initial awareness raising achieved through KAP, the approach moved to implementation of VCT at the workplace and supporting by all means possible the prevention of mother to child transmission (PMTCT).

Data collection concentrated on key performance indicators such as VCT uptake per delegation, PMTCT and financial data.

Results

Geographical expansion

The Table 2 illustrates the growing expansion of the programme, starting with two pilot projects in Kenya 2004 and Senegal in 2005. Finding local actors for KAP

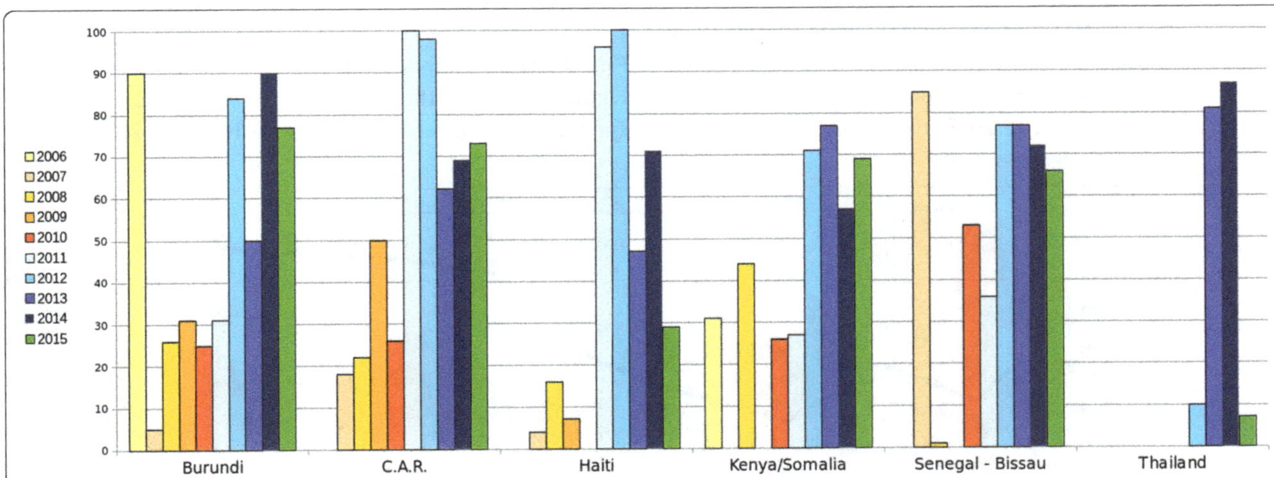

Fig. 1 Annual VCT uptake in percentage of staff from 2006 to 2015; choice of countries

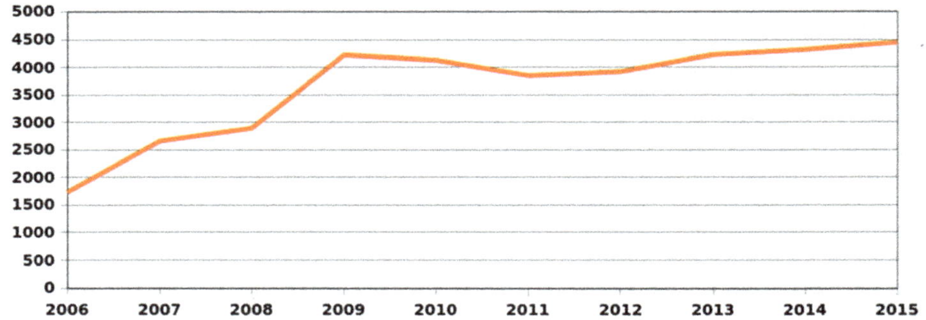

Fig. 2 Number of ICRC staff covered by the HIV WPP since its beginning

and VCT partnerships in respect of national policies was the main challenge of the first years. The numbers reported are percentages of staff knowing their HIV status on an annual basis. The HIV WPP started in 2004, so 2006 data are cumulative ones for 2004 to 2006. We put 0 for HIV WPP present without VCT. Mali and Niger were one single delegation originally, but became two separate delegations in 2014. The South Africa 2014 results were not communicated by the health insurance agency according to national WPP protocols. Some delegations (e.g. Angola) were closed as a result of conflict ending. Figure 3 illustrates the results from a selection of these countries.

Staff coverage and VCT uptake

Figure 1 illustrates different dynamics in representative delegations.

Burundi was an early successful programme thanks to the personality of the HFP, sharing his/her HIV positive status. Erosion is visible from 2007 to 2011, when the offering of testing and health coverage of other conditions boosted the VCT.

Continuum of care from VCT to access to treatment was offered in the Central African Republic, the HFP being a doctor working in both services. The leadership of the HIV-positive Head of Delegation boosted the VCT of 2011 and 2012.

The drop of VCT in Haiti is due to a security incident affecting the delegation in 2013, then a drastic reduction of staff in 2015. Awareness and mobilization were extremely country specific, with, for example, Haitians expressing themselves about HIV with a striking freedom.

The figures from the regional delegations of Kenya/Somalia and Senegal/Guinea Bissau illustrate the difficulties of keeping annual VCT mobilization. The family days were parties attended by numerous employees but very few VCT were taken during these events. The combination of VCT with other tests at the workplace during working hours is the reason for the visible increase in 2012.

The prevalence of HIV being low in Thailand, it was virtually impossible to interest the staff in knowing their status without a combination with other tests. While this approach was validated, the VCT uptake increased rapidly and was maintained in 2015.

Figure 2: The increase is due to growing number of countries involved and regular increase of staff.

Figure 3: 2006 VCT values are persons tested since the beginning of the programme (2004 to 2006) while 2007–2015 values are a calculation of annual VCT uptake. In order to avoid discrimination, we proposed that persons living with HIV should queue with their colleagues and receive, in the privacy of the medical consultation, a free voucher for CD4/viral load (VL) testing. The lowest annual VCT uptake was 9 % while 60 % was reached in 2015.

Prevention of mother to child transmission

Figure 4 shows that access to PMTCT for staff and spouses rose from 67 % in 2007 to 100 % in 2015.

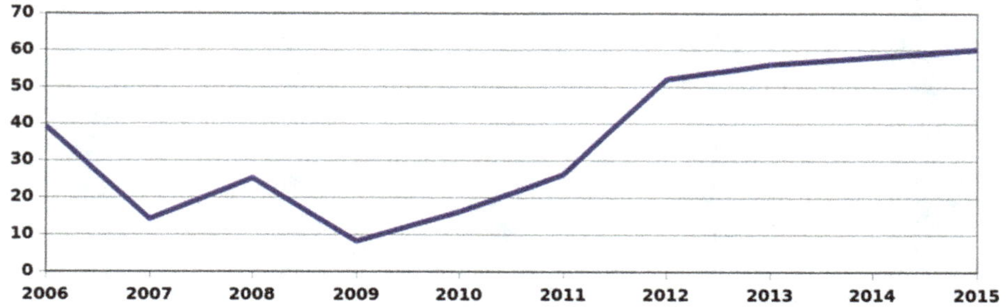

Fig. 3 Annual VCT uptake in percentage of ICRC staff since the beginning of the HIV WPP

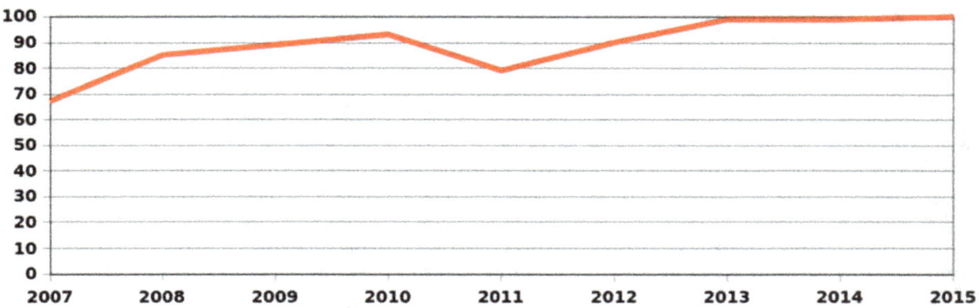

Fig. 4 Percentage of pregnant women knowing their HIV status on annual basis since the beginning of the HIV WPP

HFP reinforced the anchorage of the programme in national health policies, which were developing at their own pace.

Financial split

Figure 5 shows that since 2011, we aimed to decrease the cost of awareness (social events, material) in favour of testing (HIV testing, VL, CD4, hepatitis B vaccination, other screening tests) and ART.

Discussion

The HIV WPP had to overcome unique challenges, similar to those facing multinational companies [23], due to the geographical disparity of the settings in which the programme took place. For example, in 2014,

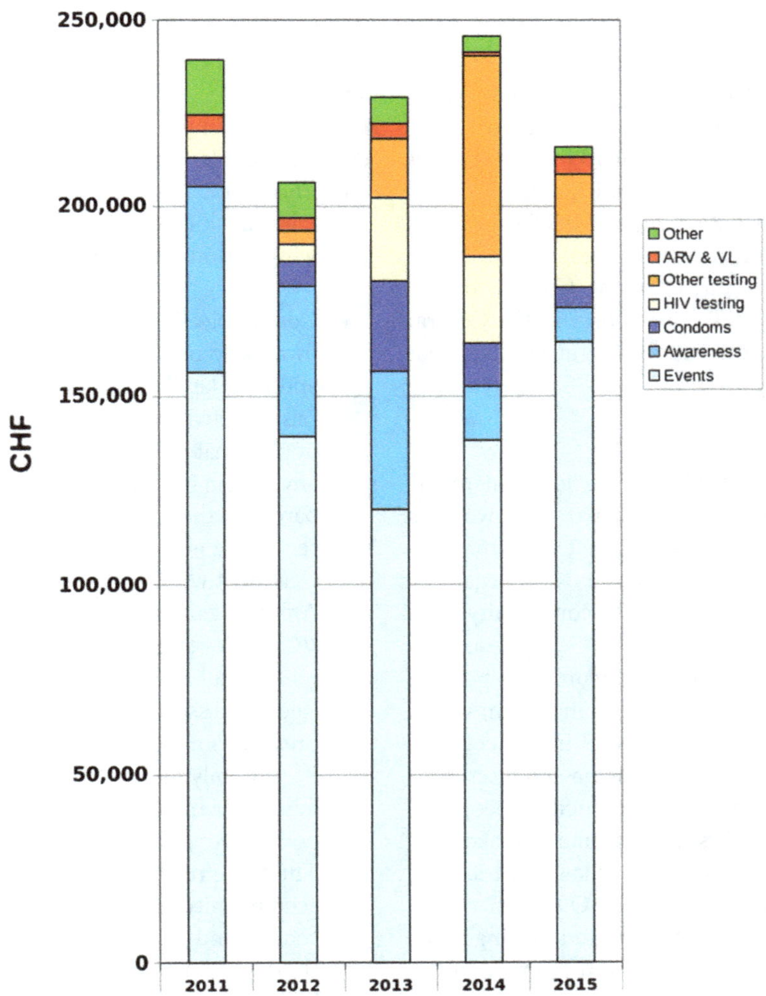

Fig. 5 HIV WPP financial split

Table 2 Expansion of the HIV WPP by its annual VCT uptake in percentage of staff

	2006	2007	2008	2009	2010	2011	2012	2013	2014	2015
Burundi	90	5	26	31	25	31	84	50	90	77
Cameroun	44	44	13	38	84	100	81	100	57	43
Eritrea	60	16	13	0	8	18	33	63	26	40
Ethiopia	46	25	21	17	6	36	37	18	53	53
Ivory Coast - Togo - Faso	0	24	47	15	4	36	68	91	77	67
Kenya/Somalia	31	0	44	0	26	27	71	77	57	69
Rwanda	83	0	0	5	0	3	36	33	69	71
Tanzania	61	0	16	44						50
Uganda	14	6	73	41	15	8	76	76	48	41
Zambia	9	0								
Zimbabwe	31	8	13	7	50	47	79	89	46	51
C.A.R.		18	22	50	26	100	98	62	69	73
Congo Brazza	0	40	0	0	46	12	83	88	89	100
D.R.Congo	0	1	8	5	23	15	63	54	78	63
Haiti		4	16	7	0	96	100	47	71	29
Liberia	0	13	19	17	48	51	100	100	83	98
Senegal - Bissau	0	85	1	0	53	36	77	77	72	66
Sierra Leone	0	76								
Angola			26							
Guinea Conakry			2	1	39	95	67	87	69	75
Nigeria		0	69	0	60	92	100	100	73	70
Chad				0	7	66	82	100	87	0
Mali/Niger				0	43	37	64	30		
Mali									60	65
Niger									84	71
Sudan			0	0	0	1	2	37	10	0
Madagascar						0	90	75	61	90
South Africa		She was caught during productive time for her bre				0	76	52	n/a	50
South Sudan							24	38	37	57
Thailand				0	0	0	10	81	87	7
Cambodia							0	100	100	0
Laos								0	100	100

0 for HIV WPP present without VCT
Mali and Niger were one delegation, became 2 in 2014
South Africa 2014 results not communicated by health insurance in 2014 according to national WPP protocols

767 employees in the Democratic Republic of the Congo were spread across eight locations, while in South Africa the 24 employees all worked in the capital, Pretoria.

Another challenge is related to working in conflict zones. In the last three years, we anticipated and prevented national or regional stock outs of ART drugs (e.g. in Burundi), HIV tests or access to annual CD4 count (e.g. in the Democratic Republic of the Congo), or destruction and looting of ART centres (e.g. in the Central African Republic). This increased drastically the trust placed in the programme by staff.

External mainstreaming

An indirect effect of the WPP was the external mainstreaming conducted by sensitized and trained workers in their communities with a positive effect on communities in terms of knowledge and attitude. In Senegal, for example, proactive outreach in the community was undertaken in collaboration with the Senegalese Red Cross to prevent HIV/AIDS in migrant women. A positive effect on the communities was also seen in Sudan, where the ICRC's HIV WPP was the first WPP in the country. This contributed to the fight against stigma and discrimination, in disseminating information and inciting people to test for HIV. It was also the first programme to make condoms available, while respecting national law, contributing to the reduction of HIV transmission. Outreach of the programme to families with adolescents and making treatment available, which drastically reduce the spread of the virus when ART is correctly taken, played a positive role in HIV prevention.

The success of de-stigmatization of HIV testing over the last years

Due to a low initial VCT uptake, mainly due to the belief that people taking an HIV test put themselves at risk or are promiscuous, we introduced in 2010 three different strategies as incentives and rewards for testing, after reviewing various strategies in the literature [24, 25]:

(a) Communication campaigns for developing people's ownership of their own health: "Be responsible for you and your family" was the motto of all awareness-raising activities (posters, talks, online articles). This implies that you do not take an HIV test on suspicion any longer, but do so as a responsible person or parent so that if you are negative you can work at remaining negative and if you are positive, early treatment will be offered to you at no cost.

(b) Annual health status screening packages including VCT. We reviewed the literature in order to select meaningful and contextualized screening tests (blood pressure, body mass index, cervical smear, breast examination, fasting blood sugar and hepatitis B). We only did these tests in contexts where follow-up and care would be provided in case of positive results.

(c) The three regional coordinators, on request, accompanied colleagues living with HIV to the ART centres and during hospitalization. Covering ART shortages for ICRC staff and their families increased WPP acceptance and continuum of care because confidentiality was always maintained.

Evolution of monitoring and evaluation (M&E)

While reviewing eight major studies based in the workplace, the Cochrane Collaboration [26] illustrated the numerous risks of bias and the difficulties in comparing indicators, despite previous literature urging that M&E operational challenges be addressed [27, 28].

We regularly assessed the quality of testing, tools, methodology and confidentiality in each delegation. We introduced key performance indicators, in respect of ILO standards, to document mortality, morbidity, infections related to HIV, medical costs and absenteeism. Nonetheless, the diversity of ICRC settings, the respect of patient confidentiality and the proven long-term benefit of VCT and ART in the literature [17, 18, 29–32] and the documented effectiveness of WPP [15, 23, 33–36] made these indicators of reduced interest with time. It was then proven by others that it is more efficient to implement an HIV WPP than to lose and to replace people.

Due to confidentiality concerns and the policy of referring people to existing external ART services, ART uptake and retention and treatment adherence could not be documented consistently in the 35 contexts. In exceptional cases, at the request of the family, the HFP was called in to persuade PLHIV to start or continue with treatment.

Since 2009, we decided to provide annual VCT at the workplace and encountered initial resistance despite its recognized benefits [37]. Afraid of social turmoil, or convinced that the national programmes were "so well in place in the country", some line managers, who had to address competing operational priorities in conflict zones, had to be convinced before accepting the implementation of this strategy in their place of work. This internal resistance, also documented in other organizations [38], contrasted with the involvement of the line manager in the Heineken brewery in Bukavu, who led by example in HIV testing, knowledge of condom use etc., with condoms being available on his own desk.

Regular visits to the main HIV stakeholders in the different countries (ministries of health, Global Fund, UNAIDS representatives, PLHIV groups and the main VCT-ART providers) allowed the sharing of experiences, adaptation of the programme, and benchmarking.

External evaluations were done in 2005 and 2010, resulting in regular proposed improvements. Benchmark visits generated changes in 2011 and 2012.

The ICRC HIV workplace policy was compared to ISO 26000 standards on corporate social responsibility [13] by four masters students from Zurich University in early 2014 [Haering A, Mayer I, Sager R, Sayer S. A Framework for HIV Workplace Programs based on Social responsibility Issues. Switzerland: University of Zurich; 2014. Unpublished master manuscript], which compared the ICRC WPP with the ILO standards in the world of work [9, 39], finding no substantial missing points.

Conclusions

The ICRC HIV WPP shows the feasibility of running such a programme in an operational institution working in conflict zones. This success has been possible through leadership and commitments at different levels, from the ICRC Assembly to the staff benefiting from the programme, and has been maintained despite the relatively high turnover of staff within the ICRC. Positive results of external mainstreaming of the WPP are strong arguments to develop more WPP and contribute to the UNAIDS Fast-Track 90-90-90 objectives.

After years of awareness rising, we have been able to implement VCT uptake in the workplace, and to expand geographically (to 25 countries in 2013) and thematically to promote health on a larger scale.

Indeed, the HIV WPP has to continuously adapt to evolving contexts, and keep in mind the safety of staff (Primum Non Nocere). The 2015 VCT uptake results (60 %) might be difficult to reach in the future due to political turmoil in many countries. In 2014, the Ebola crisis in Liberia and in Guinea jeopardized the blood sampling of VCTs. New interreligious (e.g. Central African Republic) and/or interethnic (e.g. South Sudan) conflicts have created new boundaries within countries and restricted access of ICRC staff to HIV care.

As part of the ICRC's social responsibility commitments, we aim to replicate the HIV WPP structure in other ICRC operational contexts (e.g. in the Syrian Arab Republic and Iraq) within the framework of the ICRC's duty of care, which in some cases in such contexts focuses other health priorities, like chronic conditions and mental health, rather than on HIV.

Abbreviations

AIDS: Acquired Immune Deficiency Syndrome; ART: Antiretroviral therapy; CAR: Central African Republic; CD4: Lymphocytes type CD4; GIZ: Deutsche Gesellschaft für Internationale Zusammenarbeit: German society for International Cooperation; HFP: Health Focal Point; HIV: Human Immunodeficiency Virus; HR: Human Resources; ICRC: International Committee of the Red Cross; IFRC: International Federation of Red Cross and Red Crescent Societies; ILO: International Labour Organization; KAP: Knowledge, Attitude and Practices; M&E: Monitoring & Evaluation; PE: Peer Educators; PLHIV: People Living with HIV; PMTCT: Prevention Mother to Child Transmission; STI: Sexually Transmitted Infection; UNAIDS: United Nations for AIDS; VCT: Voluntary Counselling (Confidential) Testing; VL: Viral Load; WPP: Workplace Programme.

Acknowledgement

The authors would like to thank the reviewers for their constructive comments, which enabled this article to be improved. All authors were under ICRC contract while working on the programme and its documentation.
The authors thank M. Leo Vita-Finzifor editing the English text.

Authors' contributions

SDM shared with SM and CS the conception, design, acquisition of data, analysis and interpretation of data, and the three of them carried out the HIV

WPP in the field. SDM drafted the manuscript while SM edited the first manuscript. Based in Geneva, LN and SAP supervised the HIV WPP and helped to draft and edit the manuscript. All authors read and approved the final manuscript.

Competing interests

The authors declare that they have no competing interests.

References

1. Suthar, AB, Ford N, Bachanas PJ, Wong VJ, Rajan JS, Saltzman AK, Baggaley RC. Towards Universal Voluntary HIV Testing and Counselling: A Systematic Review and Meta-Analysis of Community-Based Approaches. PLoS Med. 2013;10(8). doi:10.1371/journal.pmed.1001496
2. Liu Y, Canada K, Shi K, Corrigan P. HIV-related stigma acting as predictors of unemployment of people living with HIV/AIDS. AIDS Care: Psychological and Socio-medical Aspects of AIDS/HIV. 2012;24(1):29–135. doi:10.1080/09540121.2011.596512.
3. UNAIDS. UNAIDS report shows that 19 million of the 35 million people living with HIV today do not know that they have the virus. Geneva: UNAIDS; 2014. Retrieved from http://www.unaids.org/en/resources/presscentre/pressreleaseandstatementarchive/2014/july/20140716prgapreport.
4. Setswe G. Best practice workplace HIV/AIDS programmes in South Africa: A review of case studies and lessons learned. Afr J Prm Health Care Fam Med. 2009;1(1):82–7. doi:10.4102/phcfm.v1i1.30.
5. Taylor K, DeYoung P, Boldrini F. Business and HIV/AIDS: A Global Snapshot. World Economic Forum. 2004. Retrieved from http://www.popline.org/node/239437
6. Research Symposium University of the Witwatersrand. HIV/AIDS in the Workplace. 2004:3. Retrieved from http://www.wbs.ac.za/article/2004_publications
7. Sidibé M. The end of AIDS begins in the workplace. Geneva: UNAIDS; 2013. Retrieved from http://www.unaids.org/sites/default/files/en/media/unaids/contentassets/documents/speech/2013/06/20130606_SP_EXD_launch-VCTWork_en.pdf.
8. ICRC. Overview of operations. ICRC. 2014;p.13. Retrieved from https://www.icrc.org/eng/assets/files/other/icrc_overview_2004.pdf. International Federation of Red Cross and Red Crescent Societies. (2009).
9. International Labour Organization. An ILO code of practice on HIV/AIDS and the world of work. International Labour Organization. 2001. Retrieved from http://ilo.org/aids/Publications/WCMS_113783/lang–en/index.htm
10. International Labour Organization. Implementing the ILO Code of Practice on HIV/AIDS and the world of work: an education and training manual. International Labour Organization. 2002. Retrieved from http://www.ilo.org/global/publications/ilo-bookstore/orderonline/books/WCMS_PUBL_9221134628_EN/lang—en/index.htm
11. Hodges J. Guidelines on addressing HIV/AIDS in the workplace through employment and labour law. International Labour Organization. 2014. Retrieved from http://www.ilo.org/aids/Publications/WCMS_116658/lang–en/index.htm
12. International Labour Organization. Recommendation Concerning HIV and AIDS and the world of work. International Labour Organization. 2010. Retrieved from http://ilo.org/aids/WCMS_142706/lang–en/index.htm
13. International Organization for Standardization. ISO 26000, Guidance on social responsibility. 2011. Retrieved from http://www.iso.org/iso/catalogue_detail?csnumber=42546
14. Bakuwa R, Mamman A. Factors hindering the adoption of HIV/AIDS workplace policies: evidence from private sector companies in Malawi. The International Journal of Human Resource Management. 2012;23(14):2917–37. doi:10.1080/09585192.2012.671511.
15. Charalambousa S, Innesa C, Muirheada D, Kumaranayakeb L, Fielding K, Pemba L, PChurchyard GJ. Evaluation of a workplace HIV treatment programme in South Africa. AIDS. 2007;21 Suppl 3:S73–8. Retrieved from http://www.ncbi.nlm.nih.gov/pubmed/17666964.
16. Chimbetete M, Gwandure C. Impact of a Workplace-based HIV and AIDS Risk Reduction Training Intervention. J Hum Ecol. 2011;35(1):11–9. Retrieved from http://www.krepublishers.com/02-Journals/JHE/JHE-35-0-000-11-Web/JHE-35-1-000-11-Abst-PDF/JHE-35-1-011-11-2184-Chimbetete-M/JHE-35-1-011-11-2184-Chimbetete-M-Tt.pdf.
17. Feeley FG, Collier AC, Richards SC, Van den Borght SF, Rinke de Wit TF. A Successful Workplace Programme for Voluntary Counseling and Testing and Treatment of HIV/AIDS at Heineken, Rwanda. Int J Occup Environ Health. 2007;13:99–106. doi:10.1179/107735207800244910.
18. Gavin G. Workplace ART programmes: Why do companies invest in them and are they working? African Journal of AIDS research. 2006;5(2):179–88. Retrieved from http://www.ajol.info/index.php/ajar/article/view/7209.
19. Lim VK. Managing HIV, at the Workplace: An Empirical Study of HIV and HR Managers in Singapore. J Occup Health Psychol. 2003;8(4):235–46. doi:10.1037/1076-8998.8.4.235.
20. Population Council. Addressing HIV/AIDS Stigma and Discrimination in a Workplace Program: Emerging Findings. Population Council/Horizons. 2002. Retrieved from http://www.popcouncil.org/uploads/pdfs/horizons/eskombslnsum.pdf
21. Sexual Health Exchange. Addressing stigma. 2004. Retrieved from http://healthlink.org.za/uploads/files/she__2_04.pdf
22. Standards for HIV peer education programmes. IFRC. Retrieved from https://ifrc.org/Global/Publications/Health/hiv_peer_education-en.pdf
23. Brink B, Pienaar J. Business and HIV/AIDS: the case of Anglo American. AIDS. 2007;21 Suppl 3:S79–84. Retrieved from http://www.ncbi.nlm.nih.gov/pubmed/17666965.
24. Horwitz JR, Kelly BD, DiNardo JE. Wellness Incentives in The Workplace: Cost Savings Through Cost Shifting To Unhealthy Workers. Health Aff. 2013;32(3):468–76. doi:10.1377/hlthaff.2012.0683.
25. Weihs M, Meyer-Weitz, A. A lottery incentive system to facilitate dialogue and social support for workplace HIV counselling and testing: A qualitative inquiry. Journal of Social Aspects of HIV/AIDS. 2014. doi:10.1080/17290376.2014.937739
26. Ojo O, Verbeek JH, Rasanen K, Heikkinen J, Isotalo LK, Mngoma N, Ruotsalainen E. Interventions to reduce risky sexual behaviour for preventing HIV infection in workers in occupational settings. Cochrane Database Syst Rev. 2001;Issue 12. doi:10.1002/14651858.CD005274.pub3
27. Rispel LC, Peltzer K, Nkomo N, Molomo B. Evaluating an HIV and AIDS Community Training Partnership Programme in five diamond mining communities in South Africa. Evaluation and Programme Planning. 2010;33:394–402. doi:10.1016/j.evalprogplan.2010.02.001. Elsevier.
28. Vember HF. An Evaluation of the Influence of an HIV/AIDS Peer Education Programme at a Higher Education Institution in the Western Cape (Doctoral dissertation). Stellenbosch University, South Africa. 2003. Retrieved from http://scholar.sun.ac.za
29. Riviello ED, Sterling TR, Shepherd B, Fantan T, Makhema J. HIV in the Workplace in Botswana: Incidence, Prevalence, and Disease Severity. AIDS Res Hum Retroviruses. 2007;23(2):1453–9. doi:10.1089/aid.2007.0132.
30. Van der Borght SF, Rinke de Wit TF, Janssens V, van der Schim Loeff MF, Rijckborst H, Lange JM. HAART for the HIV-infected employees of large companies in Africa. Lancet. 2006;368:547–50. doi:10.1016/S0140-6736(06)69165-4.
31. Van der Borght SF, Clevenbergh P, Rijckborts H, Nsalou P, Onyia N, Lange JM, van der Schim Loeff MS. Mortality and morbidity among HIV type 1-infected patients during the first 5 years of a multicountry HIV workplace programme in Africa. Antivir Ther. 2009;14:63–74. Retrieved in http://www.researchgate.net/publication/24233127_Mortality_and_morbidity_among_HIV_type-1-infected_patients_during_the_first_5_years_of_a_multicountry_HIV_workplace_programme_in_Africa/file/79e4150e826d8205cd.pdf.
32. Van der Borght SF, van der Schim Loeff MF, Clevenbergh P, Kabarega JP, Kamo E, van Cranenburgh KP, de Rinke Wit TF. Long-term voluntary counseling and testing (VCT) uptake dynamics in a multicountry HIV workplace programme in sub-Saharan Africa. AIDS Care: Psychological and Socio-medical Aspects of AIDS/HIV. 2010;22(2):195–205. doi:10.1080/09540120903111486.
33. George G, Surgey G, Gow J. South Africa's Private Sector Investment in Training and its Erosion as a Results of HIV and AIDS. SAJEMS. 2014;2:109–23. Retrieved from http://reference.sabinet.co.za/sa_epublication_article/ecoman_v17_n2_a1.
34. Scott K, Campbell C, Skovdal M, Madanhire C, Nyamukapa C, Gregson S. What can companies do to support HIV-positive workers? Recommendations for medium- and large-sized African workplaces. International Journal of Workplace Health Management. 2013;6(3):174–88. doi:10.1108/IJWHM-12-2010-0043.
35. Thomas EP, Colvin M, Rosen SB, Zuccarini C, Petzer S. HIV Prevalence Study and Costing Analysis undertaken for the development of an HIV/AIDS

Workplace Strategy for Buffalo City Municipality. The Medical ResearchCouncil. 2005. Retrieved from http://wiredspace.wits.ac.za/handle/10539/3939
36. Connelly P, Rosen R. Treatment for HIV/AIDS at South Africa's largest employers: myth and reality. S Afr Med J. 2006;96:128–33. Retrieved from http://www.ncbi.nlm.nih.gov/pubmed/16532081.
37. Mooketsi ML. Factors Preventing the Uptake of HIV Counseling and Testing (HCT) Programmes: The Case of the Industrial Development Corporationin Johannesburg, South Africa (Master's thesis). Stellenbosh University, South Africa.2014. Retrieved from http://scholar.sun.ac.za
38. George G, Quinlan T. 'Health Management' in the Private Sector in the Context of HIV/AIDS: Progress and Challenges Faced by Company Programmes in South Africa. Sust. Dev. 2008. doi: 10.1002/sd.366
39. Ishikawa J. Key Features of National Social Dialogue: A Social Dialogue Ressource Book. International Labour Organization. 2003. Retrieved from http://www.newunionism.net/library/internationalism/ILO%20-%20A%20Social%20Dialogue%20Resource%20Book%20-%202003.pdf

16

A case of Methyl Ethyl Ketone Peroxide poisoning and a review of complications and their management

Isurujith K. Liyanage[1,2*], Mitrakrishnan R. Navinan[1], A C A Pathirana[1], H R I S Herath[1], Jevon Yudhishdran[1], Nilesh Fernandopulle[1] and Aruna Kulatunga[1]

Abstract

Methyl Ethyl Ketone Peroxide (MEKP) is a highly toxic clear liquid used as a solvent. It is a strong oxidizing agent and a corrosive. Acute and chronic toxicity can occur as an occupational hazard. Ingestion is associated with corrosive burns leading to stricture formation, inhalational pneumonitis, acidosis, liver failure and renal failure. In this paper we present a case of a young patient who intentionally ingested MEKP. The patient developed multiple complications including proximal intestinal obstruction, acidosis and acute kidney injury. He was managed conservatively and recovered after a prolonged hospital stay. He had multiple inflammatory strictures on esophageal endoscopy, which improved over 3–6 moths.

Keywords: Methyl Ethyl Ketone Peroxide, Management of corrosive gastrointestinal burns, Occupational safety

Background

Methyl Ethyl Ketone Peroxide (MEKP) is used as a hardener in manufacture of resins, synthetic rubber and other petrochemical plastics. It is an ingredient of paints, varnishes and paint removers. MEKP is also used in fiberglass and plastics industry as a curing agent. It is an organic peroxide, which is explosive in its pure form. Hence it is commercially available as a 40-60 % solution with stabilizing agents such as dimethyl phthalate, cyclohexane peroxide, or diallyl phthalate [1, 2].

MEKP is listed as a highly toxic substance and is categorized into United Nations Hazard class 5.2. [3]. Its colorless nature and minimal odor has led to accidental ingestion both among adults and children [4, 5]. Several cases of intentional ingestion for self-harm or suicide have been reported [6]. In addition, poisoning by inhalation and spillage to eyes leading to corrosive damage has also been reported. Unprotected workers are victims of chronic exposure and toxicity [7].

Commercially available preparations of MEKP are strong oxidizing substances. They are known to produce alkylperoxyl radicals upon contact with metal ions, a process accelerated by the presence of iron in the heme molecule in biological systems. Tissue damage is believed to be caused by these free radicals, which denature organic molecules, including peroxidation of lipids. Further toxicity is caused by the acidity of the chemicals produced [8].

In a case report and review of literature, van Enckevort et. al described the clinical features of acute intoxication in four categories. These include inflammation and ulceration of exposed gastrointestinal tract, acute oxidative liver injury, complications of formation of organic acids including metabolic acidosis and secondary acute complications. Secondary complications include acute renal failure secondary to rhabdomyolysis, ventilator assisted pneumonia, myocarditis and acute respiratory distress syndrome [9].

Acute gastrointestinal (GI) injury has been observed in all documented case reports. It can lead to bleeding or perforation of the GI tract which is potentially fatal [10]. Severe pain due to chemical burns will develop soon after ingestion. The extent of injuries visible on mouth and oropharynx are known to be poor predictors of distal injuries. The presence of stridor, odynophagia (pain on swallowing), abdominal guarding and rigidity however, indicate the presence of distal GI injuries [11]. Long

* Correspondence: isurujith@gmail.com
[1]National Hospital of Sri Lanka, Colombo 10, Sri Lanka
[2]Department of Pharmacology, Faculty of Medical Sciences, University of Sri Jayewardenepura, Nugegoda, Sri Lanka

term problems such as esophageal strictures requiring multiple endoscopic dilatations has been reported [5]. Liver failure due to oxidative hepatocyte injury is the most significant single cause of mortality in the previous case reports [4, 9, 12, 13]. Reversible acute kidney injury (AKI) has been reported in almost a third of published case studies. This is mainly attributed to rhabdomyolysis and myoglobinuria [14]. MEKP can be aspirated resulting in proximal airway edema and obstruction, pneumonitis or acute respiratory distress syndrome [15]. Respiratory complications have been seen frequently (38 %) and has also been a direct cause for documented fatality [9].

Case report

The patient was a 31-year-old healthy male who is self-employed in the shipping industry as a repairman of fiberglass boats. After consuming half a bottle of locally produced arrack (alcohol 38 % W/w) he ingested an estimated volume of 150 ml of MEKP containing solvent (60 % MEKP in phthalate solution) as an act of deliberate self-harm. He was unaware of the level of toxicity of the substance.

The patient developed severe throat and epigastric discomfort soon after ingestion. He was admitted to a regional hospital where he was given activated charcoal. A nasogastric tube was inserted in anticipation of erosive complications. Over the next 24 hours, his symptoms progressed with worsening irritation of the throat, development of abdominal pain, difficulty in breathing and noticeably reduced urine output. He was transferred to our tertiary care unit for further management of progressive multi organ involvement.

On general examination he was alert and coherent with Glasgow coma scale score of 15. There were multiple ulcerations in his mouth and oropharyngeal region. Nasogastric tube contents revealed coffee ground aspirate. Respiratory examination revealed rapid shallow breathing with a respiratory rate of 40 per minute. Auscultation of the lungs was unremarkable and oxygen saturation was 99 % on room air on pulse oxymetry. He was tachycardic (heart rate:104 beats per minute) with normal blood pressure and adequate peripheral perfusion. Severe guarding and tenderness over the epigastrium was present in examination of the abdomen. Bowel sounds were sluggish.

Preliminary investigations revealed progressively rising serum creatinine and blood urea. He had a neutrophil leukocytosis (Table 1). Arterial blood gas analysis showed a high anion gap metabolic acidosis with a pH of 7.21. Serum potassium was elevated at 6.4 mmol/L, which persisted through the first week of hospital stay. Ultrasound scan of the abdomen showed normal sized kidneys with evidence of acute renal failure. Subsequent complete blood counts showed a reducing trend in hemoglobin and platelets. Bite cells, Heinz bodies and fragmented red cells were also seen. Serum lactate dehydrogenase level was elevated. Direct Coombs test was negative. The reticulocyte count was 1.5 % showing an inadequate bone marrow response. Hemolysis settled by the second week of the illness.

The patient was managed in the ward. Acute management included intravenous sodium bicarbonate to correct acidosis and medical management of hyperkalemia. Urgent hemodialysis was followed by regular renal replacement therapy for the next four weeks. Repeated blood transfusions (8 units during the first week) were required to maintain hemoglobin levels.

Gastric protection was instituted with intravenous proton pump inhibitors. Parenteral feeding was initiated due to intolerance of oral feeds. On third day the patient developed large volume coffee ground aspirate through

Table 1 Basic investigations

	Reference range	D2	2nd week	3rd week	D28
Creatinine (umol/L)	60-120	366	706	800	253
Hemoglobin (g/dl)	-	12.2	4.4	7.5	12.1
Platelets $10^3/mm^3$	150-450	49	87	170	245
White cell count $10^3/mm^3$	4-11	12.9	22.2	5.3	8.2
AST (U/l)	10-35	611	212	24	29
ALT (U/l)	10-40	527	252	8	19
ALP (U/l)	100-360	105	143	129	-
Total Bilirubin (umol/L)	5-21	29	18	8	-
Direct Bilirubin	<3.4	25	14	5	
Urine RBC /hpf	-	>100		10 to 15	0
Urine pus cells /hpf	-	4 to 6		Field full	2 to 3
LDH (U/L)	140-280		812	643	343
Creatine Kinase (U/L)	25-174	457			

AST Aspartate transaminase, *ALT* alanine transaminase, *ALP* alkaline phosphatase, *RBC* red blood cells, *hpf* high power field, *LDH* Lactate dehydrogenase

the NG tube, which later became bilious. This heralded distal duodenal obstruction, which was confirmed by a gastrografin study. This resolved after 2 weeks and liquid feeds were gradually started as tolerated. However, he had persistent odynophagia. Upper gastrointestinal endoscopy performed on day 28 revealed inflammatory lesions extending from upper esophagus to duodenum. There were slough, exudate and fibrotic bands but significant stricture formation was not seen (Fig. 1).

The patient was discharged on the 29th day. He was tolerating semisolid diet despite having persisting odynophagia. He had lost 4.7 kg during his hospital stay. His follow up plan included a repeat endoscopic assessment in 3 months time, psychiatric assessment and follow up with the medical unit. He was also referred to the dietitian for nutritional support and supervision.

By his first review in 2 weeks the renal functions had returned to baseline. First follow up endoscopy at 3 months revealed slough, which was cleared by the passage of the endoscope. This resulted in temporary relief of odynophagia. However it recurred and the odynophagia persisted for six months. At 6-month review he was tolerating normal feeds with only slight discomfort. He has lost further 7 kg (weight on admission 68 kg) but features of other nutritional deficiencies were not present. One year after ingestion, he was asymptomatic and was gaining weight.

Discussion

Lethal limit of MEKP is estimated to be 50–100 ml for adults (Lethal dose in rats: 65 mg/kg) [16]. The patient in this case study consumed a lethal dose of MEKP and developed most of the local and systemic complications of ingestion. Different management strategies have been tried in the past for acute poisoning. Almost all of these have been supportive until tissue damage and organ dysfunction recovers spontaneously.

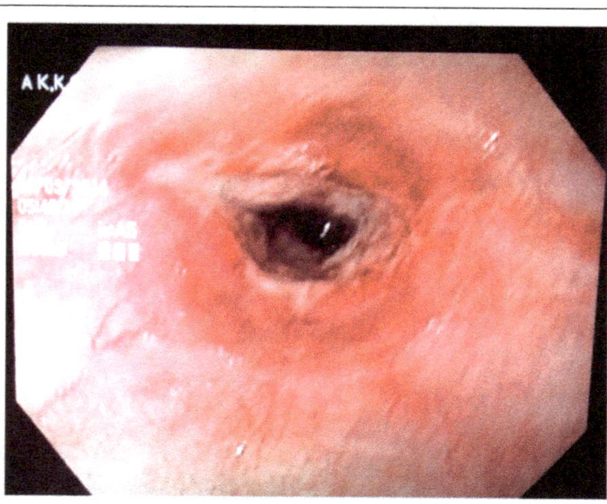

Fig. 1 Fibrotic bands seen in upper gastrointestinal endoscopy on the 28th day

MEKP is a potent oxidizing agent and antioxidant properties of vitamin E has been shown to be of benefit in rat models [17]. However there are no clinical data to support their use in acute poisoning [14].

Following ingestion of MEKP, the mouth should be rinsed with water. Drinking large volumes of milk or water to dilute the gastric contents has been practiced. It is advisable to continue of oral feeds as tolerated unless perforation is suspected [14]. Baseline investigations recommended are full blood count, renal functions, liver functions, arterial blood gas analysis, creatine kinase and coagulation profile. First line imaging includes plain X-ray films of the neck, chest and abdomen as clinically indicated. Intraluminal air shadows, air in the fascial planes, pleural effusions, and gas under diaphragm are X-ray features supporting gastrointestinal perforation [18]. Endoscopic evaluation is recommended within the first 24 hours of ingestion and may be beneficial up to 96 hours [19, 12]. After the initial 48–96 hours however, upper gastroesophageal endoscopy (UGE) should be avoided until after 2 weeks due to wound softening which can lead to perforation [11]. If perforation is suspected oral water soluble contrast studies (gastrografin) can be used to confirm and locate the site [18]. If perforated and severe continuous leakage of bowel contents is present surgical intervention may be needed.

This patient developed acute transient proximal intestinal obstruction, which spontaneously resolved over the first two weeks. This could have been due to mucosal edema due to the injuries. In the absence of esophageal perforation, insertion of nasogastric tube before the onset of edema was useful in managing this patient. It helped to identify obstruction when continuous bilious aspiration was noted. It also allowed continuation of enteral feeding when persistent odynophagia prevented the patient from tolerating oral feeds. Hence we recommend early insertion of a nasogastric tube within the first 24 hours unless severe edema or ulceration precludes its use. To prevent further GI injury, proton pump blockers should be used.

Delayed fibrosis and stricture formation leading to intestinal obstruction is one of the main long-term complications of corrosive ingestion as seen in this case of MEKP poisoning. This can occur up to one year after ingestion. This patient had multiple inflamed areas of sloughing in the first esophageal endoscopy, which indicated the possibility of long-term fibrosis and luminal narrowing. Endoscopic dilatation is needed to relieve the strictures if present. Further, endoscopic intra-lesional steroid injections are postulated to augment the affects of endoscopic dilatation and may reduce further fibrosis [13, 20]. However, evidence for use of steroid injections is minimal and recommendations vary widely. As the lesions were superficial, the gastroenterology team decided not to give intra-lesional steroid injections to our patient. Patients should be followed up after discharge to monitor for features of obstruction. In our patient, the follow up endoscopic examination itself cleared the inflammatory fibrotic bands producing dramatic improvement of his swallowing difficulty.

If swallowing difficulty is present, providing adequate long-term nutrition under the supervision of a specialist nutritionist is recommended. This patient had significant weight loss despite being on high protein diet until dysphagia and odynophagia improved. A weight gain was only noted after 9 to 12 months. If swallowing difficulty persists and impedes nutritional supplementation, endoscopic esophageal dilatation or esophageal resection is recommended [14].

Oxidative liver injury can be theoretically minimized or prevented by administration of N-acetyl cysteine (NAC) [21]. This should be administered within the first 24 hours of ingestion. One case study reports successful use of NAC as a liver protective agent [9]. However further evidence is needed to confirm its effectiveness.

Aspiration and other respiratory complications can be minimized by not inducing emesis. Aspiration if occurs should be managed symptomatically with supportive measures. Acute renal failure may necessitate repeated renal replacement therapy. There is minimal evidence to compare continuous renal replacement therapy with conventional dialysis and both methods have been used successfully [22].

Hematological complications such as bleeding, hemolysis and disseminated intravascular coagulation have been reported [9, 6]. Anemia in this patient was multifactorial, contributed by hemolysis, inadequate bone marrow response and gastrointestinal bleeding. Although continuing hemolysis was a possibility, coffee ground like NG aspirate and very low hemoglobin with symptoms of anemia warranted transfusions during the first weeks of treatment.

Conclusions

MEKP is a potentially lethal industrial chemical. Acute poisoning can occur due to accidental or intentional ingestion. Ingestion can affect multiple organ systems, leading to short and long term morbidity. These include gastrointestinal burn injuries with stricture formation, acute liver failure, rhabdomyolysis, renal failure and metabolic acidosis. Management is mainly supportive. Careful monitoring for these complications with prompt intervention when they occur can save lives. Users of these chemicals may be unaware of the potential hazards. There is a need to increase the awareness on potential toxicity and safety measures among the handlers of these uncommon toxic substances.

Consent

Informed written consent has been obtained from the patient for publication of this article and associated data and images.

Competing interests
Authors of this case study do not have competing interests.

Authors' contributions
This paper is written by the medical team who managed this patient. All authors contributed in literature review and case discussion. AK was the consultant physician (MD, FRCS) and team leader who supervised this case study. NF (MD, MRCS) is the consultant gastroenterologist. All authors read and approved the final manuscript.

References

1. Gooch JW. Methyl Ethyl Ketone Peroxide. Encyclopedic Dictionary of Polymers. 2011:458-.
2. Barbalace K. Chemical Database: Methyl ethyl ketone peroxide. Environmental Chemistry com. 2009.
3. Eller PM, Cassinelli ME. NIOSH manual of analytical methods. DIANE Publishing; 1994.
4. Prez-Martnez A, Gutirrez-Junquera C, Gonzlvez-Piera J, Marco-Macin A, Rubio-Guijarro J, Moya-Marchante M. Oesophageal stenosis in a child caused by ingestion of methyl ethyl ketone peroxide. European journal of pediatrics. 1997;156(12):976.
5. Bates N, Driver CP, Bianchi A. Methyl ethyl ketone peroxide ingestion: toxicity and outcome in a 6-year-old child. Pediatrics. 2001;108(2):473–6.
6. Mittleman RE, Romig LA, Gressmann E. Suicide by ingestion of methyl ethyl ketone peroxide. Journal of forensic sciences. 1986;31(1):312–20.
7. Brigham CR, Landrigan PJ. Safety and health in boatbuilding and repair. American journal of industrial medicine. 1985;8(3):169–82.
8. Akaike T, Sato K, Ijiri S, Miyamoto Y, Kohno M, Ando M, et al. Bactericidal activity of alkyl peroxyl radicals generated by heme-iron-catalyzed decomposition of organic peroxides. Archives of biochemistry and biophysics. 1992;294(1):55–63.
9. Van Enckevort C, Touw D, Vleming L-J. N-acetylcysteine and hemodialysis treatment of a severe case of methyl ethyl ketone peroxide intoxication. Clinical toxicology. 2008;46(1):74–8.
10. Moon SW, Lee SW, Choi SH, Hong YS. Gastric emphysema after methyl ethyl ketone peroxide ingestion. Clinical toxicology. 2010;48(1):90–1. doi:10.3109/15563650903478315.
11. Jain AL, Robertson GJ, Rudis MI. Surgical issues in the poisoned patient. Emergency medicine clinics of North America. 2003;21(4):1117–44.
12. De Jong A, Macdonald R, Ein S, Forte V, Turner A. Corrosive esophagitis in children: a 30-year review. International journal of pediatric otorhinolaryngology. 2001;57(3):203–11.
13. Kochhar R, Ray JD, Sriram PV, Kumar S, Singh K. Intralesional steroids augment the effects of endoscopic dilation in corrosive esophageal strictures. Gastrointestinal endoscopy. 1999;49(4):509–13.
14. Farrow C. Guy's and St Thomas' Hospital Trust. Chemical Incident Response Service. The chemical incident management handbook. Chemical incident management series. London: Stationery Office; 2000.
15. Bozdemir M, Yildiz M, Seyhanlı E, Gurbuz S, Kilicaslan I, Karlidag T. Narrowing of airway caused by ingestion of methyl ethyl ketone peroxide. Human & experimental toxicology. 2011;30(12):2002–6.
16. Patnaik P. A comprehensive guide to the hazardous properties of chemical substances. John Wiley & Sons; 2007.
17. Litov R, Matthews L, Tappel A. Vitamin E protection against in vivo lipid peroxidation initiated in rats by methyl ethyl ketone peroxide as monitored by pentane. Toxicology and applied pharmacology. 1981;59(1):96–106.
18. Kaman L, Iqbal J, Kundil B, Kochhar R. Management of esophageal perforation in adults. Gastroenterology Research. 2011;3(6):235–44.
19. Erdoğan E, Eroğlu E, Tekant G, Yeker Y, Emir H, Sarimurat N, et al. Management of esophagogastric corrosive injuries in children. European journal of pediatric surgery: official journal of Austrian Association of Pediatric Surgery [et al] = Zeitschrift fur Kinderchirurgie. 2003;13(5):289–93.

20. Anderson KD, Rouse TM, Randolph JG. A controlled trial of corticosteroids in children with corrosive injury of the esophagus. New England Journal of Medicine. 1990;323(10):637–40.
21. Chyka PA, Butler AY, Holliman BJ, Herman MI. Utility of acetylcysteine in treating poisonings and adverse drug reactions. Drug safety. 2000;22(2):123–48.
22. Goodman JW, Goldfarb DS, editors. The role of continuous renal replacement therapy in the treatment of poisoning. Seminars in dialysis; 2006: Wiley Online Library.

17

Hepatitis C among healthcare personnel: secondary data analyses of costs and trends for hepatitis C infections with occupational causes

Claudia Westermann[1*], Madeleine Dulon[2], Dana Wendeler[2] and Albert Nienhaus[1,2]

Abstract

Background: Hepatitis C infection is a global public health issue. Chronic hepatitis C infection is associated with significant morbidity and mortality. The aim of this study is to describe the costs for occupationally-cased hepatitis C infections based on data from an accident insurance carrier.

Methods: This study is a secondary analysis based on the Database of a German Institution for Statutory Accident Insurance. The analysis is based on a sample of insured parties whose hepatitis C infections were recorded as occupational diseases between 1996 and 2013. The analysis is based on recognised hepatitis C cases and incorporates records registered between 1 January 2000 and 31 December 2014.

Results: Within the study period, the number of reported and recognised hepatitis C cases declined by 73 and 86% respectively. The majority of recognised hepatitis C cases ($n = 1.121$) were female, older than 40 years and were active in a medical nursing profession. In the study period, the costs came to a total of € 87.9 million, of which 60% was attributable to pension payments (€ 51,570,830) and around 15% was attributable to pharmaceutical and medicinal products (€ 12,978,318). Expenses for drugs exhibited heavy increases in 2012 (from around € 500,000–800,000 to € 1.7 million) and 2014 (to € 2.5 million) in particular. Pension payments came to € 1.6 million in 2000 and rose continuously to over € 4 million in 2014. Expenses for occupational rehabilitation accounted for less than 1%.

Conclusions: For hepatitis C infections as an occupational disease, a considerable increase in costs has been observed in recent years, while the number of reports has declined heavily. This rise in costs is explained by the increase in pension payments and, since 2012, by a rise in the costs for drugs. The high costs of anti-viral therapies is offset by the potential for considerable treatment benefits. Healing the infection is expected to generate long-term cost savings for statutory accident insurance carriers, and also for social security systems.

Keywords: Hepatitis C virus, Occupational disease, Healthcare personnel, Burden of disease, Secondary data analysis

* Correspondence: c.westermann@uke.de
[1]University Medical Center Hamburg-Eppendorf (UKE), Center of Excellence for Health Services Research in Nursing (CVcare), Hamburg, Germany
Full list of author information is available at the end of the article

Background

The viral disease hepatitis C (HCV) is globally one of the most common infectious diseases. The hepatitis C RNA virus is transmitted from person to person, primarily through contact with infected blood while the skin or mucosa is also injured [1]. Healthcare personnel are at greater risk of HCV infection due to the nature of their occupational duties [2]. The progression of the infection is often non-specific, which is why the infection often remains undetected. Up to 85% of infections are chronic (HCV-RNA positive longer than six months). According to data from the World Health Organisation (WHO), around 150 million people globally have chronic hepatitis C (CHC); 700,000 people die each year as a result [1, 3, 4]. CHC is associated with a high level of morbidity and a diminished quality of life. Up to 68% of patients suffer from symptoms including fatigue, exhaustion, limited performance and subclinical cognitive impairment. CHC is also associated with an increased risk for developing cirrhosis of the liver and hepatocellular carcinoma [4, 5]. A variety of extrahepatic manifestations may also develop. The development of depression symptoms, diabetes mellitus and malignant lymphoproliferative disorders such as follicular non-Hodgkin lymphoma are associated with HCV. Several studies have also indicated impairment of certain central nervous functions and neurotransmission [4]. US scientists have calculated the costs for the US healthcare system associated with CHC on the basis of data from a private health insurance company. They (retrospectively) studied the insurance data of 53,796 CHC patients over a period of eight years (2002–2010), according to which the average cost attributable to CHC per patient, per year was $ 24,176 (approx. € 21,776). Stratified according to stages of the disease, these costs increase as the disease progresses, reaching their peak in patients with terminal cirrhosis of the liver ($ 59,995/€ 53,880 per patient, per year) [6]. According to estimates, the share of patients with manifest liver disease will quadruple over the next 20 years without effective treatment [7]. Due to the potentially severe progression of the disease and the high associated costs, successful treatment of CHC is important [3, 6, 7]. The use of second-generation direct anti-viral agents (DAAs) today provide promising treatment combinations. Treatment of a CHC infection is considered successful if RNA viruses (HCV-RNA) can no longer be detected in the blood between 12 and 24 weeks after treatment is concluded [4, 5, 8]. As initial publications have shown, interferon-free DAA treatments have achieved substantial sustained virological response rates (SVRs) of over 90% in both treatment-naive and treatment-experienced patients with CHC infections. Such treatments are shorter than previous interferon-based therapies, have fewer side effects, and are currently a recommended course of treatment for HCV infections [3, 4].

The purpose of this study is to illustrate the costs for occupational hepatitis C infections based on data of the Institution for Statutory Accident Insurance and Prevention in the Health and Welfare Services (Berufsgenossenschaft für Gesundheitsdienst und Wohlfahrtspflege, BGW) for the period from 2000 to 2014.

Methods

This study is reported in line with A Consensus German Reporting Standard for Secondary Data Analyses, Version 2 (STROSA) [9].

Secondary data from BGW were used to analyse the costs of occupational HCV infections. BGW's occupational disease routine data records (BK-DOK) were used as a data source.

Occupational disease procedure

In Germany, if there is reasonable cause to suspect an occupational disease (OD), physicians are required to submit a report. Reports of suspected ODs may also be submitted by health insurers, employers, representatives of company interests or parties insured with the statutory accident insurance carriers. The statutory accident insurance carriers will follow an investigative procedure to determine whether a disease is an OD as defined by the Occupational Disease Ordinance (*Berufskrankheiten-Verordnung*, BKV) (Section 9, para. 1 & 2 of the German Social Security Code VII). A fully documented connection must be established here between the insured activity and the damaging exposure. The disease must also be fully documented. There must be a probable causal relationship between the exposure and the disease.

In the case of infectious diseases, the exposure is often difficult to identify, which is why it is sufficient to prove that duties have been performed that are associated with an elevated risk of infection. The performance of surgery and contact with blood would be an example of such a hazardous activity with an elevated risk for blood-borne viral diseases. An occupational infectious disease can either be classified as an insurance claim without entitlement to pension disbursement (if the reduced work ability –RWA- is less than 20%), or an entitlement to pension disbursement can be recognised. If there is already a 10% RWA from a previous insurance claim, a new 10% RWA can give rise to a pension disbursement entitlement. In cases where the OD suspicion has not been proven, a rejection is issued.

Documentation of OD reports

The key features of an OD suspicion report are registered in a standardised fashion in BK-DOK. OD suspicion reports are fundamentally registered as reportable if there are indications of an infection. This applies irrespective of which decision is taken under insurance law in the investigative procedure later. Because the investigative procedure is time-consuming and a decision may not be taken in the year of the OD report, the cases ruled upon in a given reporting year can contain suspicion reports from previous years.

Analysis

The analysis of the BK-DOK is based on data from insured parties whose HCV infections were reported as suspected ODs between 1996 and 2013. The sample was acquired from the "Insurance Claims" database, which contains not only fundamental personal data but also other details (including sociodemographic features such as sex, year of birth, industry, profession, diagnostic information, year of registration, first and most recent decision, year of decision, OD-triggering circumstances, insurance claim reference number, etc.) The "Compensation Payments" database provided data on expenses incurred on behalf of the insured for drugs and benefits related to medical and occupational rehabilitation.

Analysis of reduced work ability [RWA]

The RWA classification may change over the course of the disease, depending on the severity of the disease at any given time. The level of impairment and the dates on which it starts and ends are documented for each change in RWA. The analysis of the RWA is based on data from 1996 to 2014 and relates to the first established RWA and the current RWA (as of 31 December 2014). For the presentation of changes in the RWA, CHC patients were sorted according to the current RWA (as of the analysis date) and grouped according to the year of registration of the OD (in five-year groups). Distribution of current RWAs in the respective accident registration periods is presented using percentiles.

Because data on compensation payments have only been collected and processed since 2000, only registrations falling between 1 January 2000 and 31 December 2014 are reflected. The registration titles were grouped and reduced from 100 down to nine categories. In order to represent changes in compensation payments, we have allocated costs to medical rehabilitation (medicines, pharmaceuticals, inpatient and outpatient treatment), occupational rehabilitation (phased return, retraining, etc.) and pension payments (Fig. 2). The results are presented descriptively (absolute and relative frequencies), and the incurred costs are added together over a reporting period of 15 years.

Data on insured parties is provided from within BGW by the Rehabilitation Coordination department. It is derived from the standardised occupational diseases records and is analysed in anonymised form. Data were acquired

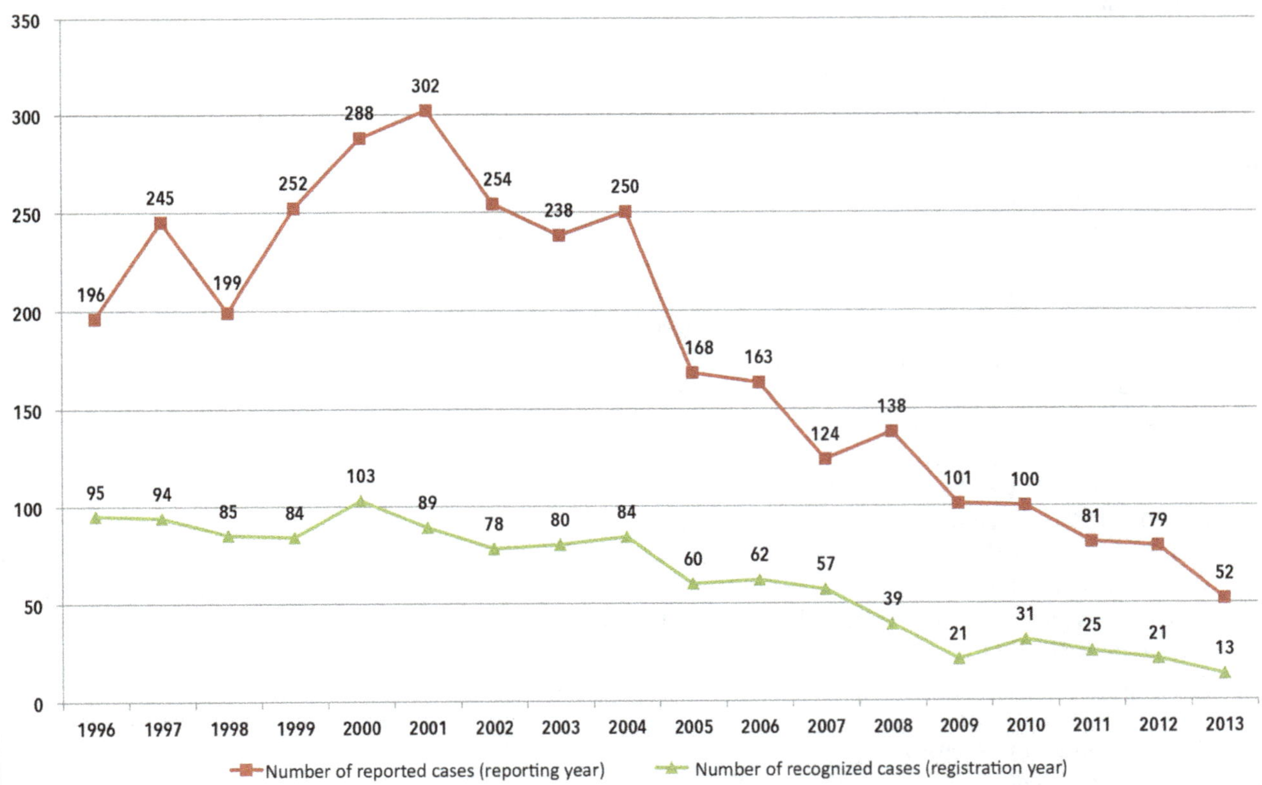

Fig. 1 Changes in mandatory reports for suspected hepatitis C and in recognised hepatitis C cases according to registration/reporting year (1996–2013, BGW data)

in accordance with data protection regulations and with the agreement of the BGW Data Protection Officer. The data was analysed using the statistics software SPSS version 23.

Results

In 1996 to 2013, a total of 3230 reports of suspected cases of occupational HCV diseases were registered with BGW. In the same period, infections were recognised as ODs for 1121 insured parties. Across the study period, the number of reported and recognised cases declined by 73 and 86% respectively (Fig. 1).

Description of the sample (OD cases)

OD reports identified 1121 insured parties with an occupational HCV. Mainly affected were female, older than 40 years of age and employed in hospitals. Over 90% of the insured were engaged in a medical or nursing occupation at the time that they developed the disease (Table 1).

In the period under analysis, 42 deaths were recorded as the result of an OD. Of those, one person was under 30 years of age, 16 (43%) were between 30 and 60 years of age, while 25 (55%) were over the age of 61. The majority of them (67%) were employed in hospitals, with just 21% working in doctor's practices and 11% in residential geriatric care or rehabilitation clinics (no table).

Table 1 Description of the sample of insured parties with a recognised hepatitis C infection according to sociodemographic characteristics and the degree of reduced work ability (RWA) first established ($n = 1121$)

Characteristics	N	%
Sex, female	838	75
Age (years)[a]		
< 20	17	1
21–40	335	30
41–60	646	58
> 61	123	11
Field of work		
Clinic/hospital	510	46
Doctor's practice	341	30
Geriatric care/nursing	131	12
Outpatient/social welfare services	79	7
Administration	60	5
Occupation		
Physician	195	17
Nurse	473	42
Medical assistant	266	24
Geriatric care assistant	84	8
Medical personnel	31	3
Administration	36	3
Social worker	19	2
Domestic services	17	1
RWA as %[b]		
No RWA	342	30
RWA <20	3	0.4
RWA 20	493	63.2
RWA 30	127	16.3
RWA 40	64	8.2
RWA 50	35	4.5
RWA 60–80	37	4.7
RWA 100	20	2.6
Total	1121	100

[a]Age at the time of registration of the ODs reports
[b]Values relate to RWA as first established

Reduced work ability [RWA]

A total of 70% of insured parties ($n = 779$) had an initial documented RWA in the analysis period from 1996 to 2014. The distribution of the degrees of RWA is shown in Table 1. In 57% of cases, the RWA did not increase during the period of their disease. In just under 40% of cases, there were between two and four changes; only a few had more than five changes. In one case, the RWA changed twelve times.

Of 1121 cases, 75% had no RWA (as of the analysis date of 31 December 2014) (Table 2). These include insured parties who died in the period under analysis (1996 to 2013, $n = 52$). A RWA was established for 779 insured parties over the course of the disease, although a RWA was only in effect for 279 insured parties on the analysis date, showing that 64% of the CHC patients only had a temporary RWA (500 of 779). Breaking down the entire reference period into four intervals shows only minor differences in the RWA grade. Only the 95th percentile and the maximum RWA are higher for cases registered before 2011 than for cases between 2011 and 2013 (40 versus 30% and 100 versus 50%).

Description of changes in expenses

Table 3 lists the payments and number of postings registered. For 98% of the recognised HCV cases, at least one posting was registered during the period of 15 years ($n =$ 1097). Most postings were attributable to outpatient treatments (40%) and pension disbursements (37%). In the period under analysis, compensation payments came to € 87.9 million, of which just under 60% were attributable to pension payments (€ 51,570,830) and around 15% to expenses for pharmaceuticals and other medicines (€ 12,978,318).

Compensation payments for medical rehabilitation (pharmaceuticals and other medicines), occupational rehabilitation (phased returns, retraining, etc.) and pensions

Table 2 Documented reduced work ability (RWA) as of the analysis date 31 December 2014 grouped by period of occupational disease (OD) registration

RWA as %	Year of OD registration (grouped)									
	1996 to 2000		2001 to 2005		2006 to 2010		2011 to 2013		Total	
	N	%	N	%	N	%	N	%	N	%
No RWA[a]	357	77	289	74	154	73	42	71	842	75
010	1	0	0	0	1	0	0	0	2	0
020	58	13	53	14	26	12	11	19	148	13
030	15	3	20	5	13	6	4	7	52	5
040	9	2	7	2	5	2	0	0	21	2
050	9	2	5	1	7	3	2	3	23	2
060	4	1	7	2	1	0	0	0	12	1
070	5	1	4	1	0	0	0	0	9	1
080	1	0	1	0	1	0	0	0	3	0
100	2	0	5	1	2	1	0	0	9	1
Total	461	100	391	100	210	100	59	100	1,121	100
P 75	0		20		20		20		0	
P 95	40		40		40		30		40	
Max	100		100		100		50		100	

[a]Total deaths $n = 52$, of which 42 resulting from occupational disease (1996–2000 $n = 18$; 2001–2005 $n = 14$; 2006–2010 $n = 8$; 2011–2013 $n = 2$); not resulting from occupational disease (1996–2000 $n = 6$; 2001–2005 $n = 3$; 2006–2010 $n = 1$)

have developed differently over the 15-year period under review (Fig. 2). Annual expenses rose from € 2.6 million to € 6.3 million between 2000 and 2005, remaining at an annual € 6 million between 2005 and 2010 before then rising to € 7.3 million and € 8.3 million in 2012 and 2014 respectively. In all years except 2014, payments for medical rehabilitation accounted for around one third, while expenses for pensions accounted for around two thirds of the costs. In 2014 on the other hand, expenses for medical rehabilitation accounted for around half of expenditure. Pension payments came to € 1.6 million in 2000 and rose continuously to over € 4 million in 2014. Benefits aimed at enabling involvement in working life (occupational rehabilitation) accounted for less than 1% in all years.

Drugs for the treatment of hepatitis C

For the sample of recognised HCV cases, expenses for drugs of € 255,730 in 2000 first rose continuously to around € 1 million and remained at this level until 2010, with the exception of 2007 (Fig. 3). A clear rise in expenses for drugs was recorded for 2012 (to around € 1.7 million) and 2014 (to around € 2.5 million). Relative to

Table 3 Accounting entry descriptions (grouped) according to number of cases, number of postings and expenses for recognised HCV cases – added together from 2000 to 2014; sorted by percentage share of total costs

Entry descriptions	Number of cases	Number of entries (%)	Expenses in	
			€	%s
Pensions	862	69,585 (37)	51,570,830	59
Pharmaceuticals and other medicines from pharmacies	619	9,897 (5)	12,978,318	14
Injury compensation, care allowances and other treatment costs	586	10,397 (6)	8,461,788	10
Inpatient treatment	543	1,669 (1)	5,460,608	6
Outpatient treatment (including treatment costs by physician)	921	74,376 (40)	4,812,063	6
Diagnosis costs	1,050	14,910 (8)	3,576,946	4
Benefits aimed at enabling involvement in working life (occupational rehabilitation)	49	1,310 (1)	730,423	1
Costs for resources	78	345 (0)	206,087	0
Reports	631	4,492 (2)	60,564	0
Total[a]	5,339[b]	186,981 (100)	87,857,627	100

[a]Does not include combined invoices and payments received for rehabilitation ($n = 19,445$, 9%), [b]Cases may arise in more than one posting description (e.g., costs for treatments, reports and pharmaceuticals)

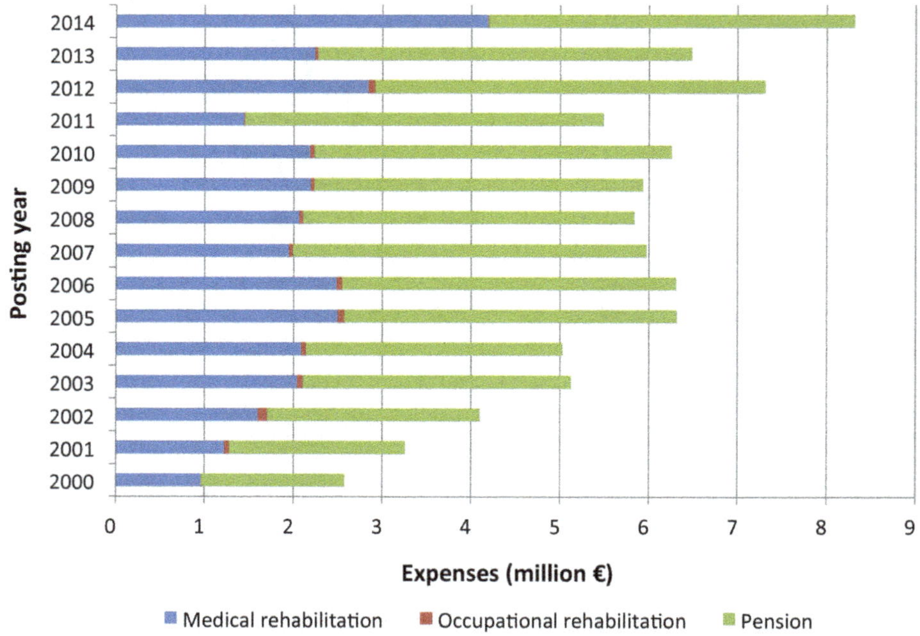

Fig. 2 Payments for medical, occupational rehabilitation and pensions for recognised HCV cases; 1097 cases between 2000 and 2014

the annual costs incurred for the years 2005 to 2010, the increase in costs for drugs was over 70% in 2012 and over 120% in 2014.

Discussion

Among German healthcare personnel workers, both reported and recognized occupational HCV infections decreased over the study period, yet costs associated with HCV increased. The majority of claims was represented by females aged 40 years and older who were employed as nurses in hospitals. The anti-HCV prevalence in the general population in Germany is estimated to be stable at a low level (0.3%) [10]. The number of reported OD cases among healthcare personnel in Germany declined over the time possibly due to improved blood-borne pathogen handling practices. Guidelines have been issued since 2000 that aim to prevent exposure to blood, for example, from NSI [11]. In the mid-1990s it came to a strong increase in reported ODs, probably in many cases linked to old cases, as a result of increased investigations since the mid-1990s in Germany [12]. In addition, the number of reported and recognized ODs may not reflect the real number of HCV infection cases among healthcare personnel. Needlestick injuries (NSI) are the most frequently reported occupational accidents in healthcare [13]. The results of epidemiological studies indicate that most of HCWs (80%) have been affected by NSI, and many such injuries remain unreported [11].

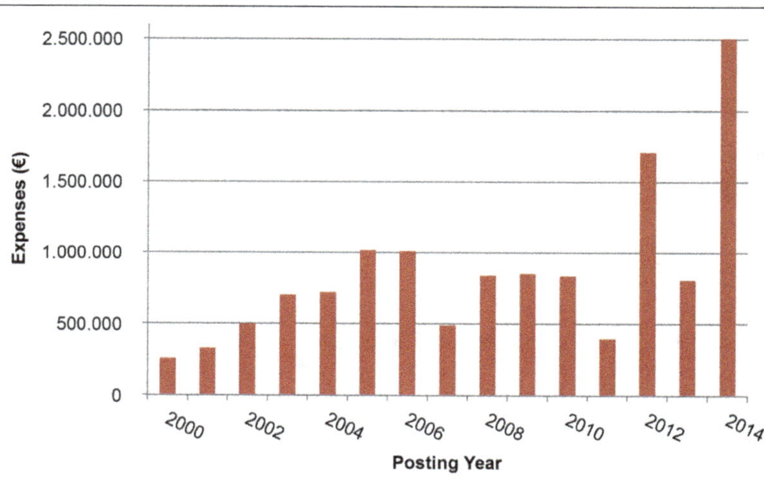

Fig. 3 Expenses for drugs for the sample of recognised HCV cases listed by posting year

Despite lower OD HCV prevalence, the costs related to occupational exposure have increased. The costs for CHC are largely defined by the rising expenses for pensions. In 2012 to 2014, however, there was a strong rise in each case in costs for drug therapy. This likely associated with expenses for triple combinations of pegylated interferon, ribavirin and one of the two first-generation protease inhibitors, boceprevir and telaprevir in 2012. The rise in expenses in 2014 is probably attributable to the use of new direct antiviral agents (DAAs, second-generation protease inhibitors) for the treatment of HCV infections.

Initial research results on the new DAAs indicate sustainable SVR rates with shorter treatment periods and a tendency for fewer side effects [4]. DAAs initially involve higher expenses, but may reduce long term treatment costs as reported by Nevens et al. [14]. SVR rates are associated with a reduction in CHC-caused (hepatic and extrahepatic) morbidity and mortality [15, 16]. Functional improvements in the cirrhosis were observed through the SVRs, as were sustained successes in the treatment of extrahepatic complications [4, 8]. CHC remains the most frequent indication for liver transplantation [17]. Preoperative treatment to achieve an SVR at the time of transplantation sustainably reduces the risk of the transplanted organ being infected with the HCV [15, 17]. Early identification of an infection is a key factor in enabling the patient to recover as fully as possible. The treatment of patients in less severe stages of the disease using DAA therapy is costly, but is likely to be successful in preventing future advanced liver diseases that are also associated with high expense [6]. Nevens et al. also observed a considerable reduction in the costs in cases where an SVR was achieved in the mild, less pronounced phases of CHC [14]. In the long term, the high costs of this treatment are likely to pay off by allowing early treatment of CHC infections to reduce morbidity and mortality rates. The case figures presented here do not provide a complete picture of the costs for occupation HCV infections in Germany. The BGW database used here only contains OD reports on employees from non-government institutions. Those restrictions that generally apply for secondary data apply to this register data. The data is not clinical in nature, but rather administrative with limited sociodemographic characteristics present. As in table one reported, nurses are the largest represented demographic group among the healthcare professionals with an HCV infection as OD. This data was not corrected for the total population because it was not possible to get the necessary information, with the same corresponding to the age groups presented. Although this lack of data adjustment is an inherent limitation of our study, a positive feature of this data is that it provides a longitudinal perspective, enabling the claiming of insurance benefits as relevant outcome (e.g., in the form of compensation payments) to be observed over a sufficiently long period of time.

Conclusions

For hepatitis C infections as an OD, a considerable increase in costs has been observed, while the number of cases has declined heavily. These costs are explained by the increase in pension payments and, since 2012, by a rise in the costs for drugs. The use of DAA treatments is currently fundamentally changing disease management for CHC patients. The high costs of the treatments might be offset by the potentially considerable benefits. The optimum solution is successful therapy at as early a stage in the disease as possible in order to preserve the health-related quality of life of the insured as fully as possible, thereby also preserving their ability to work. The resultant reduction in concomitant hepatic and extrahepatic diseases will potentially result in lower RWA gradings in the long term among the overall insured population. In the long run, maintaining the ability to work would generate overall cost savings for accident insurers and also for the other social security systems.

Abbreviations

BGW: Berufsgenossenschaft für Gesundheitsdienst und Wohlfahrtspflege; BK-DOK: BGW's occupational disease routine data records; CHC: Chronic hepatitis C; DAA: Direct anti-viral agent; HCV: Viral hepatitis C; OD: Occupational disease; RWA: Reduced work ability; STROSA: A consensus German reporting standard for secondary data analyses; SVR: Sustained virological response; WHO: World health organisation

Acknowledgements

We would like to thank the Rehabilitation Coordination Department (BGW) for their support.

Funding

No special funds were received for this study. However, the Institute for Health Services Research in Dermatology and Nursing of the University Medical Centre Hamburg-Eppendorf (UKE) receives an unrestricted fund from the Institution for Statutory Accident Insurance and Prevention in the Health and Welfare services (BGW) on an annual basis to maintain the working group at the UKE. The funds are provided by a non-profit organization that is part of the social security system in Germany. The funder had no role in study design, data collection and analysis, decision to publish, or preparation of the manuscript.

Authors' contributions

MD, CW and AN developed the study design. DW and MD conducted the data analysis. The interpretation of the data was made by MD, DW, CW and AN. CW wrote the manuscript, with significant contribution from the other authors. Uncertainties were discussed between the authors regularly. AN revised the manuscript critically for important intellectual content and gave final approval for the version to be published. All authors read and approved the final manuscript.

Competing interests

The authors declare that they have no competing interests.

Ethics approval and consent to participate

The study was not submitted to an ethic commission as only anonym routine data of an insurance were used and no personal data were collected and no medical test was performed in the scope of the study. However, the study was accepted by the data protection board of the insurance which provided the data. In accordance with the Professional Code for Physicians in Hamburg (Art. 15, 1., Status of 10.03.2014) and the Chamber Legislation for Medical Professions in the Federal State of Hamburg (HmbKGH) it is only necessary to obtain advice on questions of professional ethics and professional conduct from an Ethics Committee if data which can be traced to a particular individual is being used in a research project.

Author details

[1]University Medical Center Hamburg-Eppendorf (UKE), Center of Excellence for Health Services Research in Nursing (CVcare), Hamburg, Germany. [2]Institution for Statutory Accident Insurance and Prevention in the Health and Welfare Services (BGW), Department of Prevention and Rehabilitation Principles (GPR), Hamburg, Germany.

References

1. Askarian M, Yadollahi M, Kuochak F, Danaei M, Vakili V, Momeni M. Precautions for health care workers to avoid hepatitis B and C virus infection. Int J Occup Environ Med. 2011;2:191–8.
2. Westermann C, Peters C, Lisiak B, Lamberti M, Nienhaus A. The prevalence of hepatitis C among healthcare workers: a systematic review and meta-analysis. Occup Environ Med. 2015;72:880–8.
3. WHO. WHO Guidelines Approved by the Guidelines Review Committee. Geneva: Guidelines for the Screening Care and Treatment of Persons with Chronic Hepatitis C Infection: Updated Version. 2016. (http://www.ncbi.nlm.nih.gov/pubmed/27227200. Accessed 14 Jun 2016).
4. Sarrazin C, Berg TP, Buggisch MM, Dollinger H, Hinrichsen H, Hofer DH, et al. Aktuelle Empfehlung zur Therapie der chronischen Hepatitis C S3 guideline hepatitis C addendum. Z Gastroenterol. 2015;53:320–34.
5. WHO. Hepatitis C - Fact sheet Geneva: N°164. 2014. (http://www.who.int/mediacentre/factsheets/fs164/en/. Accessed 4 Feb 2016).
6. Gordon SC, Pockros PJ, Terrault NA, Hoop RS, Buikema A, Nerenz D, et al. Impact of disease severity on healthcare costs in patients with chronic hepatitis C (CHC) virus infection. Hepatol (Baltimore, Md). 2012;56:1651–60.
7. Younossi ZM, Singer ME, Mir HM, Henry L, Hunt S. Impact of interferon free regimens on clinical and cost outcomes for chronic hepatitis C genotype 1 patients. J Hepatol. 2014;60:530–7.
8. Westbrook RH, Dusheiko G. Natural history of hepatitis C. J Hepatol. 2014;61 Suppl 1:58–68.
9. Swart E, Bitzer EM, Gothe H, Harling M, Hoffmann F, Horenkamp-Sonntag D, et al. A consensus German reporting standard for secondary data analyses, version 2 (STROSA-STandardisierte BerichtsROutine fur SekundardatenAnalysen). Gesundheitswesen (Bundesverband der Arzte des Offentlichen Gesundheitsdienstes (Germany). 2016;78(SO1):e145–260.
10. Poethko-Muller C, Zimmermann R, Hamouda O, Faber M, Stark K, Ross RS, et al. Epidemiology of hepatitis a, B, and C among adults in Germany: results of the German health interview and examination survey for adults (DEGS1). Bundesgesundheitsblatt, Gesundheitsforschung, Gesundheitsschutz. 2013; 56(5–6):707–15.
11. Elseviers MM, Arias-Guillen M, Gorke A, Arens HJ. Sharps injuries amongst healthcare workers: review of incidence, transmissions and costs. J Ren Care. 2014;40(3):150–6.
12. Dulon ML B, Wendeler D, Nienhaus A. Occupational infectious diseases in healthcare workers 2014. Data from the institution for statutory accident insurance and prevention in the health and welfare services. Zentralbl Arbeitsmed Arbeitsschutz Ergon. 2015;65:210–6.
13. Nienhaus A, Kesavachandran C, Wendeler D, Haamann F, Dulon M. Infectious diseases in healthcare workers - an analysis of the standardised data set of a German compensation board. J Occup Med Toxicol. 2012;7(1):8.
14. Nevens F, Colle I, Michielsen P, Robaeys G, Moreno C, Caekelbergh K, et al. Resource use and cost of hepatitis C-related care. Eur J Gastroenterol Hepatol. 2012;24:1191–8.
15. Gonzalez-Grande R, Jimenez-Perez M, Gonzalez Arjona C, Mostazo TJ. New approaches in the treatment of hepatitis C. World J Gastroenterol. 2016;22:1421–32.
16. Tada T, Kumada T, Toyoda H, Kiriyama S, Tanikawa M, Hisanaga Y, et al. Viral eradication reduces all-cause mortality in patients with chronic hepatitis C virus infection: a propensity score analysis. Liver Int. 2016;36(6):817–26.
17. Fagiuoli S, Ravasio R, Luca MG, Baldan A, Pecere S, Vitale A, et al. Management of hepatitis C infection before and after liver transplantation. World J Gastroenterol. 2015;21:4447–56.

18

Do overweight workers profit by workplace health promotion, more than their normal-weight peers? Evaluation of a worksite intervention

Stefanie Mache[1*], Sarah Jensen[3], Stefan Linnig[2], Reimo Jahn[4], Mirco Steudtner[5], Elke Ochsmann[5] and Geraldine Preuß[2]

Abstract

Background: Worksite health promotion programs have been identified as strongly effective in decreasing body weight and increasing awareness and change in health behavior. Aim of this study is to determine the effects of a multi-component intervention in workplace health promotion.

Methods: In a controlled study trail, 1,573 workers of a logistics company had the chance to participate in a one year worksite health promotion program. Main elements of the multi-component intervention were physical activity training in combination with nutrition counseling. Employees completed a questionnaire at baseline and then again after twelve month. Main outcome variables were changes in body weight and health behaviors. Secondary outcomes were subjective health indicators.

Results: Our results showed preliminary improvements in physical activity and eating behavior among normal weight and overweight/obesity weight groups. No significant weight reduction could be found, only a minimal reduction of BMI. The reduction was larger in the overweight group. Workers considered overweight or obese showed significantly greater body weight loss and changes in eating behavior than workers with a normal weight status. Workers with obesity/overweight scored their general health status significantly lower than their colleagues with normal weight status. No significant improvements were found for overall perception of health status between baseline and follow-up in the BMI-groups.

Conclusion: This 12-month intervention-control study suggests that a well-implemented multi-component workplace health promotion program may support substantial change in health behavior (e.g. nutrition and physical activity). It is indicated that overweight employees may especially profit from such worksite health promotion. An investigation of long-term effects of this multi-component intervention is strongly recommended.

Keywords: Health behavior changes, Physical activity, Prevention of overweight, Weight gain program, Workplace health promotion

* Correspondence: s.mache@uke.de
[1]Institute for Occupational Medicine and Maritime Medicine (ZfAM), University Medical Center Hamburg-Eppendorf, Seewartenstrasse 10, 20459 Hamburg, Germany
Full list of author information is available at the end of the article

Background

Obesity, health and economic costs

During the past decades, the prevalence of overweight and obesity has increased to epidemic proportions in developed countries. In Europe, the prevalence of overweight is currently in the range of 50 - 60 % and the prevalence of obesity about 20 % [1, 2].

Obesity is strongly associated with higher rates of coronary heart disease (CHD), stroke, shorter life expectancy and CHD risk factors (e.g., diabetes) [3, 4]. In consequence, overweight and obesity are associated with an increased risk of morbidity and reduced life expectancy [3, 5] and therefore are correlated with increased healthcare and medical costs [6].

In developed countries, about 2-10 % of the overall health care costs are directly attributable to overweight and obesity [2, 7, 8]. In addition, indirect costs associated with sick leaves and working days lost, lower levels of work productivity, individual (psychological) problems and a reduced quality of life are even greater [9, 10].

Therefore, a persistent need for obesity management strategies to address the increasing prevalence of overweight is present these days [11].

The development of overweight and obesity is the result of a complex interaction of behavioral, environmental, social and economic as well as genetic factors [12–14]. The current environment is characterized by a situation whereby food is plentiful and physical activity levels are low [15]. So, overweight and obesity are most often the result of a continuing body weight gain that is triggered by an imbalance between energy expenditure (e.g. low physical activity) and energy intake (e.g. unhealthy dietary behavior) [16].

Increasing physical activity has therefore become an important public health concern. It is important to understand physical activity patterns and health behavior among normal weight but especially among overweight and obese adults in order to develop implement and evaluate successful health interventions.

Obesity and worksite health promotion

As long-term consequences of overweight and obesity are burdensome for individuals, employers and society, it is necessary to target health behavior such as physical activity and dietary behavior in worksite health promotion interventions [17]. The workplace is considered a central setting to implement programs and strategies both to promote physical activity and to prevent body weight gain and obesity [18, 19]. Moreover, the place of employment represents a relatively controlled environment and a substantial proportion of the adult population can be reached through worksite interventions [20]. Studies evaluating the effect of worksite health promotion interventions targeting physical activity have shown that physical activity levels can be increased [21]. For example, evidence of this effect was found for exercise training and sport interventions [22, 23]. A recently published review shows evidence for limited to moderate positive effects of educational, environmental and multi-component interventions on dietary behavior [24]. For employers, the possibility of increasing productivity may represent a strong incentive for the implementation of worksite programs [25].

Aim of this study

The aim of the present study was to evaluate the effectiveness of a one-year worksite multi-component intervention related to body weight groups (normal weight vs. overweight) on weight gain, physical activity, perception of health status, eating behavior and health attitude among workers of a logistics company.

We hypothesize that between baseline (t0) and the end of the intervention (follow-up, t2) there will be:

1. Significant differences in the primary outcomes: "body weight"/"body mass index" (BMI) and "perceived health status" and
2. Significant differences in secondary outcomes: "physical activity during leisure time", "food consumption", "behavioral eating attitudes" and "stages of readiness to change dietary behavior" between the normal weight group and the overweight group.

Methods

Study-Design

The success of the worksite health intervention was assessed in a controlled study trial. Participants' ratings were measured at baseline (t0), after six months (t1, process evaluation), and after twelve months (follow-up; t2) (see Fig. 1).

Outcome evaluation

The data was evaluated at baseline (t0) and at 12 months (t2). Preliminary results of the worksite health intervention related to body weight groups have been assessed on the following types of outcome variables:

1. Participation in training,
2. Satisfaction with training and trainer,
3. Physical activity during leisure time,
4. Changes in weight and body mass index,
5. Nutrition behavioral outcomes (changes in eating behavior, attitudes and stages of readiness to change dietary practices),
6. Perceived health status

Participants

Throughout the entire year of 2013, 1,573 workers of a German logistics company were invited to participate in

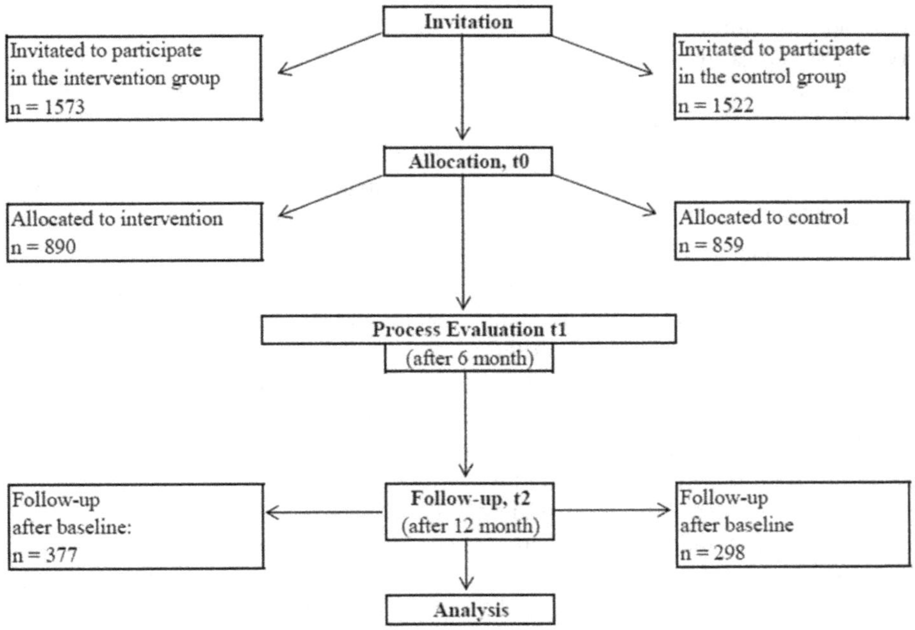

Fig. 1 Flow chart

multi-component health promotion training (intervention group; ig). In addition, a control group (cg) of 1,522 employees of the same company – comparable to the intervention group in socio-demographic and work-related variables (e.g. gender, age, job description etc.) – has been invited to participate. Groups of workers have been randomized to either the intervention or control group.

In summation, 890 workers of the intervention group (response rate = 58 %) and 859 workers of the control group were involved at baseline (response rate = 56 %). At follow-up (twelve month later), 793 employees of the intervention group and 697 workers of the control group filled-out the survey (response rates of 50 % versus 46 %). Questionnaire data at baseline and follow-up were matched afterwards: It was found, that 377 workers (ig) or 298 (cg), respectively, answered both questionnaires (at baseline and follow-up).

Worksite Intervention

One of the main aims of this worksite intervention was to encourage health behavior changes in employees, including:

1. fostering motivation towards physical activity,
2. eating healthy food and
3. achieving or maintaining a healthy BMI (<25.0 kg/m^2).

Secondary goals targeted health behavior and attitude changes.

Participants in the intervention group received a twelve-months health promotion intervention. The training sessions took approx. 30 to 60 minutes every week/fortnight and were held, for example, in a room at the worksite in a group setting of several participants or as an individual coaching. Employees participated during paid working hours; the timetable was set considering the working hours of the staffs (e.g. before working hours, around lunch time and after working hours).

A trainer provided educational information and advice on healthy eating, physical activity, or performed other health promotion activities (e.g. personalized nutrition counseling). Additionally, free fruit and vegetables were provided and physical exercise was included in the sessions at the workplace. Physical activity training focused on general body strength training and included exercises to ease and strengthen muscles at the back, shoulders and arms. Training sessions included practice with flexi bars, barbells, balls and work related objects.

Measurement/Questionnaires

Participation in intervention

Frequency of participation in the intervention was assessed by the following question "How often did you take part in the multi component intervention?"; response options were "frequently" (up to once per week), "irregularly" (two or three times per month) or "never" (no attendance at all).

Satisfaction with the intervention/trainer

Participants were asked to rate their overall satisfaction on a five-point Likert-type scale: "All in all, how satisfied are you with the training/trainer?" (1 = very satisfied, 2 = satisfied, 3 = neither...nor, 4 = dissatisfied, 5 = very dissatisfied). High scores correspond to high values on the dimensions.

Physical activity during leisure time

In addition, physical activity during leisure time was assessed in the survey. The regularity of physical (sports) activities was specified by categories: regularly (>2 h/week), regularly (≤1-2 h/week), irregularly (≤1 h/week), and no (or almost no) activity.

Eating behavior/Dietary intake

In order to evaluate individual health behavior, the German version of the *Questionnaire for the Assessment of Health Behaviour*, the FEG (Fragebogen zur Erfassung des Gesundheitsverhaltens), developed by Dlugosch [26] was used. The survey includes several scales and items measuring health risk behavior, health behavior and attitudes towards a healthy diet, smoking, physical activity and the perception of personal well-being. For example, participants are asked to report on frequency of key health behaviors that were emphasized in the program.

In addition, fruit intake was assessed by a short food questionnaire consisting of six questions. Also the intake frequency of fruit, vegetables, sweets (chocolate, cake etc.), fast food, meat products and soft drinks (e.g. cola or lemonade) were assessed by utilizing categorical response options (1 = several times a day, 2 = daily, 3 = several times a week, 4 = seldom, 5 = never) for each category [26]. The survey has been checked for reliability, validity and objectivity by Dlugosch [26].

Stage of readiness to change eating behavior

The assessment of stage to change eating behavior which is represented by ordered categories of motivational readiness to change (pre-contemplation, contemplation, preparation, action, maintenance) was based on the recommendations by Prochaska and colleagues [27]. For practical reasons, the stages of readiness to change were condensed to four categorical variables of *pre-contemplation, contemplation, preparation*, and *action/maintenance*. Response options for this question were : "I do not want to change anything/I have no plans to start" (pre-contemplation), "considering a change" (contemplation), "making plans to change" (preparation), "I started doing this" (action, maintenance) [27].

Eating-related attitudes

Eating-related attitudes and behaviors were measured by the *Questionnaire for the Assessment of Eating-and Weight-Related Attitudes and Behaviors* [28]. Two scales of this questionnaire were included. One of these scales (titled: Attitudes towards healthy eating) consists of 14 items (for example: "I eat lots of vegetables"; "I am very conscious of how much fat is in the food I eat"). Items can be rated on a four-point Likert-type scale (1 = strongly disagree, 2 = disagree, 3 = agree, 4 = strongly agree). Psychometric qualities were acceptable at all measurements (e.g. range of Cronbach's $\alpha = 0.65$ to 0.71) [28].

Employees' perceived health status

The German version of the *Copenhagen Psychosocial Questionnaire* (COPSOQ) was used to assess employees' self-rated health status and well-being. Subjective health status was scored on a ten-point rating scale based on the EQ-5D and was transformed to a scale ranging from 0 ("worst health status score") to 100 points ("best health status score"). Previous investigations successfully proved the quality criteria of the COPSOQ [29]. High scores correspond to high values on the respective dimensions. Thus, in most cases high levels represent a "good" or, in this case, "healthy" status.

Covariates

At baseline, data on potential effect modifiers and confounders were assessed including age, gender, marital status (assessed in the categories of married; partnership; single; divorced; widowed). Body height and body weight were also measured. Weight status has been evaluated based on three categories of Body Mass Index (BMI): healthy body weight BMI (<25 kg/m^2); overweight BMI (≥25 kg/m^2) and obesity BMI (≥30 kg/m^2). BMI is calculated by dividing body weight in kilograms by the square of the body height in meters and has been measured from self-reported height and weight at baseline (t0) and follow-up (t2).

Statistical analyses

Descriptive statistics were used to characterize baseline demographics as well as behavioral, cognitive and weight loss outcomes. Normal distribution has been proved by the Shapiro-Wilk test of normality. Chi-square and t-tests revealed significant differences in and associations of socio-demographics, eating behaviors, health attitudes and subjective health status with weight status (i.e., normal weight vs. overweight/obese). In addition, linear mixed effect models were performed with the outcome measures as the dependent variable, group (intervention vs. control group) as independent variable and time of follow-up measurements (t2: follow up at twelve months) as fixed factor, while adjusting for the baseline levels of the outcome measure. A p-level of < 0.05 was considered to indicate statistical significance. All statistical analyses were performed using IBM SPSS (Version 21).

Results

Baseline characteristics of the study participants

Table 1 presents the characteristics of the participants divided into bodyweight groups. Most of the participants in the intervention group were in the age groups between 41 and 60 years (73.4 %) (see Table 1). Mean age

Table 1 Selected demographic characteristics of matched participants

Characteristic	Matched sample participants[a] (Normal weight[b]) (n = 201)	Matched sample participants (Overweight[c]) (n = 169)	Matched sample control group (Normal weight[b]) (n =158)	Matched sample control group (Overweight[c]) (n = 135)
Age, years, %				
21-30	6.0	8.3	8.2	3.0
31-40	17.4	18.9	12.7	12.6
41-50	44.3	30.8	47.5	45.2
51-60	29.4	39.1	30.4	38.5
>60	1.0	1.2	1.3	0.7
Sex, %				
Male	36.8	43.5	24.1	32.6
Female	58.7	51.8	74.7	63.7
BMI[1], kg/m^2				
T0: Mean (SD[1])	22.6 (1.6)	28.6 (2.5)	22.3 (1.8)	28.6 (2.1)
T2: Mean (SD)	22.7 (1.8)	28.1 (2.9)	22.6 (1.7)	28.7 (2.4)

[1]Abbreviations: BMI - body mass index; SD - standard deviation
[a]Matched sample participants represent the workers identified by code, age, sex, and height with a completed assessment at baseline and follow-up
[b]Normal weight = BMI ≤ 24.9 kg/m^2
[c]Overweight = BMI ≥ 25.0 kg/m^2

of the participants was 44 years (SD = 10.26). Gender distribution of the whole sample was approximately equally divided in the groups: 45 % were female, 55 % were male workers. The majority of intervention group (ig) had a normal body weight, with mean BMI being 25.9 (SD = 3.6) and mean BMI of the control group being 25.6 (SD = 3.4). At baseline, 55 % of the participants (ig) or 52 % (cg), respectively, had a normal weight status; 34 % were overweight (cg: 35 %) (BMI > 25 kg/m2); 12 % were obese (cg: 11 %). Chi-square tests show that no significant difference exist between the intervention group (ig) and control group (cg) at baseline with regard to age, gender or other relevant socio-demographic factors.

Participation in the worksite intervention

Body weight groups did not differ significantly with regard to participation in the intervention program (P = .38). 36.9 % of the overweight group (n = 169) reported that they "frequently" participated in the intervention program (n = 62); 37.5 % participated "irregularly" (n = 63). Only 24.4 % did not participate in the intervention program at all (n = 41). In comparison, 37.9 % of the normal weight group (n = 201) reported that they took part "frequently", 41.0 % (n = 76) "irregularly". 21.0 % of these participants reported that they did not take part in the intervention program at all (n = 42).

Satisfaction with training and trainer

The overweight group showed a mean of 1.89 (SD = 1.23) for satisfaction with the training in total and a mean of 2.15 (SD = 1.73) for satisfaction with the trainer. In comparison, the normal weight group evaluated the training also with a mean of 1.89 (SD = 1.25) and mean of 1.90 (SD = 1.47) for satisfaction with the trainer. No significant difference was found between body weight groups with regard to satisfaction with the intervention (P = 0.79) or trainer (P = 0.57).

Physical activity during leisure time

As illustrated in Table 2, improvements have been found regarding regularity of physical activity during leisure time between the weight groups.

Participants in both weight groups reported a more regular physical activity rate at follow-up than at baseline measurement (P = .01).

Weight Loss: Changes in body weight and body mass index

Results of measurements at baseline and after twelve-month show that both body weight groups (normal and overweight weight status) in the intervention group did not significantly lose body weight with regard to baseline measurement data. Age- and gender-adjusted BMI changes for the nw-group were −0.21 (CI (95 %) -0.49; −0.15) kg/m^2 and for the overweight group: −0.32 (CI (95 %) -0.55; −0.12) kg/m^2 at follow-up. After twelve months, 35 % of the participants (ig) were overweight (cg: 32 %), 12 % were obese (cg: 14 %), 52 % had a normal weight (cg: 53 %).

Changes in dietary intake and specific eating attitudes

We evaluated changes in eating behaviors between baseline and follow-up. Table 3 shows changes (means and standard deviations at baseline and follow-up measurements) for the targeted dietary intake and eating behaviors among body weight groups. With regard to changes in dietary intake, it was found that participants

Table 2 Physical activity during leisure time

	Matched sample participants[a] (Normal weight[b]) (n = 201) baseline (%)	Matched sample participants (Overweight[c]) (n = 169) baseline (%)	Matched sample participants (Normal weight[b]) (n =201) follow-up (%)	Matched sample participants (Overweight[c]) (n = 169) follow-up (%)
Physical activity				
no activity	46.2	54.1	39.6	45.2
almost no activity	11.8	15.1	14.2	19.2
irregularly≤1 h/week	4.1	1.4	17.8	8.2
regularly 1–2 hours per week	26.0	17.8	11.2	10.3
regularly, more than 2 hours per week	11.8	11.6	17.2	17.1

[a]Matched sample participants represent the workers identified by code, age, sex, and height with a completed assessment at baseline and follow-up
[b]Normal weight = BMI ≤ 24.9 kg/m^2
[c]Overweight = BMI ≥ 25.0 kg/m^2

with normal weight status (BMI < 25) differ from participants with overweight status (BMI > 25). As illustrated in Table 3, participants who are overweight/obese showed greater improvements in consumption of fruit/vegetables and fast food between t0 and t2 than workers who had a normal weight. In general, both groups showed several significant improvements differences in food consumption between baseline and follow-up measurement (P > 0.05).

In addition changes in eating attitudes have been analyzed (see Tables 4 and 5). At baseline, attitudes to healthy eating were similar in both body weight groups (intervention and control group). At follow-up, few significant differences and improvements in health attitude between the body weight groups (baseline (t0) and follow-up (t2)) were found (see Tables 4 and 5).

Stage of readiness to change for healthy eating among body weight groups

Significant differences between participants with normal weight (nw; n = 201) and overweight (ow; n = 170) were found regarding stage of readiness to change for health eating.

As illustrated in Table 6, for participants with normal weight, 21 % of the workers were in the preparation stage and 7 % were in the action or maintenance stage at baseline. At follow-up, the percentage of participants in the preparation stage increased to 32 % and the percentage in the action or maintenance stage increased to 14 % (P = 0.001).

For workers in the overweight group, 35 % were in the preparation stage and 8 % were in the action or maintenance stage at baseline. At follow-up, the percentage of participants (ow) in the preparation stage increased to 53 %; the percentage in the action or maintenance stage increased to 12 % (P = .001).

Subjective health status

At baseline, participants rated their subjective health status with a mean of 6.36 (SD = 1.90). Correlation analysis showed a significant negative correlation between BMI and subjective health status (r = –.18, P = 0.01). Workers with overweight and obesity rated their perceived health status worse than did workers with a normal weight status. In line with that, stratification showed a significant difference in health status between employees with normal weight status (t0: M = 6.5; SD = 1.9; t2: M = 6.6; SD = 1.8) and employees with overweight status (t0: M = 6.0; SD = 1.8; t2: M = 6.1, SD = 1.9) in the intervention group (P = 0.01).

For the total study population, we found no significant improvements in perceived health status between baseline and follow-up, neither in the intervention nor in the control group (intervention group: M = 6.30, SD = 1.9 vs. M = 6.4, SD = 1.9; P = 0.53; control group: M = 6.17, SD = 1.77 vs. M = 6.21, SD = 1.78, P = 0.69). No interaction between intervention and baseline health status was noted (P > .05).

Discussion

This study focused on differences among body weight groups regarding changes of body weight, nutrition behavior and health perceptions after a one-year worksite health promotion program that includes physical exercise training in combination with educational nutrition counseling during working time. In total, we found preliminary effects twelve months after the beginning of the intervention, as discussed in the following part.

Weight gain among BMI-groups

In the beginning, over 40 % of the 890 workers were overweight or obese. This situation indicated a strong need for workplace health promotion. We assumed a significant weight loss after a twelve-month worksite health promotion in both body weight groups. However, body weight did not decrease significantly in both weight groups. Only

Table 3 Statistical differences between weight status groups (normal weight vs. overweight/obese)

How often do you eat or drink . . . ?	% at Baseline normal weight (n = 198)	% at Baseline overweight/obese (n = 170)	% at Follow-up normal weight (n = 198)	% at Follow-up overweight/obese (n = 170)	*P* -Value[a]
Vegetables					
several time a day	3.1	3.0	8.6	4.7	P(nw[b]) = .05 P(ow[c]) = .01
daily	28.0	29.8	33.8	44.7	
several times a week	47.7	53.0	48.0	40.6	
less often	13.0	7.1	8.1	8.8	
never	0	0	0	0	
Fruits					
several time a day	8.3	9.5	14.1	14.2	P(nw) = .04 P(ow) = .01
daily	37.3	35.7	40.4	44.7	
several times a week	29.0	24.4	26.8	28.2	
less often	16.6	22.6	16.7	11.8	
never	1.0	1.8	1.5	0.6	
Sweets					
several time a day	6.7	3.0	6.1	4.7	P(nw) = .00 P(ow) = .32
daily	24.4	19.6	22.7	18.8	
several times a week	35.8	42.9	41.4	44.1	
less often	24.3	28.0	26.8	28.8	
never	1.0	0.6	1.5	0.6	
Meat					
several time a day	8.3	9.5	7.1	4.1	P(nw) = .00 P(ow) = .00
daily	31.6	41.7	42.9	46.5	
several times a week	43.0	35.7	36.4	34.7	
less often	7.8	6.0	12.1	12.9	
never	1.0	0.6	1.5	0.6	
Fast Food					
several time a day	0	0	0	0	P(nw) = .00 P(ow) = .00
daily	0	0.6	0	0	
several times a week	5.7	7.7	7.6	7.1	
less often	76.2	78.0	78.3	84.1	
never	9.3	7.1	12.1	8.8	
Soft drinks (coca-cola, limonade)					
several time a day	3.0	3.5	3.5	0.6	P(nw) = .34 P(ow) = .53
daily	12.1	10.6	7.1	10.6	
several times a week	13.6	19.4	15.7	20.0	

Table 3 Statistical differences between weight status groups (normal weight vs. overweight/obese) *(Continued)*

less often	46.5	43.5	43.4	42.4	
never	22.2	22.4	27.3	24.7	

Notes: $\chi2$ test used for unadjusted comparisons between baseline and one-year follow-up,
[a]P < .05 is significant
[b]nw - normal weight
[c]ow - overweight/obese

few participants reported a sizeable weight loss in the overweight group. In comparison to studies targeting similar participants or using comparable intervention methods our findings show comparable results [30, 31]. However, other workplace health promotion studies aiming at weight loss in different body mass index groups illustrated weight losses from 0.5 to 4.0 kg [32–34].

In sum, our results indicate that a worksite health program may lead to weight loss and support former recommendations of combining diverse initiatives for successful weight loss [17]. However, the long-term effects of this combined intervention remain to be investigated. As reported by van Berkel and colleagues, long term effectiveness in weight loss should be central for health interventions, since reaching and maintaining a changed behavioral pattern is challenging, especially for weight loss [35, 36]. To increase long-term success in weight loss, workplace health promotion should be integrated as an inherent part in the company.

Physical activity among BMI-groups

Our results demonstrate an explicit improvement in physical activity among the BMI-groups as a result of the intervention. Moreover, results indicated that especially overweight employees took advantage of the training: a more regular physical activity is one of their health benefits.

Our findings are comparable to other studies which have also shown an increase in physical activity especially in overweight employees [37–40]. The current public health recommendations advocate regular physical activity as a key component in the prevention and treatment of excess body weight [41]. However, the promotion and modification of physical activity requires an understanding of current activity patterns among normal-weight and overweight adults. Our study provides insight into important issues of how employees spent time in physical activity that can be used to develop programs towards those activities, intensity levels and periods of the week that are especially concerning overweight and/or obese individuals. In addition, our results indicate that the time spent in sport activity differs across BMI categories, suggesting that these should continue to be targets for interventions. However, from a clinical point of view, extreme sport activity should not be prescribed to individuals

Table 4 Changes in eating attitudes between participants with normal weight vs. overweight

What do you want to change ...	at Baseline (M/SD)[1] normal weight (n = 198)	at Baseline (M/SD) overweight/obese (n = 170)	at Follow-up (M/SD) normal weight (n = 198)	at Follow-up (M/SD) overweight/obese (n = 170)	*P* Value[a]
1...eating less.	1.54 (1.70)	2.12 (2.11)	1.91 (1.57)	2.16 (2.20)	P(nw[b]) = .01
					P(ow[c]) = .83
2... eating more regularly.	1.69 (2.64)	2.62 (2.21)	1.95 (2.50)	2.55 (2.36)	P(nw) = .17
					P(ow) = .98
3... eating less snacks between the meals.	1.0(2.14)	2.46 (2.24)	1.38 (2.20)	2.39 (2.30)	P(nw) = .02
					P(ow) = .86
4...taking more time for my meals.	1.70 (2.7)	2.41(2.27)	2.12 (2.61)	2.76 (2.35)	P(nw) = .03
					P(ow) = .04
5...eating healthier.	1.60 (2.61)	2.81 (2.23)	1.91 (2.49)	2.65 (2.33)	P(nw) = .11
					P(ow) = .60
6...loose weight.	1.10 (2.02)	2.99 (2.38)	1.11 (2.12)	2.79 (2.45)	P(nw) = .06
					P(ow) = .50

[1]Abbreviations: M- mean; SD- standard deviation
[a]P < .05 is significant
[b]nw - normal weight status
[c]ow - overweight/obese status

Table 5 Selected attitudes related to eating behavior: differences between weight groups at baseline and follow-up

Which statements are correct for you?	at Baseline (M/SD)[1] normal weight (n = 198)	at Baseline (M/SD) overweight/obese (n = 170)	at Follow-up (M/SD) normal weight (n = 198)	at Follow-up (M/SD) overweight/obese (n = 170)	P Value[a]
1. With nutrition I avoid everything that could affect/damage my health.	2.57(0.74)	2.51(0.76)	2.67(0.73)	2.46(0.86)	P(nw[b]) = .11 P(ow[c]) = .37
2. I always eat healthy and are on a balanced diet.	2.73(0.72)	2.52(0.72)	2.70(0.73)	2.56(0.72)	P(nw) = .64 P(ow) = .55
3. I place great value on healthy food.	2.68(0.78)	2.61(0.76)	2.73(0.84)	2.65(0.76)	P(nw) = .47 P(ow) = .46
4. I can say for myself that I eat healthy.	2.75(0.69)	2.58(0.73)	2.78(0.77)	2.57(0.89)	P(nw) = .56 P(ow) = .85
5. I barely eat unhealthy things.	2.59(0.78)	2.37(0.78)	2.49(0.87)	2.46(0.83)	P(nw) = .17 P(ow) = .28
6. I eat lots of vegetables.	2.90(0.78)	2.76(0.85)	2.91(0.77)	2.81(0.84)	P(nw) = .80 P(ow) = .49
7. I eat lots of fruits.	2.81(0.93)	2.79(1.01)	2.79(0.93)	2.71(0.92)	P(nw) = .67 P(ow) = .26
8. A low fat diet is important to me.	2.65(1.06)	2.61(0.89)	2.58(1.00)	2.58(0.93)	P(nw) = .34 P(ow) = .77
9. I pay attention for my daily diet to have lots of vitamins and minerals.	2.70(0.78)	2.60(0.79)	2.67(0.85)	2.70(0.70)	P(nw) = .53 P(ow) = .09

[1]Abbreviations: M - mean; SD - standard deviation
[a]P < .05 is significant
[b]nw – normal weight status
[c]ow – overweight/obese status

who are obese and/or not used to exercise [42]. A good approach seems to be to integrate activity into the daily routine, for example by substituting sedentary/sitting and light activities for moderate activities. Moreover, training should be adapted to meet individual needs and preconditions/requirements.

Changes in nutrition behavior among BMI groups

Furthermore, we hypothesized significant changes in eating behavior after twelve months of worksite health intervention. As a result, we found significant differences between baseline and follow-up, for example, fruit and vegetable consumption increased during the intervention. Other

Table 6 Percentage of participants (intervention group) in stages of readiness to change model from baseline to follow-up by eating behavior

	Stage of change				
	Pre-contemplation	Con-templation	Preparation	Action/maintenance	P Value
Intervention group					
Normal weight (BMI < 25) (n = 198)					
Baseline (%)	41.3	25.9	20.9	7.0	P = .000
Follow-up (%)	38.3	13.4	31.8	14.4	
Overweight (BMI > 25) (n = 170)					
Baseline (%)	17.1	34.1	35.3	8.2	P = .000
Follow-up (%)	15.9	17.6	52.9	12.4	
Controll group					
Baseline (%)	35.6	29.9	24.2	6.0	P = .003
Follow-up (%)	32.2	15.8	41.3	7.4	

Notes: $\chi 2$ test used for unadjusted comparisons between baseline and one-year follow up. P < .05 is significant. Amount of missing values are not described: thus percentages across columns do not add up to 100 percent

desirable behaviors (eg. decreasing intake of fats or sweets) were also directly rewarded by the program. Moreover, we found that food consumption did differ between normal weight and overweight employees and healthy eating behaviors in the overweight group improved more than in the normal weight group.

These findings are in line with those of a meta-analysis of studies performed in different countries revealed that overweight adults quite frequently have a more unhealthy diet (fat, sweets) than normal weight adults [43]. In contrast, Ortega and colleagues also report that food consumption between overweight and normal weight adolescents did not differ [44].

Although not all of the results reached statistical significance, we demonstrated improvements after a twelve-month follow-up. In that regard, previous evaluation studies demonstrate a high effectiveness and importance of prevention programs on healthy lifestyle changes [19, 33, 45]. However, further investigation is needed on how to achieve change in the broader range of dietary behaviors.

Subjective health status

In addition, this study's results do not show any effects on subjective health status neither in overweight nor in normal weight peers which is in line with other studies showing that the effects of health promotion programs increase only over time [46, 47].

This study also suggests that long-term changes in subjective health status require more than physical activity and dietary counseling, including extensive attendance of therapists. It further supports the idea that long-term health prevention in workers may be a more cost- and time effective approach [48].

Implications for research and practice

This study, aiming at health promotion for employees at a logistics company, did show initial effects. For the future development of worksite health promotion interventions, given the complexity of overweight and obesity, it is recommended to address dimensions other than physical training and combine environmental and individual components in an intervention.

Furthermore, it is recommended for multi-component intervention studies to perform intermediate measurement to gain insight in the possible attrition of effects, if present. In addition, it is suggested to develop and validate more reliable questions in order to conduct differentiated measurements on health behavior at work.

Moreover, long-term results of this study may show the efficacy of a multilevel physical activity program on changes in health behavior and weight gain in (overweight) employees.

Therefore, continuation of this worksite health program is strongly recommended.

Limitations

This study analyses preliminary results of a worksite intervention targeting physical activity and eating behaviors. This investigation does have some limitations. First, this was not a randomized study. The group was self-selected which may limit the generalizability of results on program effectiveness. This evaluation study is further limited by the nature of the data, which were self-reported. However, with having a twelve months' time-lag between baseline and follow-up the self-report bias may have been minimized because it can be assumed that participating workers were not able to remember the questions and their responses of the baseline questionnaire. In addition, we collected self-reported height and weight data from the respondents in order to categorize BMI groups. As reported in several studies, self-reports overestimate height and underestimate weight [49, 50]. Consequently, the prevalence of obesity based on self-reported data is underestimated. This may induce a potential bias in our study results. However, distribution of height and weight in this study sample is comparable to that of the population from which the sample was drawn [51], therefore the risk of bias is limited. Due to practical reasons self-reported measurement was the only feasible way of data collection in this large study sample.

Conclusion

Our findings from the one-year pilot of the intervention program suggest that a worksite health prevention program may improve health behaviors of employees. The program encourages health behavior changes. In conclusion, this study at a logistics company showed that physical activity training combined with nutrition counseling can be implemented successfully during working hours on a long-term basis with initial effects on health behavior changes. Effects on body weight decrease were minimal. Our findings highlight the need for worksite health promotion strategies that provide increased motivation, support and skills to enable employees living their life in a healthy way. Similarly, the results suggest a need to promote time-efficient physical activity options and alternatives. Additional strategies that recognize the perceived barriers to physical activity and healthy eating faced by employees are particularly required.

Competing interest
The authors declare that no conflicts of interest exist.

Authors' contribution
SM, GP, EO designed the study. SM, SJ, GP, SL, MS, EO performed the investigation. SM and SJ analyzed the data. SM wrote the manuscript. SM, SL, RJ, MS, SJ, EO, GP interpreted the data and contributed substantially to its revision. All authors read and approved the final manuscript.

Sources of funding
Sources of funding for this research study include institutional support.

Author details
[1]Institute for Occupational Medicine and Maritime Medicine (ZfAM), University Medical Center Hamburg-Eppendorf, Seewartenstrasse 10, 20459 Hamburg, Germany. [2]Institute of Occupational Medicine, Charité – Universitätsmedizin Berlin, Free University and Humboldt University, Thielallee 69-73, 14195 Berlin, Germany. [3]Bremen International Graduate School of Social Sciences, Wiener Straße/Ecke Celsiusstraße, 28359 Bremen, Germany. [4]Institute of Technology & Innovation Management, Helmut Schmidt University, Hamburg, Holstenhofweg 85, 22043 Hamburg, Germany. [5]Institute of Health Care Management, University of Applied Sciences Zwickau, Dr.-Friedrichs-Ring 2a, 08056 Zwickau, Germany.

References

1. Finucane MM, Stevens GA, Cowan MJ, Danaei G, Lin JK, Paciorek CJ. National, regional, and global trends in body-mass index since 1980: systematic analysis of health examination surveys and epidemiological studies with 960 country-years and 9.1 million participants. Lancet. 2011;377:557–67.
2. World Health Organization W. Obesity: preventing and managing the global epidemic: report of a WHO consultation. Geneva: World Health Organization; 2000.
3. Peeters A, Barendregt JJ, Willekens F, Mackenbach JP, Al Mamun A, Bonneux L. Obesity in adulthood and its consequences for life expectancy: a life-table analysis. Ann Intern Med. 2003;138:24–32.
4. Bray GA. Risks of obesity. Endocrinol Metab Clin North Am. 2003;32:787–804.
5. Graf C, Ferrari N, Eiser S. Obesity- status quo and therapeutic approaches. MMW Fortschr Med. 2013;155:91–4.
6. World Health Organization W. Global health risk: mortality and burden of disease attributable to selected major risks. Geneva: World Health Organization; 2009.
7. Berghoefer A, Pischon T, Reinhold E. Obesity prevalence from a European perspective:a systematic review. BMC Public Health. 2008;8:200.
8. Mensink GBM, Schienkiewitz A, Haftenberger M, Lampert T, Ziese T, Scheidt-Nave C. Overweight and obesity in Germany, Results of the German Health Interview and Examination Survey for Adults (DEGS1). Bundesgesundheitsbl. 2013;56:786–94.
9. Gates DM, Succop P, Brehm BJ, Gillespie GL, Sommers BD. Obesity and presenteeism: the impact of body mass index on workplace productivity. J Occup Environ Med. 2008;50:39–45.
10. Van Duijvenbode DC, Hoozemans MJM, Van Poppel MNM, Proper KI. The relationship between overweight and obesity, and sick leave: a systematic review. Int J Obes. 2009;33:807–16.
11. Soeliman FA, Azadbakht L. Weight loss maintenance: A review on dietary related strategies. J Res Med Sci. 2014;19:268–75.
12. French SA, Story M, Jeffery RW. Environmental influences on eating and physical activity. Annu Rev Public Health. 2001;22:309–35.
13. Faith MS, Kral TVE: Social Environmental and Genetic Influences on Obesity and Obesity-Promoting Behaviors: Fostering Research Integration. National Academies Press (US): Washington; 2006.
14. Hill JO, Wyatt HR, Reed GW, Peters JC. Obesity and the environment: where do we go from here? Science. 2003;1:299–853.
15. Peters JC, Wyatt HR, Donahoo WT, Hill JO. From instinct to intellect: the challenge of maintaining healthy weight in the modern world. Obes Rev. 2002;3:69–74.
16. Hill JO. Understanding and addressing the epidemic of obesity: an energy balance perspective. Endocr Rev. 2006;27:750–61.
17. Beresford SA, Locke E, Bishop S, West B, McGregor BA, Bruemmer B, et al. Worksite study promoting activity and changes in eating (PACE): design and baseline results. Obesity. 2007;1:4S–15S.
18. Bamberg E, Ducki A, Metz A. Handbuch Betriebliche Gesundheitsförderung. Verlag für Angewandte Psychologie: Göttingen; 1998.
19. Harden A, Peersman G, Oliver S, Mauthner M, Oakley A. A systematic review of the effectiveness of health promotion interventions in the workplace. Occup Med. 1999;49:540–8.
20. McLellan RK, Mackenzie TA, Tilton PA, Dietrich AJ, Comi RJ, Feng YY. Impact of workplace sociocultural attributes on participation in health assessments. J Occup Environ Med. 2009;51:797–803.
21. McTigue KM, Hess R, Ziouras J. Obesity in older adults: a systematic review of the evidence for diagnosis and treatment. Obesity (Silver Spring). 2006;14:1485–97.
22. Proper KI, Koning M, van der Beek AJ, Hildebrandt VH, Bosscher RJ. The effectiveness of worksite physical activity programs on physical activity, physical fitness, and health. Clin J Sport Med. 2003;13:106–17.
23. Vuillemin A, Rostami C, Maes L, Van Cauwenberghe E, Van Lenthe FJ, Brug J, et al. Worksite physical activity interventions and obesity: a review of European studies (the HOPE project). Obes Facts. 2011;4:479–88.
24. Maes L, Van Cauwenberghe E, Van Lippevelde W, Spittaels H, De Pauw E, Oppert JM, et al. Effectiveness of workplace interventions in Europe promoting healthy eating: a systematic review. Eur J Public Health. 2012;22:677–83.
25. Mills PR, Kessler RC, Cooper J, Sullivan S. Impact of a health promotion program on employee health risks and work productivity. Am J Health Promot. 2007;22:45–53.
26. Dlugosch GE. Gesundheitsberatung. In: Schwenkmezger P, Schmidt LR, editors. Lehrbuch der Gesundheitspsychologie. Stuttgart: Enke; 1992. p. 222–33.
27. Prochaska JO, Velicer WF, Redding CA, Rossi JS, Goldstein M, DePue J. Stage-based expert systems to guide a population of primary care patients to quit smoking, eat healthier, prevent skin cancer and receive regular mammograms. Prev Med. 2005;41:406–16.
28. Diehl JM, Staufenbiel T. Inventar zum Essverhalten und Gewichtsproblemen IEG. Klotz: Eschborn; 1999.
29. Nuebling M, Hasselhorn HM. The Copenhagen Psychosocial Questionnaire in Germany: from the validation of the instrument to the formation of a job-specific database of psychosocial factors at work. Scand J Public Health. 2010;38:120–4.
30. Kwak L, Kremers SP, Visscher TL, van Baak MA, Brug J. Behavioral and cognitive effects of a worksite-based weight gain prevention program: the NHF-NRG in balance-project. J Occup Environ Med. 2009;51(12):1437–46.
31. Brehm BJ, Gates DM, Singler M, Succop PA, D'Alessio DA. Environmental changes to control obesity: a randomized controlled trial in manufactering companies. Am J Health Promot. 2011;25:334–40.
32. Anderson LM, Quinn TA, Glanz K, Ramirez G, Kahwati LC, Johnson DB. The effectiveness of worksite nutrition and physical activity interventions for controlling employee overweight and obesity: a systematic review. Am J Prev Med. 2009;37(4):340–57.
33. Christensen JR, Faber A, Ekner D, Overgaard K, Holtermann A, Sogaard K. Diet, physical exercise and cognitive behavioral training as a combined workplace based intervention to reduce body weight and increase physical capacity in health care workers - a randomized controlled trial. BMC Public Health. 2011;11:671.
34. Franz MJ, VanWormer JJ, Crain AL, Boucher JL, Histon T, Caplan W, et al. Weight-loss outcomes: a systematic review and meta-analysis of weight-loss clinical trials with a minimum 1-year follow-up. J Am Diet Assoc. 2007;107:1755–67.
35. van Berkel J, Boot C, Proper KI, Bongers BM, van der Beek AJ. Effectiveness of a worksite mindfulness-based multi-component intervention on lifestyle behaviors. Int J Behav Nutr Phys Act. 2014;11:9.
36. Westenhoefer J. The therapeutic challenge: behavioral changes for long-term weight maintenance. Int J Obes Relat Metab Disord. 2001;25:85–8.
37. Scheers T, Philippaerts R, Lefevre J. Patterns of physical activity and sedentary behavior in normal-weight, overweight and obeseadults, as measured with a portable armband device and an electronic diary. Clin Nutr. 2012;31:756–64.
38. Simon C, Schweitzer B, Oujaa M, Wagner A, Arveiler D, Triby E, et al. Successful overweight prevention in adolescents by increasing physical activity: a 4-year randomized controlled intervention. Int J Obes. 2008;32:1489–98.
39. Brand R, Schlicht W, Grossman K, Duhnsen R. Effects of a physical exercise intervention on employees'perceptions quality of life: a randomized controlled trial. Soz Praeventivmed. 2006;51:14–23.
40. Sternfeld B, Block C, Quesenberry CP, Block TJ, Husson G, Norris JC, et al. Improving diet and physical activity with ALIVE: a worksite randomized trial. Am J Prev Med. 2009;36:475–83.
41. Young DR, Jerome GJ, Chen C, Laferriere D, Vollmer WM. Patterns of physical activity among overweight and obese adults. Prev Chronic Dis. 2009;6:90.

42. Weinstock RS, Dai H, Wadden TA. Diet and exercise in the treatment of obesity: effects of 3 interventions on insulin resistance. Arch Intern Med. 1998;158:2477–83.
43. Duvigneaud N, Wijndaele K, Matton L, Philippaerts R, Lefevre J, Thomis M, et al. Dietary factors associated with obesity indicators and level of sports participation in Flemish adults: a cross-sectional study. Nutr J. 2007;6:26.
44. Ortega RM, Requejo AM, Andres P, Lopez-Sobaler AM, Redondo R, Gonzalez-Fernandez M. Relationship between diet composition and body mass index in a group of Spanish adolescents. Br J Nutr. 1995;74:765–73.
45. Hutchinson AD, Wilson C. Improving nutrition and physical activity in the workplace: a meta-analysis of intervention studies. Health Promot Int. 2012;27:238–49.
46. Walseth LT, Abildsnes E, Schei E. Lifestyle, health and the ethics of good living, Health behaviour counselling in general practice. Patient Educ Couns. 2011;83:180–4.
47. Zinn C, Schofield GM, Hopkins WG. A "small-changes" workplace weight loss and maintenance program: examination of weight and health outcomes. J Occup Environ Med. 2012;54:1230–8.
48. Simon C, Schweitzer B, Oujaa M, Wagner A, Arveiler D, Triby E, et al. Successful overweight prevention in adolescents by increasing physical activity: a 4-year randomized controlled intervention. Int J Obes (Lond). 2008;32(10):1489–98.
49. Connor Gorber S, Tremblay M, Moher D, Gorber B. A comparison of direct vs. self-report measures for assessing height, weight and body mass index: a systematic review. Obes Rev. 2007;8:307–26.
50. Shields M, Connor Gorber S, Tremblay MS. Estimates of obesity based on self-report versus direct measures. Health Rep. 2008;19:61–76.
51. Mensink GBM, Schienkiewitz A, Haftenberger M, Lampert T, Ziese T, Scheidt-Nave C. Übergewicht und Adipositas in Deutschland – Ergebnisse der Studie zur Gesundheit Erwachsener in Deutschland (DEGS1). Bundesgesundheitsblatt. 2013;56:786–94.

19

The legislative backgrounds of workplace health promotion in three European countries

Rasa Šidagytė[1*], Maija Eglīte[2], Anne Salmi[3], Dovilė Šorytė[1], Ivars Vanadziņš[4], Leila Hopsu[5], Jaana Lerssi-Uskelin[5], Laima Bulotaitė[6], Lāsma Kozlova[4], Svetlana Lakiša[4] and Sigita Vičaitė[1,7]

Abstract

Background: This article investigates the legal database and theoretical basis of workplace health promotion (WHP) in three European countries: Finland, Latvia and Lithuania, and aims to find insights into effective WHP implementation.

Methods: In November 2013, a stakeholders' survey was carried out. The questionnaire included questions about legal documents and non-legislative measures relevant to WHP, institutions and other bodies/organizations working in the field, WHP conception/definition, and implementation of WHP activities according to the enterprises' size.

Results: Only Finland has adopted a specific law on occupational health care (separate from occupational safety). ILO conventions No. 161 (Occupational Health Services Convention) and No. 187 (Promotional Framework for Occupational Safety and Health Convention) are ratified only in Finland. In Finland, the Ministry of Social Affairs and Health acts as one ministry, while two Baltic countries have two separate ministries (one for health and another for social affairs). None of the countries has legally approved a definition of WHP. Latvia and Lithuania tend to separate WHP from other activities, whereas Finland integrates WHP into other occupational health and safety elements.

Conclusions: Finland has a more extensive legislative and organizational background to WHP than Latvia and Lithuania. In defining WHP, all the countries refer to the Luxembourg Declaration on Workplace Health Promotion in the European Union. Finland's practice of integrating WHP into other occupational health and safety elements is important.

Keywords: Workplace health promotion, Occupational health, Enterprise, Legislation

Background

According to the European working conditions survey (EWCS) [1], employees who think that their health or safety is at risk because of their work comprise a quarter in Finland (close to the European average), nearly one third in Lithuania and almost a half in Latvia. Similar figures illustrate the proportion of working people who think that their work mainly affects their health negatively. However, work can also affect the health of working people in a positive way. EWCS revealed that 28.7 percent of Finnish employees think that their work mainly affects their health positively. The Latvian rate for this question was 8.8 percent, and the Lithuanian rate was 6 percent, and the rates of these two countries are around the European average (7.3 percent). Thus employees' opinions on working conditions and their effect on health seem to be better in Finland than in the two Baltic countries.

Together with other occupational health services, workplace health promotion (WHP) can contribute significantly to the health of the working population. The *Luxembourg Declaration on Workplace Health Promotion in the European Union* [2] defines WHP as "the combined efforts of employers, employees and society to improve the health and well-being of people at work".

* Correspondence: rasa.sidagyte@hi.lt
[1]Occupational Health Centre, Institute of Hygiene, Didžioji str. 22, Vilnius, Lithuana

Experts notice that occupational health services are not delivered to all the workers due to gaps in implementation, coverage, content and capacity. These gaps are seen particularly in small enterprises [3]. Countries may have different experiences in developing occupational health services and also different backgrounds for WHP. This article thereafter investigates the legal database and theoretical basis of WHP in three European countries: Finland, Latvia and Lithuania, and aims to find insights into effective WHP implementation.

Methods

In November 2013, a stakeholders' survey was carried out using a questionnaire which was prepared and agreed on in all the participating countries. The questionnaire consisted of five sections (each section having several questions): Section A – legal documents and other measures relevant to WHP; Section B – WHP conception/definition; Section C – institutions and other bodies/organizations working in the field of WHP, specific networks and training courses for specialists; Section D – implementation of WHP activities; Section E – research area relative to WHP. The stakeholder institutions were: the Finnish Institute of Occupational Health (Finland), the Institute of Occupational Safety and Environmental Health of Riga Stradins University (Latvia) and the Institute of Hygiene, Occupational Health Centre (Lithuania). Stakeholders chose the appropriate excerpts from the legislative documents for the questionnaire. Then, descriptive analysis of the gathered questionnaires' content was performed and comparisons made where possible.

The questionnaire elicited the stakeholders' opinion on the implementation of various WHP activities in the different sized enterprises. In accordance with European Commission Recommendation 2003/361/EC [4] and the Eurostat Glossary [5], a small enterprise is defined as an enterprise that employs fewer than 50 people, a medium-sized enterprise is defined as an enterprise that employs fewer than 250 people and a large enterprise is defined as an enterprise that employs 250 people or more.

Results

Legislation concerning WHP

Council Directive 89/391/EEC of 12 June 1989 on the introduction of measures to encourage improvements in the safety and health of workers at work [6] is adapted by all the three countries. The main International Labour Organization (ILO) conventions regarding occupational health issues, *Occupational Health Services Convention No. 161* [7] and *Promotional Framework for Occupational Safety and Health Convention No. 187* [8], are ratified only in Finland. As is seen in Table 1, all the three countries have specific legislations on occupational safety and health issues, including WHP.

According to the Finnish *Occupational Safety and Health Act* [9], employers are required to take care of the safety and health of their employees while at work, and to have a policy for actions needed in order to promote safety and health and to maintain employees' work ability capacity.

The organization of occupational health services in Finland is based on the *Occupational Health Care Act* [10]. This is in line with ILO Convention No. 161. The content of occupational health care includes: making suggestions for action to improve the healthiness and safety of work, to adapt work to the needs of the employee, to maintain and promote employees' work ability and functional capacity; provision of information, advice and guidance in matters concerning the healthiness and safety of work and the health of the employees.

By enhancing co-operation between employer, employee and occupational health care provider, the Act aims to promote: 1) the prevention of work-related illnesses and accidents, 2) the healthiness and safety of work and the work environment, 3) the health, work ability capacity and functional capacity of employees at different stages of their working careers, 4) the functioning of the workplace community. According to the Act, employers must have a written occupational health care action plan.

The Latvian *Labour Protection Law* [11] includes both the occupational safety and occupational health aspects as the term "labour protection" is defined as "safety and health of employees at work". The Law defines "labour protection measures" as "legal, economic, social, technical and organisational preventive measures the objective of which is to establish a safe and harmless to health working environment, as well as prevent accidents at work and occupational diseases". Generally the Law emphasizes that employers are obligated to consult, inform and enforce the participation of employees in the process of occupational safety and health measures.

The Lithuanian *Law on Safety and Health at Work* [12] stresses that employers must ensure employees' safety and health at work in all work-related aspects. According to this Law, "occupational health" means the prevention of hazardous factors in the work environment, adapting the work environment to the physiological and psychological capabilities of workers, carrying out healthcare of workers, and implementing health strengthening measures.

In all participating countries, the law imposes several occupational safety and health obligations on both employers and employees, as parties in the legal relationship. First of all, the employer is responsible for the employees' health in general. Directly the specific functions (but not necessarily WHP as itself) are delegated to specialists, who may have a different education and professional titles. In Finland occupational health care providers should put forward initiatives and suggestions to the employer or his

Table 1 Most important excerpts of national legislation and other documents connected to WHP

Type of legislation	Finland	Latvia	Lithuania
Laws	1. Occupational Safety and Health Act No. 738/2002 (1958/2002) 2. Occupational Health Care Act No. 1383/2001 (2001)	Labour Protection Law (2002)	Law on Safety and Health at Work No. IX-1672 (2003/2007)
Other legislation	Government Decree on the Principles of Good Occupational Health Care Practice, the Content of Occupational Health Care and the Qualifications of Professionals and Experts (2001)	1. Profession Standard for Occupational Safety Specialists (2002) 2. Profession Standard for Occupational Safety Senior Specialist (2002)	1. Regulation on Enterprise Occupational Safety and Health Services (2002) 2. Regulation on Professional Requirements for Occupational Health Specialists (2008) 3. Regulation on Professional Development/Training Programme Content Requirements for Occupational Health Specialists (2010)

representative, on, for example, measures for monitoring the health of employees and different employee groups and for maintaining and promoting their health and work ability [13]. In Latvia, occupational health is included in the obligations of labour protection specialists [14,15] as their training includes various health-related aspects of occupational safety and health. However, health promotion, and specifically WHP, is not directly mentioned in their curricula. In Lithuania, occupational health specialists [16] should perform these functions in relation to WHP [17]: organize healthy lifestyle training, develop health promotion programmes for employees, and arrange their implementation.

Table 2 shows national policy programmes and strategies that come close to WHP in each country.

Non-legislative measures regarding WHP

Without the legislation (some of it described above), countries apply various non-legislative measures (recommendations, guidelines, other material) prepared by national, local authorities or other bodies. In Finland, the Occupational Safety Card [18] (2003), the Work Capacity Certificate [19] (2006; for students in vocational education) and the Well-being at Work Card [20] (2010; dedicated to everyone) are in use. The *Well-being at Work Card* is a one-day training certificate. The topics and contents of the training for the Well-being at Work Card are: some viewpoints on well-being at work; management and well-being at work; the functioning of the work community; health and work ability. In addition to these, there are a great deal of WHP recommendations in Finland.

Table 2 Most important excerpts of national policy programmes and strategies connected to WHP

Type of document	Finland	Latvia	Lithuania
Programmes/strategies specific to workers' health and safety	Government Resolution. Occupational Health 2015. Development Strategy for Occupational Health Care (2004)	National Strategy on Occupational Safety and Health 2008-2013 (2008) and its action plans for 2008-2010 and 2011-2013	Employee Safety and Health Strategy for 2009–2012 (2009) and its action plans for 2009-2010 and 2011-2012
Programmes/strategies from other areas, or general	1. Programme of Prime Minister Jyrki Katainen's Government (2011) 2. Finnish Nutrition Recommendations (2014) 3. Government Resolution on Development Guidelines for Health-Enhancing Physical Activity and Nutrition (2008) 4. On the Move. National Strategy for Physical Activity Promoting Health and Wellbeing 2020 (2013) 5. Health Promotion, Government Policy Programme 2007-2011 (2007) 6. National Action Plan to Reduce Health Inequalities 2008-2011 7. Developing Mass Catering Services. Guidelines by the Working Group to Monitor and Develop Mass Catering Services (2010)	1. Public Health Strategy for 2011 – 2017 (2011) 2. Plan of National Development for 2014 – 2020 (2014)	Mental Health Strategy (2007) and its action plan for 2011-2013

Latvia has prepared *Health promotion guidelines for local governments* (2011) [21] – some of the recommendations of which are meant for WHP. In Latvia a *Plan for preventive measures* is approved every year. This includes training and information seminars and information materials for occupational safety specialists, employers, employees and others.

Lithuania has several recommendations on different WHP topics for specialists performing occupational health care in enterprises, employers and employees.

Institutions and other organizations working in the field of WHP

In Finland, the *Ministry of Social Affairs and Health* and the *Ministry of Employment and the Economy* are responsible for policy-making in the area of occupational health and safety (Table 3). The co-ordination and provision of methodological support linked to WHP is responsibility of *Occupational safety and health administrations.* The Administrations enact laws (e.g. Occupational Safety and Health Act, Occupational Health Care Act) and provide supervision and inspection control. The *Finnish Institute of Occupational Health (FIOH)* is a research and specialist organization working in the field of occupational health and safety. It organizes qualification training for occupational health and safety professionals and experts. FIOH also organizes and participates in national and international projects and research together with various non-governmental institutions and international universities.

In Latvia, the *Ministry of Health* and the *Ministry of Welfare* are responsible for the legislation related to occupational health and safety. Both ministries, together with the *Ministry of Education and Science*, the *Institute of Occupational Safety and Environmental Health*, and the *State Labour Inspection* provide various sorts of information and materials that are to some extent attributable to WHP issues. The *Institute of Occupational Safety and Environmental Health* of *Riga Stradiņš University* organize training for specialists and are also known for their participation in national and international research projects and programmes related to WHP. The *State Labour Inspection* executes supervision and inspection control which in some respects is also linked to WHP. The functions of regional institutions belong to *local municipalities* in Latvia. The Latvian *Centre for Disease Prevention and Control* has developed a network of contact persons in local municipalities to co-ordinate health promotion activities locally and their training also includes some aspects of WHP. The Centre itself has developed Health Promotion Guidelines and various information material for local municipalities, which also includes information on health promotion in local companies.

In Lithuania, the responsibility for policy-making concerning occupational health and safety belongs to the *Ministry of Health* and the *Ministry of Social Security and Labour.* The *Occupational Health Centre* (at the *Institute of Hygiene*) and the *Centre for Health Education and Disease Prevention* also provide various recommendations and training for specialists. The *Occupational Health Centre* carries out national and international

Table 3 Governmental institutions (and their activity areas) that co-ordinate and methodically support WHP activities

Type of institutions (main functions)	Finland	Latvia	Lithuania
Ministries	– Ministry of Social Affairs and Health (regulations, enforcement, directions, inspection, monitoring, information, guidelines) – Ministry of Employment and the Economy (legislation on work contracts, annual and other leaves, equity, unemployment)	– Ministry of Health (policy-making, recommendations) – Ministry of Welfare (policy-making, recommendations) – Ministry of Education and Science (policy-making, recommendations, professional standards)	– Ministry of Health (policy-making) – Ministry of Social Security and Labour (policy-making)
Other institutions at national level	– Occupational Safety and Health Administration (inspection, guidelines and advice relating to health services) – Finnish Institute of Occupational Health (FIOH) (training, information, statements, advice, monitoring, recommendations, research, interventions, surveillance, services)	– Institute of Occupational Safety and Environmental Health (recommendations, specialist training) – State Labor Inspection (recommendations, inspection, supervision) – Riga Stradiņš University (specialist training)	– Occupational Health Centre, Institute of Hygiene (recommendations, research, specialist training, interventions) – State Labour Inspectorate (inspection, supervision, advice)
Institutions at regional level	6 Regional State Administrative Agencies (Occupational safety and health administrations) (inspection, guidelines, advise)	Local municipalities (WHP implementation)	Public health offices (WHP implementation)

research and provides expertise, consultation and information in the field of occupational health. *Public health offices* at the municipality level perform trainings and lectures for employees about healthy lifestyles, as well as various other health promotion activities for the employees.

At this moment the two Baltic countries do not have many NGOs that operate in WHP issues or have activities linked to this domain. The Finnish *Centre for Occupational Safety* provides training, information, materials, and development services based on the latest knowledge, and administrates and maitains a register of occupational safety personnel. These activities and services are planned in close co-operation with branch-related employers' and employees' organizations in sector groups. In addition, the activities of the Centre are based on the agreements and regulations concluded by Finnish labour market organizations. The Centre provides, for example, one-day training courses, which lead to either the Occupational Safety Card or the Well-being at Work Card.

Conception and elements of WHP

None of the participating countries has a legally approved definition of WHP. Describing WHP, all partner countries (stakeholder institutions) refer to *The Luxembourg Declaration*, mentioned at the beginning of this article. We can summarize that for implementing WHP at the enterprise level four tool groups are essential: 1) internal political decisions (workplace policies), 2) organizational structures (responsible departments and persons), 3) physical/technical structures (health supporting environment and facilities), and 4) health education (health information and training activities).

In Table 4 we see that in the stakeholders' opinion, WHP implementation is better in large enterprises, and that medium-sized and especially small enterprises lack WHP activities.

Rather then a separate phenomenon in the enterprise, WHP can also be considered as activities integrated into other elements of occupational health and safety. This approach is more characteristic of Finland – WHP is almost "everywhere". Latvia and Lithuania tend more to separate it from other elements, considering it an independent activity (Table 5).

Discussion

Our study revealed that there are differences between the countries as regards the backgrounds of WHP implementation. Finland has a more extensive legislative background for occupational health services and WHP implementation. All three countries have specific legislations and other documents on occupational safety and health issues, including WHP, but Finland is the only country that has adopted a specific law on occupational health care (separate to occupational safety). ILO conventions regarding occupational health issues, *Occupational Health Services Convention No. 161* and *Promotional Framework for Occupational Safety and Health Convention No. 187*, are ratified only in Finland.

Another feature of Finland's system is that the Ministry of Social Affairs and Health in this country acts as one ministry while the two Baltic countries have two separate ministries (one for health and another for social affairs). All these issues are important for organizing occupational health care. The Finnish model seems to be more extensive. Surveys show that working conditions and their affect on health according to employees' opinions, is better in Finland than in the two Baltic countries – this could be the result of the extensive legislative system. However, in saying this, we do not claim that legislation alone determines success. But legislation should be adequate to build a substantial background for occupational health services and WHP implementation. The governments of Latvia and Lithuania should consider including the provisions of ILO conventions mentioned above in their national legislation.

It is important to mention that in Lithuania, only bigger enterprises (with more than 100 or 200 employees, depending on the economic activity (i. e. risk level)), have to employ/hire occupational health specialists. In both Latvia and Lithuania in some cases (small companies) the employer himself is allowed to act as the occupational safety and health specialist – he only has to undergo basic level training for this. This is a problem in the light of WHP, because most employees work in smaller companies and this means that providing them with WHP services (and the quality of these services) depends on the employers' education, interests and resources.

The survey made it obvious that none of the participating countries has a legally approved definition of WHP. However, this is not necessary, as all three countries refer to the Luxembourg Declaration. Actually, all these countries are considered members of the *European Network for Workplace Health Promotion* (*ENWHP*) [22], but the two Baltic countries are currently not active. In our opinion, this situation shows the lack of the Baltic countries' government's attention to international collaboration in the occupational health area. Another actual problem that stakeholders mentioned is that the WHP training for specialists (dedicated directly to WHP) is very poor. Even in Finland, WHP is at the moment only one aspect of specialists' training. The current situation generally calls for a more integrative approach and understanding of WHP and the safety of workers [23].

To effectively contribute to the health of workers, WHP should be organized along with other occupational health and safety activities (occupational risk assessment, preventive health examinations etc.) which are all of equal importance. We noticed that sometimes WHP can

Table 4 Elements of WHP and their implementation according to size of enterprise

Elements of WHP	Size of enterprise								
	Finland*			Latvia			Lithuania		
	Large	Medium	Small	Large	Medium	Small	Large	Medium	Small
1. Specific internal documents approved at the enterprise	P	P	P	P	P	N	P	P	N
2. Initiative of Trade Unions	F	F	P	P	P	N	P	P	N
3. Giving incentives to the employees (contests, premiums, gifts)	P	P	P	F	P	N	P	P	P/N
4. Allocation of funds	F	F	P/N	N	N	N	P	N	N
5. Developing organizational structures in accordance with existing legal acts	F	P	P/N	P	N	N	F	P	N
6. Development of a healthy work environment, e.g. facilities: sports hall, healthy food canteen/shop, relaxation room, park for walking within the grounds of the enterprise, mothers' room etc.	P	P	P	P	N	N	P	P	N
7. Developing healthy psychosocial environment, e.g. conflict management programmes	P	P	N	P	N	N	P	P	N
8. Implementing WHP programmes	P	P	N	P	N	N	P	P	N
9. Dissemination of information about healthy lifestyles, e.g. health education (lectures, seminars), reference material (stands, booklets)	F	P	P	F	P	P	P	P	P
10. Formation of lifestyle skills that sustain and promote health, e.g. physical activity programmes	P	P	P	N	N	N	P	N	N
11. Involving employees and their families in active leisure activities (e.g. sports games for families)	P	P/N	N	P	P	P	P	N	N
12. Developing illness prevention and prophylaxis programmes	P	P/N	N	P	N	N	P	P	N
13. Improving access to health services	P/N	N	N	P	P	N	P	P/N	N

*Finnish information from Aura et al [24].
(F – fully implemented, P – partially implemented, N – not implemented).

even be integrated into these other activities. Latvia and Lithuania tend to treat WHP as a more independent activity, whereas Finland often integrates WHP into other occupational health and safety elements. Remembering the figures on how work affects employees' health in each country, we can state again that the Finnish approach to WHP may be more effective.

Table 5 Occupational safety and health activities containing WHP elements

Occupational safety and health activities and other enterprise work activities	Finland	Latvia	Lithuania
1. Occupational risk assessment	+	–	–
2. Preventive health examinations	+	+	–
3. Physical work environment	+	+	+
4. Psychosocial work environment	+	+	+
5. Monitoring of employees' health and work environment	+	–	–
6. Access to general health services	+	–	–
7. Occupational safety and health policy at the enterprise	+	–	–
8. Rehabilitation (medical, occupational, social)	+	–	–
9. Scientific activities	+	+	+
10. Independent WHP programmes (separate from other activities)	+	+	+
11. Employees consulting	+	–	–

A limitation of our survey is that the results are based only on stakeholders' opinions. There is a need to carry out an enterprise survey on the existing practical level and the needs for WHP activities. Since employers' motivation is essential for implementing WHP, it is necessary to find out what motivates them and what obstacles they face in this area. We also lack knowledge regarding the employees' WHP needs. Thus, recommendations on how to most effectively implement WHP should be prepared for decision-makers, employers, occupational and public health specialists, and human recourse specialists.

Conclusions

1. All three countries have specific legislation on occupational safety and health issues but Finland has a more extensive legislative and organizational background to WHP.
2. None of the investigated countries has a legally approved definition of WHP, but all refer to the Luxembourg Declaration.
3. WHP realization may have different approaches. Finland's practice on integrating WHP into other occupational health and safety elements is important.

Competing interests

The authors declare that they have no competing interests.

Authors' contributions

RS participated in the design of the study, participated in data collection in Lithuania, performed a primary comparative analysis and drafted the manuscript. ME critically revised the manuscript and gave the final approval for the version to be published. AS participated in data collection in Finland, and also provided important comments for the improvement of the draft. DS participated in the design of the study, participated in data collection in Lithuania and helped to draft the manuscript. IV organized data collection in Latvia and made valuable comments for the improvement of the draft. LH participated in data collection in Finland and gave insights into the design and content of the manuscript. JLU organized data collection in Finland and gave insights into the design and content of the manuscript. LB participated in data collection in Lithuania. LK and SL participated in data collection in Latvia. SV designed and co-ordinated the study, participated in data collection in Lithuania and helped to draft the manuscript. All authors read and approved the final manuscript.

Acknowledgements

The authors thank the Nordic Council of Ministers. The project and the publication of its results was financed by the Nordplus Adult programme.

Author details

[1]Occupational Health Centre, Institute of Hygiene, Didžioji str. 22, Vilnius, Lithuania. [2]Department of Occupational and Environmental Medicine, Riga Stradins University, Dzirciema str. 16, Riga, Latvia. [3]Finnish Institute of Occupational Health, Aapistie 1, Oulu, Finland. [4]Institute of Occupational Safety and Environmental Health of Riga Stradins University, Dzirciema str. 16, Riga, Latvia. [5]Finnish Institute of Occupational Health, Topeliuksenkatu 41 a A, Helsinki, Finland. [6]Department of General Psychology, Faculty of Philosophy, Vilnius University, Universiteto str. 9/1, Vilnius, Lithuania. [7]Positive Health Team, Šviesos str. 4B-7, Vilnius, Lithuania.

References

1. European Working Conditions Survey – mapping the results [http://old.eurofound.europa.eu/surveys/smt/ewcs/results.htm]
2. The Luxembourg Declaration on Workplace Health Promotion in the European Union. Version of January 2007 [http://www.enwhp.org/fileadmin/rs-dokumente/dateien/Luxembourg_Declaration.pdf]
3. Rantanen J, Lehtinen S, Iavicoli S. Occupational health services in selected International Commission on Occupational Health (ICOH) member countries. Scand J Work Environ Health. 2013;39(2):212–6.
4. European Commission Recommendation 2003/361/EC of 6 May 2003 concerning the definition of micro, small and medium-sized enterprises. OJ L 124, 20/05/2003, p. 36–41.
5. Statistics Explained. Glossary: Enterprise size [http://ec.europa.eu/eurostat/statistics-explained/index.php/Glossary:Enterprise_size]
6. Council Directive 89/391/EEC of 12 June 1989 on the introduction of measures to encourage improvements in the safety and health of workers at work. OJ L 183, 29/06/1989, p. 1–8.
7. C161 – Occupational Health Services Convention, 1985 (No. 161). Adoption: Geneva, 71st ILC session (25 June 1985).
8. C187 – Promotional Framework for Occupational Safety and Health Convention, 2006 (No. 187). Adoption: Geneva, 95th ILC session (15 June 2006).
9. Occupational Safety and Health Act No. 738/2002 [http://www.finlex.fi/fi/laki/kaannokset/2002/en20020738.pdf] (unofficial translation to English)
10. Occupational Health Care Act No. 1383/2001 [http://www.finlex.fi/fi/laki/kaannokset/2001/en20011383.pdf] (unofficial translation to English)
11. Labour Protection Law, adopted on 20.06.2001 by Latvian Parliament (Saeima) [http://www.vvc.gov.lv/export/sites/default/docs/LRTA/Likumi/Labour_Protection_Law.doc]
12. Republic of Lithuania Law on Safety and Health at Work. 1 July 2003, No IX-1672 [http://www3.lrs.lt/pls/inter3/dokpaieska.showdoc_l?p_id=455411]
13. Government Decree on the Principles of Good Occupational Health Care Practice, the Content of Occupational Health Care and the Qualifications of Professionals and Experts No. 1484/2001 [www.finlex.fi/en/laki/kaannokset/2001/en20011484.pdf] (unofficial translation to English)
14. Profesijas standarts. Darba aizsardzības speciālists [http://visc.gov.lv/profizglitiba/dokumenti/standarti/ps0094.pdf] (inLatvian)
15. Profesijas standarts. Darba aizsardzības vecākais speciālists [http://osha.lv/lv/training/ps_0100_d.a.%20vec.%20spec.dat.pdf] (in Latvian)
16. Profesinės sveikatos specialistų, galinčių dirbti įmonėse, kvalifikacinių reikalavimų aprašas. 2008 m. balandžio 8 d. Nr. V-271, Vilnius (in Lithuanian)
17. Įmonių darbuotojų saugos ir sveikatos tarnybų pavyzdiniai nuostatai (Regulation on Enterprise Occupational Safety and Health Services). 2011 m. birželio 2 d. Nr. A1-266/V-575, Vilnius (in Lithuanian)
18. Occupational Safety Card [http://www.tyoturvallisuuskortti.fi/english]
19. SAKU in a nutshell [http://www.sakury.net/?q=saku-nutshell]
20. Well-being at Work Card [http://www.tyohyvinvointikortti.fi/english]
21. Health Promotion Guidelines for Local Governments. Ministry of Health of the Republic of Latvia, Riga, 2012 [http://www.spkc.gov.lv/file_download/1229/Health_promotion_guidelines_for_local_governments.pdf]
22. The European Network for Workplace Health Promotion (ENWHP) [http://www.enwhp.org/]
23. Sauter SL. Editorial. Integrative Approaches to Safeguarding the Health and Safety of Workers. Industrial Health. 2013;51:559–61.
24. Aura O, Ahonen G, Ilmarinen J. Strategisen hyvinvoinnin tila Suomessa 2012. Helsinki: Pohjola Terveys Oy and Finnish Institute of Occupational Health; 2012.

20

New models for prediction of micronuclei formation in nuclear medicine department workers

Sanja Terzic[1*], Aleksandar Milovanovic[2,3], Jelena Dotlic[3,4], Boban Rakic[2] and Milan Terzic[3,4]

Abstract

Background: Ionizing radiation causes detrimental health effects such as cancer and genetic damage. The study aim was to determine predictors for micronuclei (MN) occurrence and frequency in peripheral blood lymphocytes of health workers professionally exposed to radiation.

Methods: Health workers, age matched, selected for the study on regular check-ups, were divided according to the radiation exposure. The exposed group involved nuclear medicine department employees (54) and the control group comprised workers from other departments (36). Data about workers characteristics and habits, received annual doses (AD), total years of service (TYS) and exposed years of service (EYS) were taken from each subject. Blood samples were taken and micronuclei (MN) number in peripheral blood lymphocytes was calculated using CBMN assay according to standard protocols.

Results: Most workers were female, technicians, with mean age of 45.67 years and EYS about 15 years. Health workers exposed to radiation had significantly more MN than controls ($p = 0.001$). Female gender, older age, higher received annual doses, longer EYS and TYS increased the MN number. Technicians and laboratory workers have higher risk for MN occurrence. Significant predictors of MN formation according to constructed model were workers age, sex, AD and EYS. One EYS year increases MN frequency 1.017 times, while receiving 0.1 mSy raises MN frequency by 26 %. EYS accurately predicts 86.30 % of MN frequencies and AD 64.60 %.

Conclusions: The model, developed for the first time in this study, showed that received annual doses and duration of exposure to radiation can be used for prediction of MN numbers.

Keywords: Professional exposure to radiation, Nuclear medicine, Micronucleus, Chromosomal damage

Background

The risk related to low doses of radiation is primarily due to stochastic effects [1]. The main target of ionizing radiation is the DNA molecule. Adverse biological effects of ionizing radiation are gene mutations, chromosomal rearrangement, cellular transformation, micronucleus [MN] formation, apoptosis, and radiation carcinogenesis [2, 3]. Medical personnel represent the group that is most consistently exposed to low doses of ionizing radiation, due to the widespread use of ionizing radiation as a diagnostic and therapeutic tool [4]. Various studies have been published showing increased frequencies of chromosomal aberrations in health workers occupationally exposed to low levels of radiation [5–7]. Testing for occurrence and frequency of micronuclei in peripheral blood lymphocytes is usually performed to evaluate cytogenetic damage in populations occupationally exposed to ionizing radiation [1, 4].

The aim of this study was to determine potential predictors for development of cell damage, i.e., the occurrence and frequency of micronuclei in peripheral blood lymphocytes of health workers professionally exposed to radiation.

* Correspondence: sanjamaricic@yahoo.com
[1]Occupational Health Department, General Health Center "Savski Venac", Pasterova 1, Belgrade, Serbia

Methods

We analyzed health status, characteristics and habits, as well as specific working places of health care workers professionally exposed to radiation. The study was approved by the Ethical Committee and the written consent for participation in the study was obtained from each subject.

According to the radiation exposure, all examined health workers were divided into the exposed and the control group. The exposed group consisted of all employees who worked with open sources of ionizing radiation at the Institute of Nuclear Medicine, Clinical Center of Serbia, under the supervision of the Radiological Protection Institute of Occupational Health of Serbia "Dr. Dragomir Karajovic". Workers from the exposed and control groups were matched by age and comparable according to other characteristics, in order to reduce probable confounding bias. The control group comprised health workers from Clinical Center of Serbia, who had regular check-ups in the Institute of Occupational Health of Serbia "Dr. Dragomir Karajovic" and were not in contact with radiation.

Detailed anamnesis, with questions about sex, age, use of nicotine, total years of service (TYS) and occupation (doctor, technician, laboratory worker and engineer), was taken from each subject. For workers exposed to radiation we also determined exposed years of service (EYS) and received annual doses (AD), based on data from their personal dosimeters that were taken from medical records of periodic examinations at the Institute of Occupational Health of Serbia "Dr. Dragomir Karajovic".

Samples of 5 ml of whole blood were taken from all subjects by heparinized vacutainer tubes, and kept at room temperature for less than 6 h. Using CBMN assay (Cytokinesis-block MicroNucleus Assay) cells were cultivated according to standard protocols [8]. The blood sample was mixed with standard serum based culture medium – RPMI 1640 medium supplemented with calf serum, l-glutamine and penicillin as well as 1.5 % phytohaemagglutinin (PHA) that is added in order to stimulate lymphocytes division [8]. The mixture is cultivated at 37 °C in a 5 % CO_2 during 72 h. Cytochalasin B was added 44 h after culture initiation. Finally, the preparation was centrifuged to collect cells [8]. Drop of this mixture was placed on the plate, fixed and dried. Cell staining was done in the traditional manner (Giemsa). Obtained preparations were analyzed under the light microscope 400× magnification (Olympus BX-51, magnification 1000 h). In each sample, a single operator examined 1000 binuclear cells with a well-preserved cytoplasm. The presence of micronuclei was registered and their number determined per 1000 binuclear cells. This analysis was performed according to the standard criteria established in the HUMN project (Human MicroNucleus Project) [9].

Obtained data were statistically analyzed using Kolmogorov-Smirnov test, $\chi 2$ test, Student's *t*-test, ANOVA to test significance of differences in patient frequencies regarding categories of evaluated parameters as well as between groups (exposed and unexposed). Spearman's correlation was used to assess the influence of investigated parameters on MN formations. We applied Receiver Operator Curve (ROC) analysis to determine potential predictors of radiation damage to cells. Poisson's regression (generalized linear modeling) was used to create model of relationship between tested parameters and MN frequency. Data were analyzed using the Statistical Package for the Social Sciences (SPSS) software (Advanced Statistics, version 17.0, SPSS Inc. - Chicago, IL, USA).

Results

Study involved 90 workers divided in two groups: exposed group with 54 persons professionally exposed to radiation and control group consisting of 36 workers that were not in contact with radiation.

The investigated workers were 45.67 years old on average (Table 1). The majority of workers were female and non-smokers, in the overall population as well as in both groups (Table 2). Furthermore, in both groups, most of

Table 1 Descriptive parameters of examined health workers in exposed and control groups

	Parameters	Overall population	Exposed group	Control group
AGE	Mean	45.67	45.67	45.67
	Standard deviation	10.48	10.48	10.48
	Minimum	28.00	28.00	28.00
	Maximum	64.00	64.00	64.00
TYS	Mean	18.80	19.31	18.03
	Standard deviation	10.39	10.83	9.78
	Minimum	1.00	1.00	3.00
	Maximum	35.00	35.00	34.00
EYS	Mean	14.98	14.98	0.00
	Standard deviation	10.03	10.03	0.00
	Minimum	1.00	1.00	0.00
	Maximum	35.00	35.00	0.00
MN per 1000 binuclear cells	Mean	13.28	18.39	5.61
	Standard deviation	10.74	10.81	3.92
	Minimum	0.00	3.00	0.00
	Maximum	59.00	59.00	14.00

MN micronucleus, *TYS* total years of service, *EYS* exposed years of service

Table 2 Frequency of examined workers in different categories of examined parameters in exposed and control groups

Patient characteristics		Overall population		Exposed group		Cont·ol group	
		No	%	No	%	No	%
Age categories - decades	3 - 20 – 29 y	8	8.90	4	7,41	4	11,11
	4 - 30 – 39 y	20	22.20	12	22,22	8	22,22
	5 - 40 – 49 y	21	23.30	16	29,63	5	13,89
	6 - 50 – 59 y	37	41.10	20	37,04	17	47,22
	7 - 60 – 69 y	4	4.40	2	3,70	2	5,55
	x^2	25.074		16.872		21.095	
	p	0.001		0.001		0.00·	
Sex	Male	26	28.90	10	18,50	16	44,44
	Female	64	71.10	44	81,50	20	55.56
	x^2	16.044		21.407		0.444	
	p	0.001		0.001		0.505	
Occupation	Technician	40	44.40	22	40,70	18	50,00
	Lab. worker	15	16.70	8	14,80	7	19,44
	Doctor	29	32.20	18	33,30	11	30,56
	Engineer	6	6.70	6	11,10	0	0
	x^2	30.089		13.259		5.467	
	p	0.001		0.004		0.046	
MN categories (intervals of 10) per 1000 binuclear cells	1 cat: 1 – 9	43	47.80	13	24,07	30	83,33
	2 cat: 10 – 19	14	15.60	8	14,81	6	16,67
	3 cat: 20 – 29	22	24.40	22	40,74	0	0
	4 cat: 30 – 39	10	11.10	10	18,52	0	0
	5 cat: 40 – 49	0	0	0	0	0	0
	6 cat: 50 – 59	1	1.10	1	1,85	0	0
	x^2	29.444		12.602		16.000	
	p	0.001		0.001		0.001	
Smoking	Yes	27	30.00	17	31,50	10	27,78
	No	63	70.00	37	68,50	26	72,22
	x^2	14.400		7.407		7.111	
	p	0.001		0.006		0.008	

Lab laboratory, *MN* micronucleus, *Cat* category; *Y* years

the workers were technicians (Table 2). Average TYS was 18.8 years, while mean EYS, assessed only in exposed workers, was 15 years (Table 1). Technicians and laboratory workers cumulated significantly more EYS than doctors and engineers ($p = 0.004$).

Investigated nuclear medicine department workers received on average 1.37 +/− 0.29 mSy (min = 0.74 mSy; max = 3.71 mSy) of radiation during one year period. The mean received annual doses for doctors was 1.02 +/− 0.33, engineers 0.86 +/− 0.42, technicians 1.95 +/− 0.67, while for laboratory workers AD were 1.69 +/− 0.51. Received annual doses of all workers were in the referral range. There were no significant differences ($p > 0.05$) between received AD between all four assessed occupations, but technicians and laboratory workers evaluated together, received significantly higher AD than doctors and engineers ($p = 0.039$).

Investigating the number of MN in the overall population we found that the mean MN number was 13.28 per 1000 binuclear cells (Table 1). The majority of workers in the overall population, as well as in the exposed and control group had 1 to 9 MN per 1000 binuclear cells. Moreover, in the control group all workers had less than 20 MN per 1000 binuclear cells (Table 2).

In order to have more bias control of the data we tested differences in distribution of male and female workers in different categories of age, occupation and MN number. As there were no significant differences regarding, we eliminated sex skewing the data as a problem (Table 3).

There was no statistically significant differences between groups (exposed and control) concerning the TYS, occupation, nicotine use and age decades of workers ($p > 0.05$). On the other hand, there was a significant difference in the number of micronuclei observed between the groups (exposed and control). Significantly more micronuclei have been observed in samples of the exposed workers compared to controls ($p = 0.001$).

There were significant differences in MN number per 1000 binuclear cells in the overall population regarding workers sex and age, AD, TYS and EYS. Women ($p = 0.012$) and older workers ($p = 0.001$) had more MN per 1000 binuclear cells. Health workers who received higher annual doses had more MN per 1000 binuclear cells ($p = 0.026$). Furthermore, workers who with longer EYS ($p = 0.001$) and TYS ($p = 0.001$) had more MN per 1000 binuclear cells. There were no significant differences in the number of MN among the various occupations of the examined health workers from both groups ($p > 0.05$).

When we examined only those health workers who were professionally exposed to radiation, the frequency of registered MN per 1000 binuclear cells was not significantly different regarding sex ($p = 0.065$), nicotine use ($p = 0.086$) and age decades ($p = 0.370$). The difference in MN was also not significant between all four occupation categories ($p = 0.931$), but technicians and laboratory workers together had significantly more MN per 1000 binuclear cells than doctors and engineers combined ($p = 0.010$).

Female sex was significantly correlated with EYS and MN number, while male sex was in correlation with nicotine use. Age was in positive correlation with AD, EYS, TYS and number of MN per 1000 binuclear cells. EYS was significantly and positively correlated with, AD, TYS and MN number. TYS was significantly and positively correlated with number of MN per 1000 binuclear cells, annual doses, nicotine use and age. Annual doses were not significantly correlated with nicotine use and workers' sex (Table 4).

EYS accurately apprehends 86.30 % of MN frequencies, TYS 69.30 %, while age predicts the occurrence MN with the reliability of 67.40 %. Received AD explain correctly the findings of MN in 64.60 % of cases. EYS

Table 3 Distribution of male and female workers in different categories of age, occupation and MN number per 1000 binuclear cells

Parameters		Overall population		Exposed group		Control group	
		Male	Female	Male	Female	Male	Female
Age categories - decades	3 - 20 – 29 y	1	7	1	4	0	3
	4 - 30 – 39 y	10	10	4	6	6	4
	5 - 40 – 49 y	8	13	2	10	6	3
	6 - 50 – 59 y	6	31	3	21	3	10
	7 - 60 – 69 y	1	3	0	3	1	0
	χ^2	9.173		4.351		8.834	
	p	0.057		0.361		0.065	
Occupation	Technician	9	31	2	20	7	11
	Lab. worker	6	9	2	6	4	3
	Doctor	9	20	4	14	5	6
	Engineer	2	4	2	4	0	0
	χ^2	1.819		2.555		0.687	
	p	0.611		0.465		0.709	
MN categories (intervals of 10) per 1000 binuclear cells	1 cat: 1 – 9	11	13	5	8	6	5
	2 cat: 10 – 19	4	11	0	8	4	3
	3 cat: 20 – 29	8	25	4	18	4	7
	4 cat: 30 – 39	3	13	1	9	2	4
	5 cat: 40 – 49	0	2	0	1	0	1
	χ^2	5.350		5.955		2.303	
	p	0.253		0.203		0.680	

Lab laboratory, *MN* micronucleus, *Cat* category, *Y* years

Table 4 Correlations of investigated parameters

Parameters		Sex	Age	Occup.	EYS	TYS	MN No	Nicotine use	Group exp/cont
Sex	ρ	1.000	0.176	−0.095	0.331	0.151	0.263	−0.257	−0.280
	p	.	0.098	0.371	0.001	0.156	0.012	0.015	0.007
Age	ρ	0.176	1.000	0.193	0.321	0.811	0.283	−0.115	−0.095
	p	0.098	.	0.069	0.002	0.001	0.007	0.281	0.372
Occup.	ρ	−0.095	0.193	1.000	0.118	0.058	0.064	−0.002	−0.152
	p	0.371	0.069	.	0.267	0.590	0.548	0.981	0.152
EYS	ρ	0.331	0.321	0.118	1.000	0.323	0.771	−0.162	−0.878
	p	0.001	0.002	0.267	.	0.002	0.001	0.127	0.001
TYS	ρ	0.151	0.811	0.058	0.323	1.000	0.304	−0.242	−0.038
	p	0.156	0.001	0.590	0.002	.	0.004	0.022	0.722
MN No	ρ	0.263	0.283	0.064	0.771	0.304	1.000	−0.130	−0.725
	p	0.012	0.007	0.548	0.001	0.004	.	0.223	0.001
Nicotine use	ρ	−0.257	−0.115	−0.002	−0.162	−0.242	−0.130	1.000	0.040
	p	0.015	0.281	0.981	0.127	0.022	0.223	.	0.711
Group exp/cont.	ρ	−0.280	−0.095	−0.152	−0.878	−0.038	−0.725	0.040	1.000
	p	0.007	0.372	0.152	0.001	0.722	0.001	0.711	.
Annual doses	ρ	0.078	0.259	0.273	0.972	0.071	0.364	0.371	−0.753
	p	0.547	0.048	0.019	0.000	0.293	0.000	0.193	0.000

MN micronucleus per 1000 binuclear cells, *TYS* total years of service, *EYS* exposed years of service, *Exp* exposed, *Cont* control, *No* number, *Occup.* occupartion

duration of 14.5 years is the best reference value with a sensitivity 86.4 % and specificity of 80.9 %. TYS duration of 20.5 years is the best reference value with a sensitivity 86.4 % and specificity of 54.4 %. If workers receive more than 1.5 mSy annually (sensitivity 57.1 % and specificity of 83.1 %), they can be expected to have more MN in their cells. Above 43 years of age more MN are produced in the cells, with a sensitivity of 90.9 % and specificity of 47.1 % (Fig. 1).

When all examined parameters were assessed together, using Poisson's regression, a statistically significant model of their impact on MN formations was

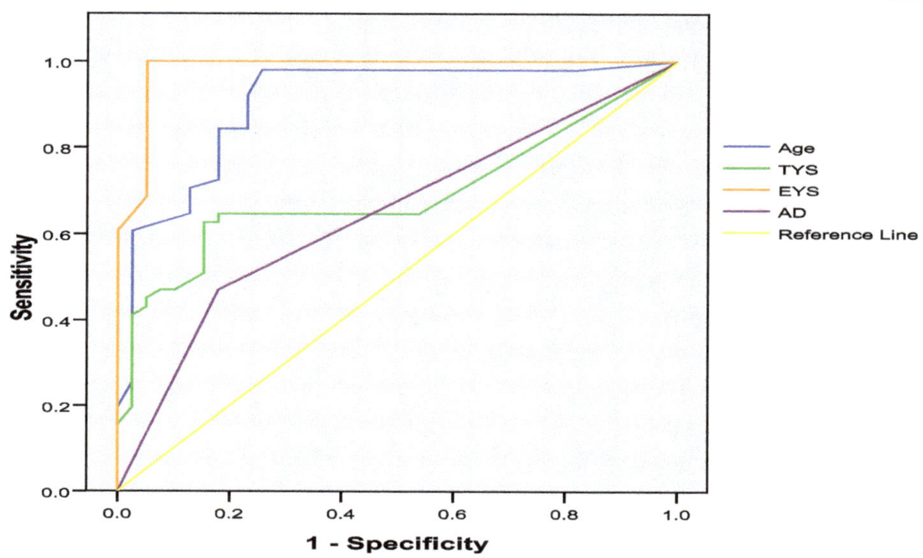

Fig. 1 ROC curve for investigated parameters (annual doses, EYS, TYS and age) showing the level to which they explain the occurrence of MN in workers exposed to radiation. Legend: ROC – Receiver Operator Curve – relation of sensitivity and specificity of investigated parameters; TYS – total years of service; EYS – exposed years of service; AD – annual doses

constructed ($\chi^2 = 471.848$; $p = 0.001$). Obtained model fits our data reasonably well (χ^2 value/df = 2.838).

$$\text{MN per 1000 binuclear cells} = 1.231 + 0.244 \times \text{AGE} + 0.301 \times \text{SEX} + 0.017 \times \text{EYS} + 0.683 \times \text{AD}$$

The model shows that older age and female sex of workers, longer duration of exposed years of service and higher annual doses increase the number of MN per 1000 binuclear cells. One EYS year increases the frequency of MN per 1000 binuclear cells 1.017 times. Furthermore, receiving 0.1 mSy raises the frequency of MN per 1000 binuclear cells by 26 %. Specific working places, TYS, workers' sex and age as well as nicotine use were not significant predictors of formation of MN.

Discussion

Application of ionizing radiation in many different fields is constantly increasing, including the use for medical purposes. Ionizing radiation is known to induce mutations and cell transformations, predominantly by causing single-strand and double-strand DNA breakage, thereby leading to chromosome instability and carcinogenesis [10]. Of all workers exposed to man-made sources of radiation, medical personnel represent the largest group, but receive relatively low doses. However, some medical uses of radiation, such as nuclear medicine and interventional procedures, may expose personnel to higher doses, and these are subjects of particular concern [11]. Cytogenetic studies report a significant increase of chromosomal damage in exposed subjects, especially interventional cardiologists, operational radiologists and nuclear medicine physicians [12, 13]. On the other hand, some studies concerning mixed population of hospital workers do not report data on cytotoxicity if the measures of prevention and protection from radiation were undertaken adequately [14].

Our study established that the incidence of MN significantly increased for health workers in nuclear medicine departments occupationally exposed to ionizing radiation in comparison to unexposed individuals. Our findings are in accordance with the most other literature data [15–17]. The novelty of this study, that sets it apart from other similar investigations, is construction of a new model for prediction of micronuclei formation in nuclear medicine department workers professionally exposed to ionizing radiation. This model showed that duration of radiation exposure and received annual doses could be used as predictors of MN frequency. Moreover, the originality of our study lies in the fact that it has taken into account the potential impact of working place and specific daily work activities of employees who are in contact with sources of radiation in nuclear medicine department. Additionally, applying the ROC analysis we have, for the first time in this study, set the cut of points of TYS, EYS, AD and age that can imply on higher risk for MN production.

Researchers usually did not find any associations between the MN frequency and the duration of employment except for interventional cardiologists, where MN values are higher in physicians with exposure >10 years in comparison with exposed physicians with hospital work lasting less than 10 years [18]. On the other hand, some authors point out that the length of exposure increases chromosomal aberrations and the number of damaged cells [19]. Moreover, an increased frequency of bi-nucleated and mono-nucleated cells with micronuclei was observed in most of the studies, based on the accumulated radiation dose: statistically significant values were observed above 10 mSv cumulative effective dose along a number of years of employment [19]. Our findings also indicate that the most important predictors for hospital personnel working with radiation sources are received annual doses and duration of EYS. Receiving more than 1.5 mSy annually significantly increases the production and frequency of MN in workers' cells. Technicians and laboratory workers are at higher risk for MN occurrence as they are generally exposed to more radiation than doctors and engineers.

Evidence in the literature shows a significant correlation of MN frequency with older age and female sex [16, 17]. These findings were confirmed by the results of our study, as well. Women had more MN in the overall population, but among the exposed personal, there were no significant differences regarding MN numbers. Persons occupationally exposed to radiation typically have less than 10 micronuclei if they were exposed for less than 5 years. This all might indicate that radiation itself is more important than workers sex. We also found that, in our population, nuclear medicine department workers aged above 43 years, with more than 20.5 years of TYS and 14.5 years of EYS have more MN. As all received doses were within referent limits, our findings might imply that older personnel should be in some way shielded from adverse effects of radiation more than younger health workers. Perhaps in the age group above 43 years, referent doses should be lowered, which might be the possible methods of preventing adverse effects of radiation in the older population of health workers.

Some studies found that smoking might increase MN numbers in cells of workers exposed to radiation [16]. Still, the majority of literature data agree that it did not affect the MN frequency if examinees consumed less than 20 cigarettes per day, while a significant effect was only registered for heavy smokers [20]. According to our results nicotine use also did not have significant influence on MN formation.

Finally, our results illustrated that low levels of chronic occupational exposure to ionizing radiation causes increased frequency of MN in cells, even when the absorbed dose is below the acceptable limit. Consequently, occupational exposure to radiation can be determined as a risk factor for genotoxicity. The main predictors of the formation and the number of MN in cells, according to our results and the model we constructed, are received annual doses and the length of exposure to ionizing radiation of staff regardless of their specific workplace. Based on the Poisson model, one EYS year increases the frequency of MN per 1000 binuclear cells 1.017 times, while receiving 0.1 mSy raises MN frequency by 26 %. The additional cofactors include age and sex, and they should be closely involved in genetic research monitoring risk assessment of chronic exposure to low doses of radiation of health workers employed in the departments of nuclear medicine. The constructed model might be useful in further research aiming on lowering the referent doses or determining a cut off value for MN in exposed personnel for whom a genotoxic risk is too high. Moreover, it could be used in clinical practice for calculating the number of MN in health workers in case that blood analyses are unavailable, while clinical parameters are known. The equation can be applied to all personnel working with ionizing radiation. It was constructed for our population, but could be used in other countries as well.

MN analysis in human lymphocytes using the cytochalasin B technique has been proposed as a valid and reliable procedure for the assessment of chromosomal damage induced by ionizing radiation. The cytokinesis-blocked micronucleus test has the advantage to detect in interphase both acentric chromosome fragments attributed to DNA breakage and chromosome loss resulting from chromosome lagging in anaphase [21]. Therefore this method was applied in our study as well. This study also demonstrates the usefulness of MN analysis for individual risk assessment in programs of medical surveillance of employees in the departments of nuclear medicine.

This study has some limitations. Although we assessed MN frequency, we did not score nuclear buds and nucleoplasmic bridges. Knowing that one dicentric chromosome manifests as one nucleoplasmic bridge, this additional scoring could provide a stronger causation between IR and potential risk for cancer in occupational settings. However, we are leaving this as well as assessment of other possible genotoxicities for further research. Moreover, currently there were not enough patients to make 5-years or 1-year age groups.

Conclusions

Parameters such as female gender of workers, older age, higher received annual doses, longer total and exposed years of service increase the number of MN in cells of health workers exposed to radiation. In our population, health workers older than 43 years, with TYS longer than 20.5 years and EYS longer than 14.5 years have significantly more MN. If workers receive more than 1.5 mSy annually, they can be expected to have more MN in their cells. The most important predictors of the micronuclei formation and frequency in nuclear medicine department workers are received annual doses and the length of exposed years of service. Technicians and laboratory workers are at higher risk for occurrence of MN than doctors and engineers, due to receiving higher annual radiation doses.

We developed a model of relationship between clinical parameters and MN numbers showing that both received annual doses and radiation exposure duration could be used as predictors of MN frequency per 1000 binuclear cells. One EYS year increases the frequency of MN per 1000 binuclear cells 1.017 times, while receiving 0.1 mSy raises MN frequency by 26 %.

Competing interests

Authors declare no conflicts of interest.

Authors' contributions

ST has written the manuscript, helped with the molecular genetic studies and treated the evaluated workers and collected the data. AM was involved in the study design and literature review. JD participated in the statistical analysis and helped to draft the manuscript. BR carried out the molecular genetic studies and literature review. MT participated in the design of the study and helped to draft the manuscript. All authors read and approved the final manuscript.

Author details

[1]Occupational Health Department, General Health Center "Savski Venac", Pasterova 1, Belgrade, Serbia. [2]Institute of Occupational Medicine and Radiological Protection, Deligradska 29, Belgrade, Serbia. [3]School of Medicine, University of Belgrade, Dr Subotica 8, Belgrade, Serbia. [4]Clinic of Obstetrics and Gynecology, Clinical Center of Serbia, Dr Koste Todorovica 26, Belgrade, Serbia.

References

1. UNSCEAR. Biological mechanisms of radiation actions at low doses. New York: United Nations; 2012.
2. Bouraoui S, Mougou S, Drira A, Tabka F, Bouali N, Mrizek N, et al. A cytogenetic approach to the effects of low levels of ionizing radiation (IR) on the exposed Tunisian hospital workers. Int J Occup Med Environ Health. 2013;26:144–54.
3. Huang L, Snyder AR, Morgan WF. Radiation-induced genomic instability and its implications for radiation carcinogenesis. Oncogene. 2003;22:5848–54.
4. Milacic S. Chromosomal aberrations after exposure to low doses of ionizing radiation. J BUON. 2009;14:641–6.
5. Morandi E, Severini C, Quercioli D, Perdichizzi S, Mascolo MG, Horn W, et al. Gene expression changes in medical workers exposed to radiation. Radiat Res. 2009;172:500–8.
6. Raja RB, Arunachalam KD. Anti-genotoxic potential of casein phosphopeptides (CPPs): a class of fermented milk peptides against low background radiation and prevention of cancer in radiation workers. Toxicol Ind Health. 2011;27:867–72.
7. Kłucinski P, Mazur B, Sędek Ł, Aptekorz M, Cieslik P, Hryczek AH, et al. Assessment of selected B cells populations in the workers of X-ray departments. Int J Occup Med Environ Health. 2014;27:467–73.

8. Fenech M. The in vitro micronucleus technique. Mutat Res. 2000;455:81–95.
9. Bonassi S, Neri M, Lando C, Ceppi M, Lin Y, Chang WP, et al. Effect of smoking habits on the frequency of micronuclei in human lymphocytes: results from the Human MicroNucleus project. Mutat Res. 2003;543:155–66.
10. Ren R, He M, Dong C, Xie Y, Ye S, Yuan D, et al. Dose response of micronuclei induced by combination radiation of α-particles and γ-rays in human lymphoblast cells. Mutat Re. 2013. doi:10.1016/j.mrfmmm.2012.12.007.
11. Mondello C, Smirnova A, Giulotto E. Gene amplification, radiation sensitivity and DNA double-strand breaks. Mutat Res. 2011;704:29–37.
12. Russo GL, Tedesco I, Russo M, Cioppa A, Andreassi MG, Picano E. Cellular adaptive response to chronic radiation exposure in interventional cardiologists. Eur Heart J. 2012;33:408–14.
13. Lucena EA, Rebelo AM, Araújo F, Sousa WO, Dantas AL, Dantas BM, et al. Evaluation of internal exposure of nuclear medicine staff through in vivo and in vitro bioassay techniques. Radiat Prot Dosimetry. 2007;127:465–8.
14. Okada T, Kashino G, Nishiura H, Tano K, Watanabe M. Micronuclei formation induced by X-ray irradiation does Not always result from DNA double-strand breaks. J Radiat Res. 2012;53:93–100.
15. Sakly A, Ayed Y, Chaari N, Akrout M, Bacha H, Cheikh HB. Assessment of chromosomal aberrations and micronuclei in peripheral lymphocytes from tunisian hospital workers exposed to ionizing radiation. Genet Test Mol Biomarkers. 2012. doi:10.1089/gtmb.2012.0111.
16. Maffei F, Angelini S, Forti GC, Lodi V, Violante FS, Mattioli S, et al. Micronuclei frequencies in hospital workers occupationally exposed to low levels of ionizing radiation: influence of smoking status and other factors. Mutagenesis. 2002;17:405–9.
17. Ishii H, Saito T. Radiation-induced response of microRNAexpression in murine embryonic stem cells. Med Chem. 2006;2:555–63.
18. Vral A, Fenech M, Thierens H. The micronucleus assay as a biological dosimeter of in vivo ionising radiation exposure. Mutagenesis. 2011;26:11–7.
19. Staaf E, Brehwens K, Haghdoost S, Nievaart S, Pachnerova-Brabcova K, Czub J, et al. Micronuclei in human peripheral blood lymphocytes exposed to mixed beams of X-rays and alpha particles. Radiat Environ Biophys. 2012;51:283–93.
20. Nersesyan A, Muradyan R, Kundi M, Knasmueller S. Impact of smoking on the frequencies of micronuclei and other nuclear abnormalities in exfoliated oral cells: a comparative study with different cigarette types. Mutagenesis. 2011;26:295–301.
21. Ropolo M, Balia C, Roggieri P, Lodi V, Concetta Nucci M, Saverio Violante F, et al. The micronucleus assay as a biological dosimeter in hospital workers exposed to low doses of ionizing radiation. Mutat Res. 2012;747:7–13.

The global variability of diatomaceous earth toxicity: a physicochemical and in vitro investigation

C. Nattrass[1], C. J. Horwell[1*], D. E. Damby[2], A. Kermanizadeh[3,4], D. M. Brown[3] and V. Stone[3]

Abstract

Background: Diatomaceous earth (DE) is mined globally and is potentially of occupational respiratory health concern due to the high crystalline silica content in processed material. DE toxicity, in terms of variability related to global source and processing technique, is poorly understood. This study addresses this variability using physicochemical characterisation and in vitro toxicology assays.

Methods: Nineteen DE samples sourced from around the world, comprising unprocessed, calcined and flux-calcined DE, were analysed for chemical and mineral composition, particle size and morphology, and surface area. The potential toxicity of DE was assessed by its haemolytic capacity, and its ability to induce cytotoxicity or cytokine release by J774 macrophages.

Results: The potential toxicity of DE varied with source and processing technique, ranging from non-reactive to as cytotoxic and haemolytic as DQ12. Crystalline silica-rich, flux-calcined samples were all unreactive, regardless of source. The potential toxicity of unprocessed and calcined samples was variable, and did not correlate with crystalline silica content. Calcium-rich phases, iron content, amorphous material, particle size and morphology all appeared to play a role in sample reactivity. An increased surface area was linked to an increased reactivity in vitro for some sample types.

Conclusions: Overall, no single property of DE could be linked to its potential toxicity, but crystalline silica content was not a dominant factor. Occlusion of the potentially toxic crystalline silica surface by an amorphous matrix or other minerals and impurities in the crystal structure are suggested to pacify toxicity in these samples. In vivo verification is required, but these data suggest that crystalline silica content alone is not a sufficient indicator of the potential DE hazard.

Keywords: Diatomaceous earth, Cristobalite, Crystalline silica, Cytotoxicity, Haemolysis, Variability

Introduction

Diatomaceous earth (DE), a sedimentary deposit of silica-rich diatom frustules, is mined globally for a range of purposes, including its commercial value in the filler and filter aid industries [1, 2]. Diatomite deposits are mainly composed of amorphous silica or opal diatom skeletons – the dominant diatom species of which can vary among deposits [2] – and can be interspersed with contaminant minerals, such as clays or carbonates [1]. Extracted material is processed by a series of grinding, calcination and classification techniques to give a wide range of end products. During this process, the diatomite deposit (unprocessed DE) is treated at ~1000 °C with (flux-calcined) or without (calcined) the presence of a fluxing agent, usually sodium carbonate [1, 3]. During calcination, the amorphous silica is converted to crystalline silica, predominantly in the form of cristobalite [2, 3]. The potential for crystalline silica to cause silicosis is well established [4–6], and quartz and cristobalite are classified as Group 1 carcinogens [7, 8]; therefore, exposure to processed DE has the potential to cause chronic respiratory disease.

* Correspondence: claire.horwell@durham.ac.uk
[1]Institute of Hazard, Risk & Resilience, Department of Earth Sciences, Durham University, Durham DH1 3LE, UK

A number of epidemiology studies assessing the respiratory DE hazard show increased mortality [9, 10], pneumoconiosis [11–14], increased risk of lung cancer [9, 10, 15] and other lung diseases [16] in DE workers, compared to unexposed populations. These findings are supported by radiographic evidence, which shows a strong relationship between exposure and the risk of opacities in chest X-rays indicative of silicosis [17]. However, these studies only focused on DE deposits from California, USA, and little is known about how the physicochemical characteristics of DE vary globally. As such, these data may not inform the health hazard of DE worldwide; the few studies at other locations are much less detailed. The largest of these studies, in Iceland, showed a non-significant increase in lung cancer for DE workers [18]. Beskow [19] and Ebina et al. [20] found signs of silicosis in DE workers in Sweden and Japan, but these were based on a small number of cases; whereas, Joma et al. [21] found no signs of pneumoconiosis in DE-exposed workers in the Netherlands, but airflow in the lung was reduced after exposure.

Some of the above studies include evidence of silicosis-type pathology [12, 19, 20, 22], or strong, positive correlations between crystalline silica content and level of observed disease [9, 17, 23]. However, other clinical and epidemiological studies have demonstrated no link between crystalline silica exposure and the pathogenicity observed in DE workers [14], and showed pathological changes in the lungs which differ from typical quartz-induced silicosis [22]. Generally, crystalline silica content is shown to be very low in unprocessed samples (0–4 wt.%), high in calcined samples (>10 wt.%), and highest in flux-calcined samples (>20 wt.%) (e.g. [9, 24]). It is often difficult to distinguish among these different types of DE exposures in epidemiological studies.

Toxicology studies allow differences between processed and unprocessed DE to be studied systematically. As with epidemiological studies, there is discrepancy among toxicological studies as to whether crystalline silica content is the determinant factor for disease. This knowledge is essential for the effective risk management of worker safety.

Many in vitro studies indicate that the cytotoxicity of DE does not correlate with crystalline silica content, as unprocessed and calcined DE exert a greater cytotoxic effect than cristobalite-rich flux-calcined DE in a number of in vitro assays on different cell lines [24–27]. However, work by Elias and co-workers has shown that cristobalite-rich DE samples (both flux-calcined and those calcined at high temperature) have increased pro-carcinogenic potential in Syrian hamster embryos compared to unprocessed DE and DE calcined at lower temperature [26, 28]. Exposure to both unprocessed and flux-calcined DE also resulted in an increase in abnormal nuclei formation (a marker of genotoxicity) in Chinese hamster ovary cells, with the damage more significant than quartz and cristobalite standards [24].

In vivo studies of unprocessed, amorphous DE show it has the potential to be pathogenic, causing acute/subacute inflammation in rats 60 days after a single intratracheal injection of 10 mg DE, an effect that decreased with time [29]. While inhalation of unprocessed DE (170 million particles per cubic foot (mppcf)) by guinea pigs for 39–44 h/week for 24 months resulted in fibrosis, calcined, cristobalite-rich DE was seen to cause more severe fibrosis more rapidly [30]. However, in a separate study, exposure via inhalation to 5–50 mppcf flux-calcined DE, consisting of 61 % cristobalite, for 30 h/week up to 30 months caused no body weight loss or pulmonary fibrosis in rats, guinea pigs or dogs [31].

Previous studies have focussed on few samples and single locations and, therefore, have not been able to investigate the source-dependent compositional and morphological variability of DE and the effect of this variability on toxicity endpoints. This study overcomes this limitation by determining the potential toxicity of DE sourced from seven quarries across the world, and investigating the physicochemical characteristics of the material to understand the properties that affect DE toxicity. Samples chosen cover a spectrum of deposit types, purities and processing techniques. Physicochemical analyses assessed sample composition, morphology, particle size and surface area. Haemolysis allowed for the assessment of particle-induced membrane damage, while cytotoxicity and cytokine release from macrophages were used to assess potential particle toxicity and the potential to induce inflammation.

Materials and methods

Nineteen DE samples were sourced from mines around the world to account for the global variability of DE deposits (Table 1). A range of DE products that encompass the spectrum of compositional characteristics and processing techniques available were selected using geochemical data obtained though the European Industrial Minerals Association (IMA-Europe). The sample set comprised unprocessed, calcined and flux-calcined samples, and included filler and filter aid grades of DE, which are determined by post-calcination size classification. Samples were chosen from a range of source deposits, including those with impurities (carbonates and clays). Unprocessed samples, and the equivalent sample post-processing, were sourced where possible in order to directly establish the effects of processing.

Separation of the fine fraction

Fine fractions (close to PM10) were separated from 5 bulk samples for toxicological assessment alongside their

Table 1 Information for diatomaceous earth samples, including: particle size distribution, surface area and chemical composition

Sample information				Particle size distribution (c.v. %)		BET surface area (m^2/g)		Chemical composition (wt.%)							
Sample ID	Source	Process	Grade	<4 μm	<10 μm	Mean	s.d.	SiO_2	TiO_2	Al_2O_3	Fe_2O_3	MgO	CaO	Na_2O	K_2O
DE_05[#a]	Spain	U	Filler	11.3	38.8	7.5	0.7	90.47	0.05	0.91	0.38	0.34	6.96	0.65	0.14
DE_11[b]	Spain	U	Filler	12.4	47.3	6.3	0.4	87.26	0.05	1.40	0.42	0.49	8.96	1.04	0.17
DE_13[c]	France	U	Filter aid	7.8	28.0	22.9	0.2	89.02	0.64	4.42	3.22	0.36	0.66	0.38	0.35
DE_15[d]	France	U	Filter aid	7.9	28.5	23.8	0.3	87.40	0.70	4.73	3.99	0.49	0.74	0.19	0.34
DE_16[d]	France	C	Filter aid	6.7	25.0	3.8	0.1	88.03	0.66	4.50	3.86	0.39	0.66	0.17	0.33
DE_18	China	C	Filter aid	7.3	28.1	3.1	0.1	93.49	0.15	3.71	1.67	0.35	0.08	−0.04	0.50
DE_20[#]	Mexico	C	Filter aid	6.8	25.3	4.0	0.1	92.00	0.24	5.07	1.95	0.34	0.30	−0.13	0.20
DE_21	USA-1[e]	C	Filter aid	6.2	21.7	5.7	0.2	87.83	0.32	6.57	1.81	1.02	0.54	0.51	1.02
DE_22	USA-1	C	Filler	25.4	71.5	10.6	0.2	93.24	0.17	3.82	1.15	0.65	0.17	0.03	0.59
DE_23	USA-1	C	Filter aid	21.8	65.5	6.8	0.2	93.88	0.15	3.03	1.05	0.69	0.30	0.21	0.47
DE_24[#]	Mexico	C	Filter aid	12.1	45.0	5.9	0.2	93.63	0.19	3.89	1.49	0.33	0.22	0.01	0.18
DE_06[a]	Spain	FC	Filler	8.5	34.4	1.1	0.1	91.27	0.03	0.67	0.35	0.27	6.25	1.00	0.09
DE_07	USA-1	FC	Filler	10.6	31.6	1.3	0.0	91.67	0.15	3.00	1.07	0.53	0.29	2.69	0.48
DE_08[#]	USA-2[e]	FC	Filler	9.2	28.7	1.3	0.1	93.07	0.06	1.12	1.99	0.51	0.30	2.89	0.03
DE_09	Chile	FC	Filler	9.8	33.4	1.5	0.1	93.04	0.10	1.82	0.95	0.23	1.29	2.15	0.34
DE_10[#]	Mexico	FC	Filler	8.7	35.3	1.7	0.1	93.64	0.10	2.05	0.80	0.14	0.32	2.59	0.12
DE_12[b]	Spain	FC	Filler	8.5	33.4	1.0	0.1	90.67	0.03	1.12	0.35	0.31	5.64	0.69	0.10
DE_14[c]	France	FC	Filter aid	6.4	17.0	1.1	0.1	87.36	0.58	4.10	2.61	0.40	0.62	3.17	0.39
DE_17	China	FC	Filter aid	4.6	11.4	1.0	0.0	91.68	0.13	3.12	1.44	0.27	0.11	2.22	0.51

Table sorted by process: *U* unprocessed, *C* calcined, *FC* flux-calcined, *c.v.* cumulative volume, *s.d.* standard deviation ($n = 3$). [#]The fine fractions of these samples were separated for use in toxicology assays. [e] Samples were sourced from two separate deposits in the USA and so are denoted as USA-1 and USA-2.[a–d] Unprocessed samples and their corresponding processed samples

bulk counterparts (Table 1). The samples, which comprise a range of crystalline silica contents, bulk impurities, and processing techniques, were separated by dry-resuspension as previously described by Moreno et al. [32]. Briefly, the sample was suspended in a horizontal rotating drum with a baffle (1.5 rpm). Airflow of 6 l/min was passed through this system, which carried suspended particles through a gravitational settling chamber, where coarser particles were deposited, and the fine fraction continued through a Negretti elutriation filter system and was collected on a polycarbonate filter. The particle size distribution of the separated fine fractions was determined by SEM image analysis.

Physicochemical characterisation

Physiochemical analyses were carried out on bulk samples (because of the mass required by some techniques). The crystalline silica polymorph and relative crystalline silica contents were measured by X-ray diffraction position sensitive detection (XRD-PSD; Bruker D8 Advance, Durham University) from 5 to 90° 2θ. Samples were ground to a fine powder and compacted into a well using the knife-edge of a spatula to ensure random crystal orientation [33]. The intensity of the primary peak (26.6 °2θ for quartz and 21.8 °2θ for cristobalite) was used as a proxy for the relative amounts of crystalline silica. To account for the different diffraction intensities of quartz and cristobalite, the peak heights of pure-phase quartz and cristobalite standards, run under the same conditions, were used to normalise the relative peak heights in the samples. This allowed the addition of peak intensities of quartz and cristobalite to give relative total crystalline silica contents amongst the samples. Bulk chemical compositions were measured by X-ray fluorescence (XRF; PANalytical Axios Advanced X-ray fluorescence spectrometer, University of Leicester). Particle sections were produced in polished resin blocks, coated with 25 nm carbon, and imaging and elemental analysis were performed by scanning electron microscopy (SEM) and energy dispersive X-ray spectroscopy (EDS) at 15 kV (Hitachi SU-70 FEG SEM, Durham University). The elemental composition of cristobalite in individual particles, and amorphous material in cristobalite-containing particles was measured in samples where these particles were clearly seen.

Particle size distributions were analysed by laser diffraction using a Coulter LS analyser (Durham University), with polarization intensity differentiation scattering (PIDS) to analyse particles in the range of 0.04–2000 μm diameter (all samples fell within this range). Data are presented as cumulative volume (c.v.) % and are an average of two 90 s measurements, analysed by Fraunhofer theory.

Qualitative analysis of dominant diatom morphology was performed on all samples by mounting particles on polycarbonate discs, which were adhered to aluminium stubs by carbon pads. These were coated with 25 nm gold/palladium and imaged at 8 kV by SEM. Quantitative assessment (1000–2000 particles per sample) of particle size and the abundance of fibre-like particles (defined by an aspect ratio >3 [34]), was conducted on the five fine fractions used in toxicology experiments and their corresponding bulk samples (DE_05, DE_08, DE_10, DE_20 and DE_24).

Surface area was analysed by nitrogen adsorption measurements at 77 K using a TriStar 3000 instrument (Durham University). Samples were dried in nitrogen gas at 120 °C overnight. The Brunauer-Emmett-Teller (BET) theory was applied to measurements at relative pressures of 0.05–0.24, and the results are the mean of three repeated measurements.

In vitro toxicology

Haemolysis is a measure of the ability of particles to rupture cell membranes, and has been shown to be a good indicator of the pro-inflammatory potential of crystalline silica [35]. Haemolysis was performed on all 19 bulk samples and 5 separated fine fractions by treating red blood cells with 63–1000 μg/ml DE powder for 1 h. A volume of 1 ml of sheep blood in Alsever's solutions (Oxoid Ltd.) was centrifuged at 5000 rpm for 2 min and the supernatant removed. Isolated red blood cells were washed three times with saline and 100 μl of cells were added to 3.6 ml saline. Particle suspensions of 1 mg/ml particles in saline were sonicated for 20 min, serially diluted to final concentrations, and 150 μl of the particle suspensions added to 96 well plates in triplicate. Next, 75 μl of the prepared blood was added to each well, the plate covered and placed on an orbital shaker for 1 h. Post-exposure, the plate was centrifuged at 250 rcf for 5 min, 100 μl of the supernatant transferred to a new plate and absorbance measured at 540 nm (SpectraMax M5, Heriot-Watt University).

Cytotoxicity was measured using alamarBlue® (a measure of mitochondrial enzyme activity) and lactate dehydrogenase (LDH; a measure of membrane integrity) assays (Heriot-Watt University). These assays were performed on the five fine fractions, their corresponding bulk samples, two bulk samples chosen due to their haemolytic potential (DE_11 and DE_22), as well as a further unprocessed bulk sample (DE_15). The samples were suspended in RPMI medium containing 10 μl/ml L-glutamine, 10 μl/ml penicillin and streptomycin, and 10 % bovine foetal serum (complete medium), and sonicated for 20 min. J774 macrophages were seeded in a 96 well plate (5×10^4 cells per well) and exposed to 100 μl of DE suspension in concentrations of 8, 16, 31, 63, 125, 250, and 500 μg/ml for 24 h at 37 °C and 5 % CO_2. Following exposure, the supernatant was removed and stored at −80 °C for LDH and cytokine analysis. A solution of 1 mg/ml alamarBlue® reagent (resazurin sodium salt; Sigma) in saline was diluted 1:10 in complete medium and 100 μl added to the cells. The plate was incubated for 4 h and fluorescence measured at excitation at 560 nm and emission at 590 nm. LDH release from macrophages was measured by adding 10 μl of cell supernatant to 50 μl 1 mg/ml NADH in 0.75 mM sodium pyruvate, incubating for 30 min at 37 °C in 5 % CO_2, adding 50 μl of 2 mg/ml 2,4-dinitrophenylhydrazine in 1 M HCl and incubating for 20 min at room temperature in the dark, before adding 50 μl 4 M sodium hydroxide and measuring the absorbance at 550 nm.

Cytokine production was measured as a marker of inflammation using BD™ Cytometric Bead Array cytokine flex sets (bead based immunoassay; BD Biosciences, Heriot-Watt University). Flow cytometry was used to discriminate between different bead populations based on size and fluorescence, according to the manufacturer's instructions. Keratinocyte chemoattractant (KC), interleukin 1β (IL-1β), tumour necrosis factor alpha (TNF-α) and interleukin 10 (IL-10) were measured for cells treated with 125 μg/ml or lower of the fine fractions of DE only. TNF-α and IL-1β are pro-inflammatory cytokines associated with silica induced toxicity [36, 37], IL-10 is an anti-inflammatory cytokine providing information on the balance between pro- and anti-inflammatory signalling, and KC induces neutrophil and macrophage chemotaxis. For samples demonstrating cytotoxicity, the LC20 concentration, two times the LC20 and half the LC20 would generally be assessed to investigate cytokine production. However, in low toxicity samples, where an LC20 was not reached, only a concentration of 125 μg/ml was chosen to evaluate the inflammatory response.

Cells treated with the five fine fractions were imaged by light microscopy. J774 cells (2.5×10^5) were treated with 600 μl of 63 μg/ml DE in a 24 well plate. Cells were scraped from the plate and 50 μl of the cell suspension diluted in 300 μl saline and centrifuged onto a microscope slide at 1160 rcf for 5 min. The treated cells were dried and stained with Diff-Quik (Fisher Scientific). Briefly, slides were dipped in methanol, then Eosin G in phosphate buffer and Thiazine dye in phosphate buffer, rinsed with H_2O and air dried.

In all assays, Triton-X was used as a positive control and untreated cells as a negative control. DQ12 was used as a positive crystalline silica standard and TiO_2 as a negative particle standard. A calcite standard was also used in the alamarBlue® and haemolysis assays, due to a high calcite content in some samples. Results are presented as the relative percentages of the positive and negative controls.

Statistical analysis

Student's *t*-test and ANOVA general linear model with a Tukey's post-hoc test were performed to determine the significance of differences among samples in the in vitro assays (Minitab 15). Pearson's correlation test was used to determine significant correlations amongst different physicochemical characteristics and toxicological results (* $p < 0.05$, ** $p < 0.01$, *** $p < 0.001$).

Results

Physicochemical characterisation

Bulk chemical composition

The bulk chemical composition was variable across deposit sources and processing technique (Table 1). All samples were predominantly SiO_2, which ranged from 87 to 94 wt.%. Samples contained up to 7 and 4 wt.% Al_2O_3 and Fe_2O_3, respectively. Fe_2O_3 content was highest in French samples and Al_2O_3 contents were lower in Spanish samples compared to other locations. Samples from Spain had CaO contents up to 9 wt.%, substantially higher than from all other locations. On average, flux-calcined samples contained significantly more Na_2O than unprocessed and calcined samples from all locations ($p < 0.001$), and contained less Al_2O_3 than calcined samples. Other elements comprised <1.3 wt.% in all samples.

Crystalline silica

Crystalline silica content varied amongst samples, but was the dominant mineral phase in flux-calcined and calcined samples (Fig. 1). Flux-calcined samples were predominantly cristobalite; though, samples from China and USA also contained small quantities of quartz (Fig. 1c). Conversely, calcined samples contained cristobalite as well as quartz, with the exception of cristobalite-only Mexican samples DE_20 and DE_24 (Fig. 1b). Quartz was the dominant crystalline silica polymorph in calcined samples DE_16 and DE_21, whereas cristobalite was the dominant phase in the other calcined samples. On average, cristobalite peak intensity was three times higher in flux-calcined samples than in calcined samples, as calcined samples retained more amorphous material and a proportion of the crystalline silica was quartz. These differences in abundance were substantiated by qualitative SEM imaging. Unprocessed samples were predominantly amorphous and only contained small amounts of cristobalite (Fig. 1a) or, rarely, quartz was observed in all four samples.

By backscatter SEM, crystalline silica appeared as dark grey patches within lighter grey matrices of amorphous material (Fig. 2). In samples that contained both quartz and cristobalite, cristobalite could often be identified by characteristic 'fish-scale' cracking, indicative of the particle having undergone the transition from the high-temperature beta form to the low-temperature alpha form [38]. By EDS analysis on cristobalite-only samples and 'fish-scale' patches in samples containing both polymorphs, Na, Al, Fe and Ca were detected in the cristobalite (Fig. 2). The amorphous matrix was enriched in impurities compared to the cristobalite, containing Na, Al, Fe, Ca, Mg, K, Ti and P (Fig. 2).

Contaminant phases

Spanish samples contained calcite (Figs. 1 and 3a); this was most prominent in the unprocessed samples (DE_05, DE_11), with only traces remaining in the corresponding flux-calcined samples (DE_06, DE_12). Calcium silicates were observed in abundance in all Spanish samples (Fig. 3b).

Clays were observed by SEM-EDS (texturally, and by their high Al contents) and were most prevalent in French samples (e.g. Fig. 3c), but were also observed in samples from USA-1, Mexico and China. Distinct clay

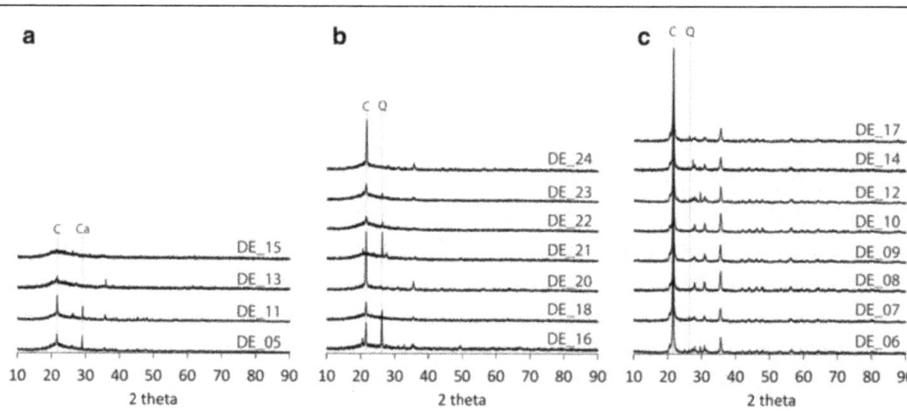

Fig. 1 XRD patterns of (**a**) unprocessed, (**b**) calcined and (**c**) flux-calcined DE. *C* cristobalite, *Q* quartz, *Ca* calcite. Only primary peaks are labelled for clarity. Quartz was not detected in unprocessed samples by XRD

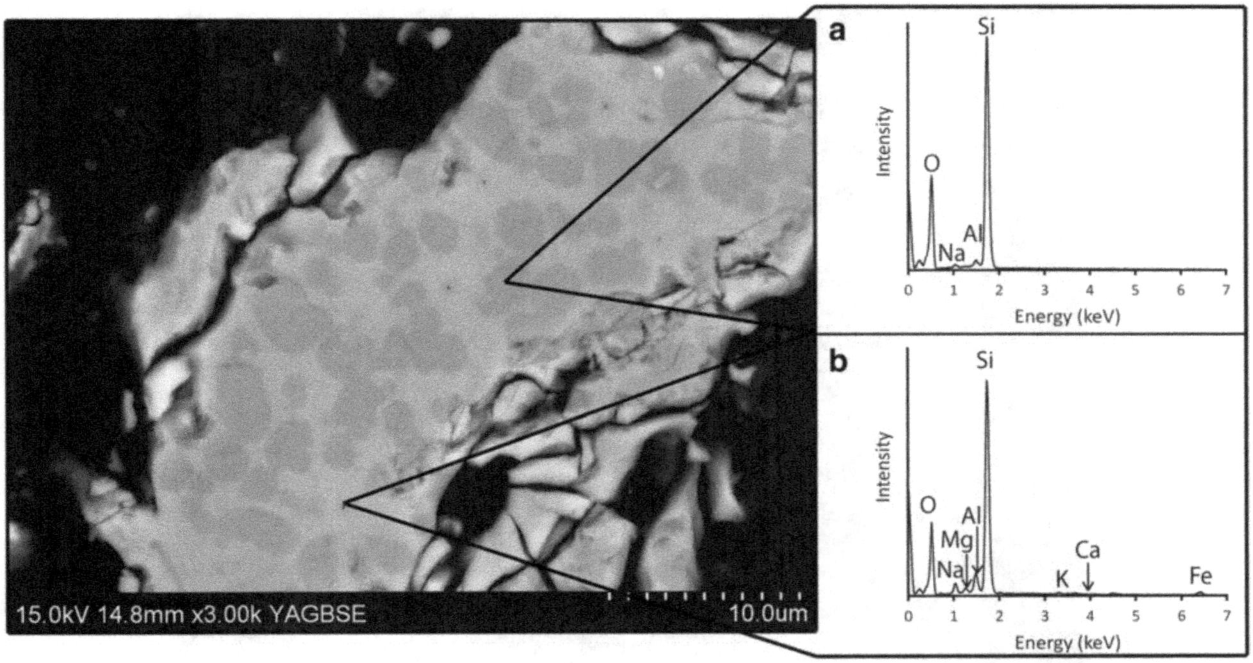

Fig. 2 Backscatter image and EDS spectra of flux-calcined DE particle. Backscatter image of DE particle in a flux-calcined sample with cristobalite patches (*dark grey*; identified by cracking and cristobalite is only crystalline phase in this sample by XRD) surrounded by an amorphous matrix (*light grey*). EDS spectra of (**a**) cristobalite patches showing Al and Na impurities and (**b**) amorphous matrix containing Na, Mg, Al, Ca, K and Fe impurities. These are representative spectra from ~800 spot analyses of cristobalite patches and amorphous matrices (400 of each). Some cristobalite patches also contained Ca and Fe, and some amorphous material also contained Ti and P

phases were not identifiable using textural features or chemical composition, and quantities were too low for detection by XRD.

In the French, unprocessed samples, iron-rich particles of up to 70 μm were observed and these were iron and titanium-rich or iron and phosphorus-rich particles (Fig. 3d). These larger particles were not observed in the calcined and flux-calcined samples from France; instead, small iron-rich patches were seen throughout particles and sometimes in cracks and pore spaces (Fig. 3e). Some of these deposits were iron and titanium-rich but were mostly iron and silicon. In calcined samples where the corresponding unprocessed samples were not available, iron-rich patches were seen throughout particles (Fig. 3f).

Physical properties

Bulk samples contained between 11 and 71 c.v. % particles <10 μm and between 5 and 25 c.v. % particles <4 μm in diameter (Table 1), analogous to the thoracic and respirable fractions, respectively [39]. Flux-calcined samples were coarser than unprocessed and calcined samples for both filler and filter aid grade samples. Calcined samples had a wide range of particle size distributions, containing between 22 and 71 c.v. % <10 μm material (Table 1). The maximum particle diameter observed in the separated fine fractions was 51 μm, reduced from 73 μm in the bulk fractions. Additionally, 83–99 % of particles, by number, in the fine fractions were <10 μm in diameter, compared to 73–96 % in the bulk samples (Table 2). The separated fraction of flux-calcined samples was coarser (median diameter 1.5–2.6 μm) than the fine fractions of calcined and unprocessed samples (median diameters 0.8 μm; Table 2). These data are not comparable to laser diffraction data, which present equivalent spherical diameter in volume % so are heavily mass-biased.

Particle morphology varied substantially amongst samples as the dominant diatom species qualitatively varied with sample source. Samples from Chile, China, Mexico and Spain contained predominantly disc-shaped diatoms, whereas samples from USA-2 and France consisted mainly of cylindrical diatoms (Fig. 4). Samples sourced from USA-1 contained a number of different diatom species and morphologies, including disc-shaped, and long, thin diatoms (Fig. 4c). Most particles were fragments of diatoms and, therefore, particle morphology varied substantially within individual samples. Processed samples contained some sintered

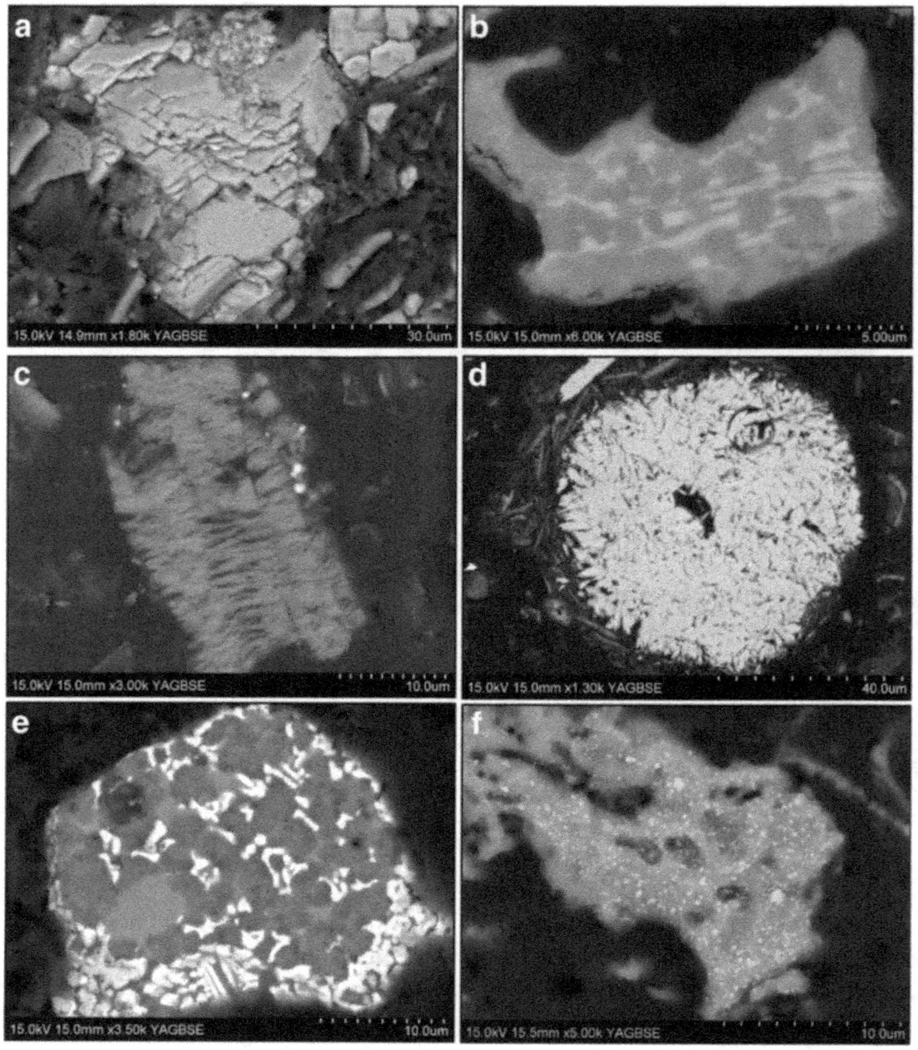

Fig. 3 Backscatter images of contaminant phases in DE. **a** a pure calcite particle in unprocessed DE from Spain (DE_05), **b** a particle containing calcium silicate (*very light grey*) and cristobalite patches (*dark grey*) in flux-calcined DE from Spain (DE_06), **c** a clay mineral particle in an unprocessed sample from France (DE_13), **d** a large iron phosphate particle in unprocessed DE from France (DE_13), and **e-f** iron-rich patches within particles in French (DE_16) and Mexican (DE_24) calcined samples

Table 2 Particle size measured by SEM image analysis

Sample	Maximum particle diameter (μm)		Median particle diameter (μm)		Particles <10 μm diameter (number %)		Fibre-like particles (%)	
	Bulk	Fine	Bulk	Fine	Bulk	Fine	Bulk	Fine
DE_05	26.9	18.5	1.7	0.8	96.6	99.2	17.9	15.4
DE_20	52.0	31.5	1.9	0.8	94.1	96.5	21.2	18.8
DE_24	47.0	17.3	1.8	0.8	96.5	99.0	17.8	16.4
DE_08	73.0	43.7	5.0	1.5	73.2	82.7	3.3	5.7
DE_10	46.2	51.3	4.1	2.6	77.9	83.0	4.9	9.8

Includes maximum particle diameter, median particle diameter, the number % of particles <10 μm, and the number % of fibre-like particles in five bulk samples and their corresponding fine fractions

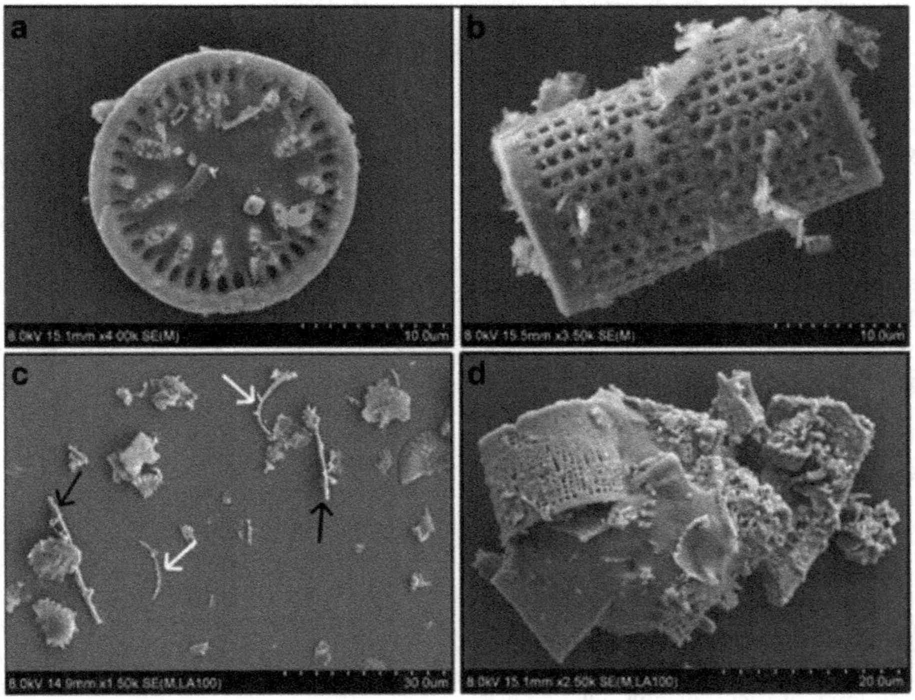

Fig. 4 SEM images of examples of DE morphologies. **a** disc-shaped DE found in Chilean, Chinese, Mexican and Spanish samples, **b** cylindrical diatoms found in French and USA-2 samples, **c** fibre-like rods (*black arrows*) and diatom rinds (*white arrows*), and **d** a large agglomeration of fused diatoms in a flux-calcined DE sample

particles and fused pores, and this was most evident in flux-calcined samples, where large agglomerates of diatoms were observed (Fig. 4d).

In the five bulk samples and equivalent fine fractions, between 3 and 21 % of particles, by number, were classified as fibre-like (Table 2). The total number of fibre-like particles was 2 to 6 times lower in flux-calcined samples than in unprocessed or calcined samples, for both bulk samples and fine fractions (Table 2).

Surface area did not vary much among flux-calcined samples and was always <1.7 m^2/g. However, in calcined and unprocessed samples, surface area varied

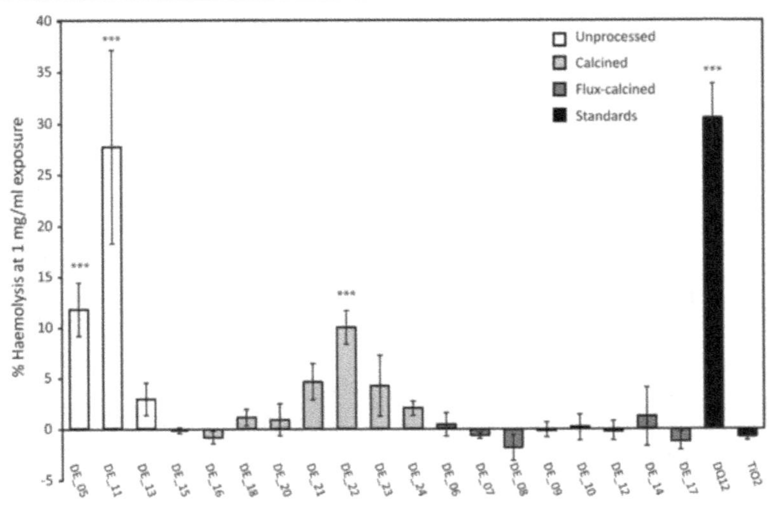

Fig. 5 Haemolytic potential of DE samples. Percent haemolysis relative to an untreated control, of sheep red blood cells post-exposure to 1 mg/ml of unprocessed (*white*), calcined (*light grey*) and flux-calcined (*dark grey*) DE and positive (DQ12) and negative (TiO_2) standards (*black*). *Error bars* represent standard error ($n = 3$), *** $p = <0.001$ difference from untreated control

substantially, ranging from 3.1 to 10.6 m^2/g in calcined samples and 6.3 to 23.8 m^2/g in unprocessed samples (Table 1).

In vitro toxicology

Haemolysis

Haemolysis results are shown in Fig. 5 for bulk samples. Haemolysis caused by the fine fractions did not differ significantly from their corresponding bulk samples and, hence, are not shown. Unprocessed samples from Spain (DE_05 and DE_11) were two of the most haemolytic samples, with DE_11 as haemolytic as DQ12. The most haemolytic calcined sample, DE_22, was one third as haemolytic as DQ12 at the highest concentration. All other samples were not significantly haemolytic at any concentration tested, including the calcite standard (data not shown).

Cytotoxicity

In the alamarBlue® assay (Fig. 6), there was no statistically significant difference in cytotoxicity of bulk DE samples and their separated fine fractions. Bulk flux-calcined samples, and DE_20 and DE_15, TiO_2 and calcite did not differ from the untreated control. All other samples exhibited a cytotoxic response and the cytotoxicity of DE_24 (bulk and fine), DE_22, DE_11 and the fine fraction of DE_05 did not differ significantly from DQ12 ($p > 0.2$). LDH release data were in broad agreement with cell viability measurements via the alamarBlue® assay, in that flux-calcined samples were less cytotoxic than unprocessed and calcined samples (Additional file 1).

Cytokine release

Only TNF-α was produced by macrophages in concentrations greater than untreated cells following exposure to the fine-fraction samples (Fig. 7, data for other cytokines given in Additional file 1). DE_05, DE_20 and DE_24 all increased TNF-α production, with DE_05 inducing the greatest TNF-α production at 125 μg/ml, which was 2.7 times greater than that released following treatment with DQ12. For the calcined samples (DE_20, DE_24), the induction of TNF-α production by treated cells was comparable to that induced by DQ12. In contrast, DE_10 and DE_08 did not enhance TNF-α production.

Cell imaging

Imaged cells treated with the fine fractions of DE and an untreated control are shown in Fig. 8. In the treated cells, there was some degree of frustrated phagocytosis, with instances of numerous cells attempting to phagocytose the same particle and particles not fully engulfed (Fig. 8b-d). Qualitatively, evidence of frustrated phagocytosis was more abundant in cells treated with calcined or unprocessed samples, compared to flux-calcined samples, but were observed in all cases.

Discussion

The variability of DE properties

DE deposits vary in composition and diatom species providing DE particles with a range of physical and chemical properties. Treatment of DE by calcination is used to optimise these properties for use in the filtration and filler industries, during which amorphous silica

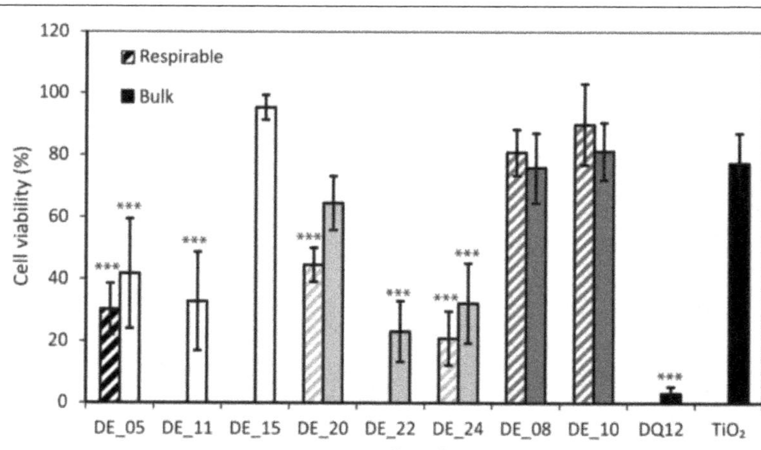

Fig. 6 Cell viability of J774 macrophages exposed to DE. Cell viability relative to an untreated control (% of untreated control–positive control), measured by the alamarBlue® assay, of J774 macrophages exposed to 500 μg/ml of bulk (*solid*) or the fine fraction (*hashed*) of unprocessed (*white*), calcined (*light grey*) and flux-calcined (*dark grey*) DE, and positive (DQ12) and negative (TiO_2) standards (*black*) for 24 h. No data for fine fractions of DE_11, DE_15 and DE_22. *Error bars* represent standard error ($n = 4$), *** $p = <0.001$ difference from untreated control

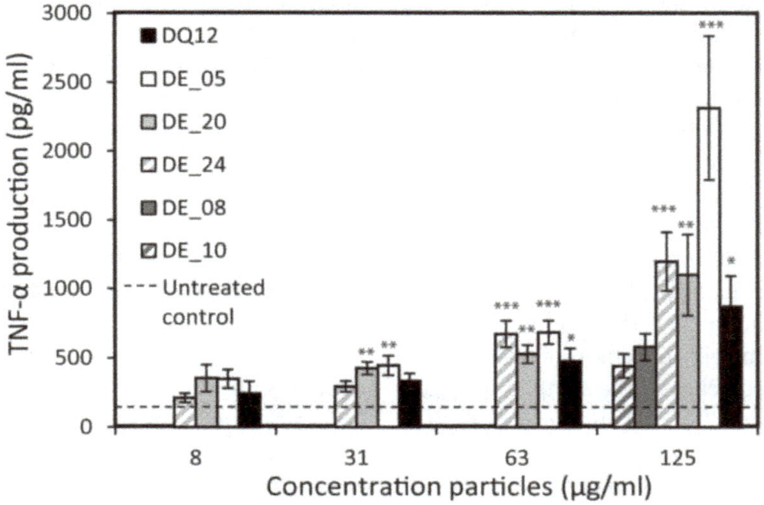

Fig. 7 TNF-α production by macrophages exposed to the fine fractions of DE. Exposure to unprocessed (*white*), calcined (*light grey*) and flux-calcined (*dark grey*) DE and a positive standard (DQ12) for 24 h. *Error bars* represent standard error ($n = 8$). * $p = <0.05$, ** $p = <0.01$, *** $p = <0.001$ compared to untreated control

crystallises [1, 2]. Here, crystalline silica contents and polymorphs varied substantially amongst DE samples from different locations, with processing playing a key role. Flux-calcined samples were the most crystalline silica-rich, and cristobalite was the dominant crystalline silica polymorph. Most calcined samples contained both cristobalite and quartz and there is some evidence that the quartz formed during calcination (based on data from the unprocessed DE_15 and calcined DE_16 samples). This distribution of crystalline silica polymorphs by processing technique has also been observed by Ghiazza et al. [27] and Elias et al. [28]. The preferential crystallisation of cristobalite in flux-calcined samples is likely due the addition of the fluxing agent: doping of

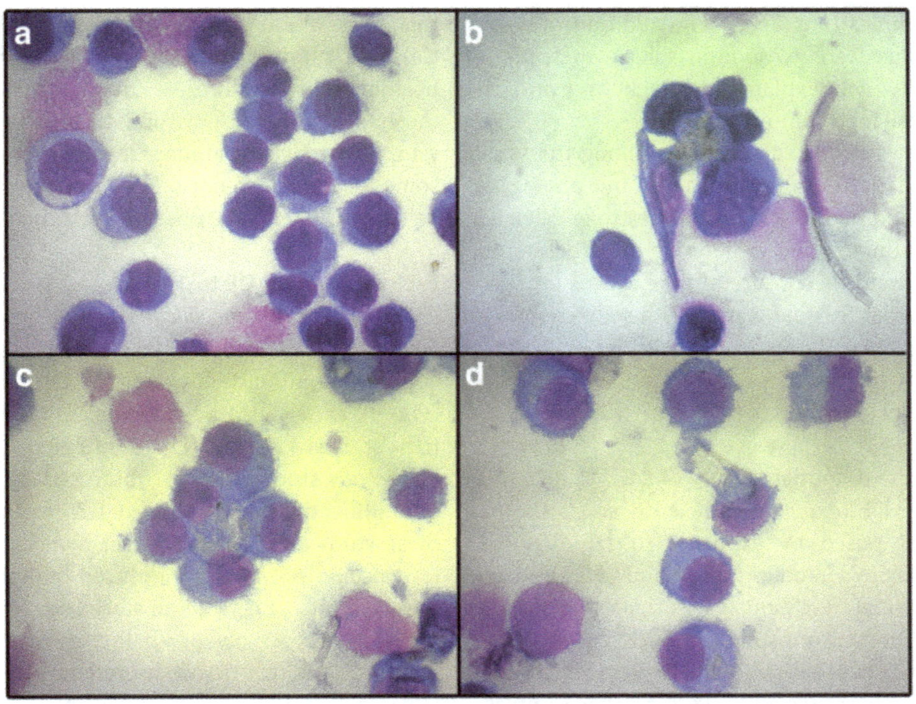

Fig. 8 Frustrated phagocytosis in macrophages treated with DE. Light microscopy image of (**a**) untreated macrophages, and (**b**-**d**) macrophages treated with DE showing indicators of frustrated phagocytosis

amorphous silica with sodium salts promotes cristobalite crystallisation instead of quartz at the temperatures used for calcination [40, 41]. It is unknown why quartz preferentially forms in some calcined samples, whereas in others only cristobalite was observed (Mexican samples DE_20 and DE_24). Unprocessed samples contained trace quantities of cristobalite and quartz; the cristobalite in unprocessed samples likely forms by diagenesis of amorphous silica over time, or is possibly from other sources, such as volcanic deposits [2].

Cristobalite formed in patches throughout particles, crystallising within a matrix of amorphous material (Fig. 2). The cristobalite patches in the samples analysed were impure, containing Al, Na, Ca and Fe (e.g. Fig. 2). Aluminium and Fe ions can substitute for Si in the silica tetrahedra, but require interstitial cations (e.g., Na or Ca) to charge balance the substitution [42], as has been discussed for volcanic cristobalite [43, 44].

Contaminant phases were observed in all samples. Spanish deposits contained calcite (DE_05, DE_11), which would thermally decompose at calcination temperatures (~1000 °C) [45], allowing Ca and Si to form calcium silicates, which were in abundance in flux-calcined samples from Spain. Clay minerals and iron-rich particles are also likely to be broken down during calcination as few individual clay mineral particles or large, iron-rich particles were seen in processed samples compared to unprocessed samples from France. As with Ca in Spanish samples, this frees Fe ions to react with Si, and precipitate in pores and cracks, which was seen in all calcined samples (Fig. 3e-f). The addition of a sodium carbonate flux leads to sodium silicate melt binding with Fe [2], which explains the lack of iron-rich particles in flux-calcined samples.

Physical properties varied substantially among the samples. Flux-calcined particles had complex morphologies, and were coarser and had lower surface area than calcined and unprocessed samples, due to sintering of particles into large agglomerates and the closure of pore spaces [3]. The morphology of diatom frustules varied with source (Fig. 4); however, the abundance of fragmented frustules in all samples meant diatom species, alone, could not be used as a good proxy for particle morphology.

The variability of the potential toxicity of DE

Previous studies of DE toxicity insufficiently constrain the respiratory hazard posed by exposure to DE deposits worldwide: epidemiology studies have mainly focussed on DE workers in a single location (California) (e.g. [9, 10, 14–17]), and are unable to distinguish between exposure to unprocessed or processed DE, while toxicology studies rarely state the sample source and investigate few samples. Therefore, variability among deposits and processing techniques has not been fully considered. Here, we show that DE is not a single entity, with a toxic potential that ranges from unreactive to as haemolytic or cytotoxic as the positive standard α-quartz (DQ12).

Unprocessed samples from Spain (DE_05 and DE_11) were haemolytic and induced significant cytotoxicity to macrophages. Furthermore, DE_05 induced a large increase in TNF-α release from treated macrophages relative to processed samples, indicating the potential for unprocessed DE to incite inflammation if inhaled. However, unprocessed samples from France did not induce any measurable haemolysis or cytotoxicity, suggesting that the potential toxicity of DE can vary by deposit source.

Flux-calcined samples all displayed low haemolytic potential, cytotoxicity and cytokine release from treated cells. This suggests that short-term exposure to flux-calcined samples may not result in toxicity or an inflammatory response. There was no variation in the reactivity of flux-calcined samples from different locations, suggesting that flux-calcination is key to dampening the adverse effects attributed to DE. This is likely due to alteration of the physicochemical properties of DE during flux-calcination and is discussed in detail below.

DE_22 from USA-1 was the only calcined sample that elicited a haemolytic response and was also one of the most cytotoxic samples analysed. This introduces the possibility that data in epidemiological studies from the USA may not be representative of likely disease outcomes worldwide. However, other calcined samples from USA-1 were non-haemolytic, emphasising the variable reactivity that exists amongst samples from a single deposit source. Calcined samples from Mexico were cytotoxic but not haemolytic. Therefore, as these assays assess different mechanisms of toxicity, and there is a disagreement in sample reactivities among the assays for samples from some locations but not others, different mechanisms may be responsible for the observed reactivity.

Factors affecting DE toxicity

Presence of crystalline silica

Here, total crystalline silica (quartz plus cristobalite) content alone did not control DE reactivity in vitro (Fig. 9), as has also been reported by other in vitro toxicity studies [24–27]. This contrasts with previous epidemiology studies that attribute observed pathologies to crystalline silica in processed DE [e.g. [9, 14]]. Some of these studies are referenced in reviews of crystalline silica toxicity [46, 47], and are used in determining safe exposure limits to crystalline silica [e.g. [48]].

The low reactivity of all flux-calcined samples agrees with previous reports on discrete samples [24, 25, 27, 31]. Ghiazza et al. [27] suggested that the low levels of cytotoxicity, lipid peroxidation and NO synthesis caused by crystalline silica-rich flux-calcined DE was due to the

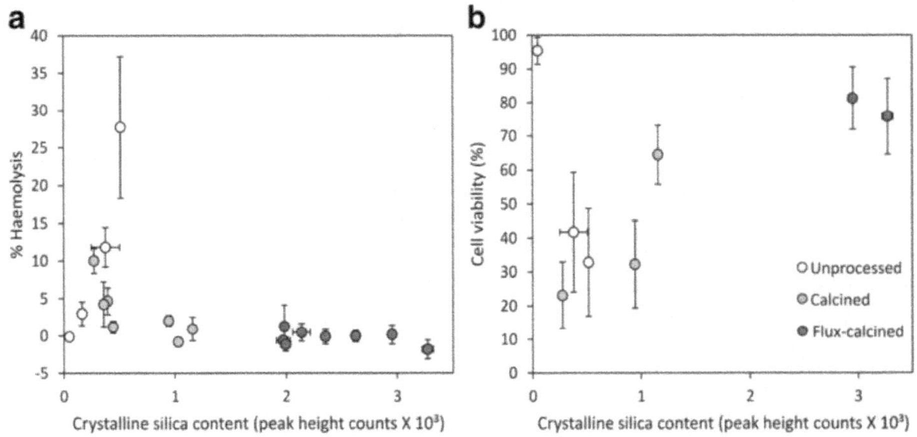

Fig. 9 Relationship between crystalline silica content and reactivity in vitro. Correlation of crystalline silica content of DE (measured by the addition of cristobalite and quartz peak heights, accounting for different diffraction power using standards) with (**a**) haemolysis post-exposure to 1 mg/ml bulk DE, and (**b**) cell viability post-exposure to 500 μg/ml bulk DE

formation of a vitreous rim during flux-calcination, which obscured cell exposure to cristobalite in these samples. No vitreous rim, per se, was observed in this study but the cristobalite is partly occluded, occurring in patches within the otherwise amorphous particles, resulting in a variable percentage of cristobalite at the particle surface. This may account for the lack of correlation between crystalline silica content and potential toxicity. The variable toxicity of crystalline-silica bearing dusts is well established [e.g. [36, 49, 50]], and the hosting of crystalline silica within heterogeneous particles has previously been suggested to explain variations in the toxic potential of quartz-rich coal dusts [49, 51], and to mask the toxicity of cristobalite in volcanic ash [44]. Here, exposure times for the cytotoxicity assays were short (24 h), and the amorphous matrix may have low bio-durability, thereby exposing more cristobalite at the surface of the particle over time. Therefore, future longer exposures and in vivo experiments may be necessary.

Toxicity of the limited surface cristobalite could be further dampened by the presence of cation substitutions (Fig. 2), as structural impurities have been hypothesised to decrease the toxic potential of cristobalite in volcanic ash [44]. Treating quartz with aluminium salts or clay extracts has also been shown to reduce its toxicity and haemolytic potential [52–55], and quartz in coal with clay mineral impurities had lower toxicity than pure, coal-sourced quartz [51]. Therefore, the production of aluminium ions via breakdown of aluminium-rich components of the DE samples could affect the cristobalite exposed at the surface of particles, decreasing the potential toxicity. Conversely, treating quartz with ferric or ferrous iron does not change its toxic potency in vivo [52] and can decrease its haemolytic potential [54]. However, Fubini et al. [56] showed iron may increase silica toxicity via production of free radicals. Therefore, the role of iron in determining DE crystalline silica toxicity remains unclear.

Reactivity of contaminant phases

Some samples with little to no crystalline silica were highly reactive, indicating contaminant phases may control the in vitro response in those samples. The presence of calcite could explain the high reactivity of Spanish (calcite-rich) unprocessed samples: Aladdin et al. [57] have shown exposure to calcite alone caused significant cytotoxic effects in human epithelial cells and inflammation in mice, and Diler and Ergene [58] showed that micronuclei and nuclei abnormalities were more common in calcite factory workers than control groups. However, as the calcite standard was non-reactive in both the haemolysis and alamarBlue® assays, it is unlikely that calcite content is solely responsible for the different reactivity of Spanish unprocessed and flux-calcined DE. The presence of clays may also have an effect, as some clays have been shown to be more haemolytic than crystalline silica [59, 60]. However, the lack of clay in processed DE samples and the low reactivity of French, unprocessed samples, suggests that clay minerals are not the cause of DE induced toxicity.

Iron has been hypothesised as a source for free radical generation in DE [26], and was measured in quantities of up to 4 wt.% here and, therefore, could be contributing to the potential toxicity. Bulk iron content did not correlate with either haemolysis or cytotoxicity (Additional file 1); however, further work would be required to determine the co-ordination of iron and its potential to produce free radicals. Calcined samples all contained iron-rich phases but had variable toxicity, suggesting total Fe does not control the reactivity of these samples. Also, previous studies have shown ferric and ferrous oxides to have low cytotoxicity [61], although exposure to ultrafine iron oxide particles has been shown to lead to oxidative stress and a pro-inflammatory response in rats [62, 63]. Soluble iron oxide has also been shown to be cytotoxic to human mesothelioma MSTO-211H cells [64]. However, as soluble components of the DE were non-cytotoxic (see Additional file 1), this is unlikely to be the case here.

Amorphous silica is generally perceived as less toxic than crystalline silica [49] but can be reactive in vitro [65, 66]. The ability of amorphous, unprocessed DE to elicit a haemolytic or cytotoxic response, or induce abnormal nuclei growth in vitro [24, 25, 29], and cause fibrosis in vivo [30], has also previously been demonstrated. Unprocessed samples from Spain, the most haemolytic of all samples, were predominantly amorphous. The cytotoxic (DE_20, DE_22 and DE_24) and haemolytic (DE_22) calcined samples also contained a substantial amount of amorphous material. It is possible that the amorphous phases of these samples are linked to their reactivity, as certain vitreous silicas have been shown to be more haemolytic than quartz [66]. However, the lack of haemolysis caused by French, unprocessed samples, which were also predominantly amorphous, means that amorphous material is unlikely the predominant control on the observed reactivity. The high levels of impurities in processed amorphous material (Fig. 2) may also play a role in its biological reactivity at the surface of the particle, but further work is needed to determine this.

Therefore, although the mineralogical and chemical compositions are likely to play a role in DE toxicity, no definitive link can be made between individual characteristics considered here and the potential toxicity measured in this study.

Physical properties

Surface area has been related to pro-inflammatory responses [67, 68], and the surface area of processed DE may be a key factor controlling toxicity. Correlations between bulk surface area of processed samples (calcined and flux-calcined) and haemolysis or cell viability were observed (Fig. 10). In flux-calcined samples, up to 27 % of particles were >10 μm (Table 2), which may account for their low surface area (Table 1) and, accordingly, their low reactivity. However, the variable particle size distributions of unprocessed and calcined DE could not be correlated to their toxic potential (Additional file 1), and the correlation between surface area and reactivity could not be extended to unprocessed samples. This suggests that other parameters are responsible for their observed toxicity.

Fibres can cause frustrated phagocytosis, where macrophages struggle to fully engulf particles [69]. Fibre-like particles, up to 21 %, in calcined and unprocessed samples, were mainly in the form of diatom 'rinds' or small fragments of diatoms. The lower abundance in flux-calcined samples is likely due to sintering of fragments into large agglomerates. Previously, DE containing fibre-like particles (aspect ratio >3) was shown to be more potent in vitro than 'non-fibrous' DE [70], suggesting that particle morphology could play a role in the observed cytotoxicity. Particle morphology is important in phagocytosis [71] and, here, frustrated phagocytosis was observed and some fibre-like particles were not phagocytised. This was most evident for calcined and unprocessed samples (which had the highest % of fibre-like particles), where TNF-α production and LDH release, potential indicators of frustrated phagocytosis [72], were also elevated above flux-calcined samples. Frustrated phagocytosis was also observed as a number of cells attempted to engulf larger, disc-shaped diatoms. This was observed after treatment of cells with all of the fine fraction samples, suggesting that large, disc-shaped particles may play a role in DE toxicity, as platelets have been recently identified as a novel respiratory hazard [73], and DE particles with a diameter >7.5 μm have previously been suggested to determine DE toxicity [24].

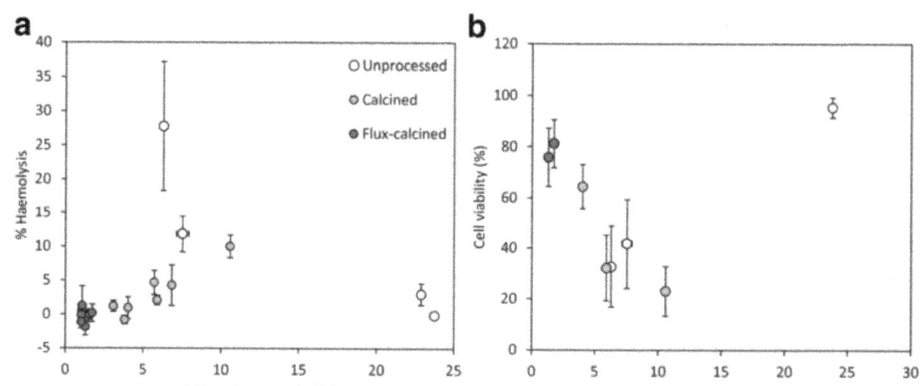

Fig. 10 Relationship between BET surface area and DE reactivity in vitro. Correlation between surface area and (**a**) haemolysis post-exposure to 1 mg/ml bulk DE, and (**b**) cell viability post-exposure to 500 μg/ml bulk DE

Conclusions

This study, the first to systematically characterise the physicochemical properties and potential toxicity of a range of globally sourced DE samples, shows that the toxic potential of DE varies by processing technique and source. Flux-calcined samples were unreactive, whereas unprocessed and calcined DE had variable reactivity.

No correlation was observed between crystalline silica content and DE's potential toxicity, despite previously being implicated in epidemiological studies of DE exposure. The dearth of crystalline silica at the particle surface, due to its crystallisation within an amorphous matrix, its presence in a heterogeneous dust, and impurities within the crystalline silica likely reduce the potential reactivity of these crystalline silica-bearing particles.

It is likely that a number of physicochemical properties play a role in DE toxicity. Calcium-rich phases may be important in the toxicity of some unprocessed samples, and iron or amorphous phases may be involved in calcined DE toxicity. Surface area, especially, was correlated to calcined and flux-calcined DE reactivity here, and the importance of surface reactivity and the unique particle morphologies of DE merits further investigation.

Although no single physicochemical property of DE considered here could be linked to its potential toxicity, a clear outcome of this study is that the crystalline silica content, alone, should not be used to determine the DE hazard, nor should it be assumed that it is the cause of disease observed in epidemiological or clinical studies without further investigation.

Abbreviations

DE: Diatomaceous earth; IMA: Industrial Minerals Association; XRD-PSD: X-ray diffraction position sensitive detection; XRF: X-ray fluorescence; SEM: Scanning electron microscopy; EDS: Energy dispersive X-ray spectroscopy; BET: Brunauer-Emmett-Teller; LDH: Lactate dehydrogenase; KC: Keratinocyte chemoattractant; IL-1β: Interleukin 1β; TNF-α: Tumour necrosis factor alpha; IL-10: Interleukin 10.

Competing interests

The research has been part-funded by IMA Europe, an umbrella organisation representing a number of diatomite companies in all non-commercial issues related to the properties and safe use of minerals. Samples were provided by one diatomite company. Neither IMA Europe nor the company had input to the experimental design or research conducted but have seen a draft version of this manuscript.

Authors' contributions

CN designed the study, performed physicochemical analyses at Durham University and in vitro toxicology assays at Heriot-Watt University, and drafted the manuscript. CJH conceived and designed the study, supervised CN, and participated in physicochemical characterisation. DED advised on study outcomes, and helped with physicochemical analyses. AK performed cytokine analysis and AK and DB participated in in vitro assays. VS and DB participated in the design of the study and VS supervised CN. All authors helped draft the manuscript, read and approved the final version.

Acknowledgements

The authors acknowledge IMA Europe and Durham University as the primary funders of this study and support provided by Horwell's NERC Postdoctoral Research Fellowship (Grant No. NE/C518081/2). Thanks to Nick Marsh, University of Leicester, for XRF analyses and to Leon Bowen, Durham GJ Russell Microscopy Facility, for assistance with SEM analyses. Thanks to Ian Chaplin for assistance with sample preparation, Kathryn Melvin, Gary Oswald and David Johnson for technical assistance with laser diffraction, XRD and BET analyses, respectively. Thanks to the Nano-Safety Group at Heriot-Watt University for technical advice regarding the toxicology assays.

Author details

[1]Institute of Hazard, Risk & Resilience, Department of Earth Sciences, Durham University, Durham DH1 3LE, UK. [2]Department of Earth and Environmental Sciences, Ludwig-Maximilians-Universität München, Munich 80333, Germany. [3]School of Life Sciences, Heriot-Watt University, Edinburgh EH14 4AS, UK. [4]Department of Public Health, Section of Occupational and Environmental Health, University of Copenhagen, Copenhagen DK-1014, Denmark.

References

1. Engh KR. Diatomite. In: Kirk-Othmer encyclopedia of chemical technology. 2000. http://onlinelibrary.wiley.com/doi/10.1002/0471238961.0409012005140708.a01/abstract; John Wiley & Sons, Inc.
2. Flörke OW, Graetsch HA, Brunk F, Benda L, Paschen S, Bergna HE, et al. Silica. In: Ullmann's encyclopedia of industrial chemistry. 2000. http://onlinelibrary.wiley.com/doi/10.1002/14356007.a23_583/abstract; Wiley-VCH Verlag GmbH & Co. KGaA.
3. Ediz N, Bentli İ, Tatar İ. Improvement in filtration characteristics of diatomite by calcination. Int J Miner Process. 2010;94(3–4):129–34.
4. Greenberg MI, Waksman J, Curtis J. Silicosis: a review. Dis Mon. 2007;53(8):394–416.
5. Leung CC, Yu ITS, Chen W. Silicosis. Lancet. 2012;379(9830):2008–18.
6. NIOSH. In: Services DoHaH, editor. Health effects of occupational exposure to respirable crystalline silica. Volume 2002–129. 2002.
7. IARC. Silica, some silicates, coal dust and para-aramid fibrils. International Agency for Research on Cancer: Lyon; 1997.
8. IARC. Arsenic, metals, fibres, and dusts. Volume 100C. Lyon: International Agency for Research on Cancer; 2012.
9. Checkoway H, Heyer NJ, Demers PA, Breslow NE. Mortality among workers in the diatomaceous earth industry. Br J Ind Med. 1993;50(7):586–97.
10. Seixas NS, Heyer NJ, Welp EAE, Checkoway H. Quantification of historical dust exposures in the diatomaceous earth industry. Ann Occup Hyg. 1997;41(5):591–604.
11. Cooper WC, Sargent EN. A 26-year radiographic follow-up of workers in a diatomite mine and mill. J Occup Environ Med. 1984;26(6):456–60.
12. Dutra FR. Diatomaceous earth pneumoconiosis. Arch Environ Health. 1965;11(5):613–9.
13. Smart RH, Anderson WM. Pneumoconiosis due to diatomaceous earth; clinical and x-ray aspects. Ind Med Surg. 1952;21(11):509–18.
14. Harber P, Dahlgren J, Bunn W, Lockey J, Chase G. Radiographic and spirometric findings in diatomaceous earth workers. J Occup Environ Med. 1998;40(1):22–8.
15. Rice FL, Park R, Stayner L, Smith R, Gilbert S, Checkoway H. Crystalline silica exposure and lung cancer mortality in diatomaceous earth industry workers: a quantitative risk assessment. Occup Environ Med. 2001;58(1):38–45.
16. Park R, Rice F, Stayner L, Smith R, Gilbert S, Checkoway H. Exposure to crystalline silica, silicosis, and lung disease other than cancer in diatomaceous earth industry workers: a quantitative risk assessment. Occup Environ Med. 2002;59(1):36–43.
17. Hughes J, Weill H, Checkoway H, Jones R, Henry M, Heyer N, et al. Radiographic evidence of silicosis risk in the diatomaceous earth industry. Am J Respir Crit Care Med. 1998;158(3):807–14.

18. Rafnsson V, Gunnarsdóttir H. Lung cancer incidence among an Icelandic cohort exposed to diatomaceous earth and cristobalite. Scand J Work Environ Health. 1997;23:187–92.
19. Beskow R. Silicosis in diatomaceous earth factory workers in Sweden. Scand J Respir Dis. 1978;59(4):216–21.
20. Ebina T, Takase Y, Inasawa Y, Horie K. Silicosis in the diatomaceous earth factories. Tohoku J Exp Med. 1952;56(3):214.
21. Joma THJM, Borm PJA, Koiter KD, Slangen JJM, Henderson PT, Wouters EFM. Respiratory effects and serum type III procollagen in potato sorters exposed to diatomaceous earth. Int Arch Occup Environ Health. 1994;66(4):217–22.
22. Vigliani EC, Mottura G. Diatomaceous earth silicosis. Br J Ind Med. 1948;5:148–60.
23. Checkoway H, Heyer NJ, Demers PA, Gibbs GW. Reanalysis of mortality from lung cancer among diatomaceous earth industry workers, with consideration of potential confounding by asbestos exposure. Occup Environ Med. 1996;53(9):645–7.
24. Hart GA, Hesterberg TM. *In vitro* toxicity of respirable-size particles of diatomaceous earth and crystalline silica compared with asbestos and titanium dioxide. 40th ed. Hagerstown, MD: ETATS-UNIS: Lippincott Williams & Wilkins; 1998.
25. Bye E, Davies R, Griffiths DM, Gylseth B, Moncrieff CB. *In vitro* cytotoxicity and quantitative silica analysis of diatomaceous earth products. Br J Ind Med. 1984;41(2):228–34.
26. Elias Z, Poirot O, Fenoglio I, Ghiazza M, Danière MC, Terzetti F, et al. Surface reactivity, cytotoxic, and morphological transforming effects of diatomaceous earth products in Syrian hamster embryo cells. Toxicol Sci. 2006;91(2):510–20.
27. Ghiazza M, Gazzano E, Bonelli B, Fenoglio I, Polimeni M, Ghigo D, et al. Formation of a vitreous phase at the surface of some commercial diatomaceous earth prevents the onset of oxidative stress effects. Chem Res Toxicol. 2009;22(1):136–45.
28. Elias Z, Poirot O, Danière MC, Terzetti F, Marande AM, Dzwigaj S, et al. Cytotoxic and transforming effects of silica particles with different surface properties in Syrian hamster embryo (SHE) cells. Toxicol In Vitro. 2000;14(5):409–22.
29. Adamis Z, Tátrai E, Honma K, Six É, Ungváry G. *In vitro* and *in vivo* tests for determination of the pathogenicity of quartz, diatomaceous earth, mordenite and clinoptilolite. Ann Occup Hyg. 2000;44(1):67–74.
30. Pratt PC. Lung dust content and response in guinea pigs inhaling three forms of silica. Arch Environ Health. 1983;38(4):197–204.
31. Wagner WD, Fraser DA, Wright PG, Dobrogorski OJ, Stokinger HE. Experimental evaluation of the threshold limit of cristobalite—calcined diatomaceous earth. Am Ind Hyg Assoc J. 1968;29(3):211–21.
32. Moreno T, Higueras P, Jones T, McDonald I, Gibbons W. Size fractionation in mercury-bearing airborne particles (HgPM10) at Almadén Spain: implications for inhalation hazards around old mines. Atmos Environ. 2005;39:6409–19.
33. Batchelder M, Cressey G. Rapid, accurate phase quantification of clay-bearing samples using a position-sensitive X-ray detector. Clay Clay Miner. 1998;46(2):183–94.
34. Ziemann C, Harrison PT, Bellmann B, Brown RC, Zoitos BK, Class P. Lack of marked cyto- and genotoxicity of cristobalite in devitrified (heated) alkaline earth silicate wools in short-term assays with cultured primary rat alveolar macrophages. Inhal Toxicol. 2014;26(2):113–27.
35. Pavan C, Rabolli V, Tomatis M, Fubini B, Lison D. Why does the hemolytic activity of silica predict its pro-inflammatory activity? Part Fibre Toxicol. 2014;11:76.
36. Mossman BT, Glenn RE. Bioreactivity of the crystalline silica polymorphs, quartz and cristobalite, and implications for occupational exposure limits (OELs). Crit Rev Toxicol. 2013;43(8):632–60.
37. Piguet PF, Collart MA, Grau GE, Sappino A-P, Vassalli P. Requirement of tumour necrosis factor for development of silica-induced pulmonary fibrosis. Nature. 1990;344(6263):245.
38. Carpenter MA, Salje EKH, Graeme-Barber A. Spontaneous strain as a determinant of thermodynamic properties for phase transitions in minerals. Eur J Mineral. 1998;10(4):621–91.
39. Quality of Urban Air Review Group. Airborne particulate matter in the United Kingdom. In: Department of the Environment, editor. Third report of the Quality of Urban Air Review Group. London, UK: Quality of Urban Air Review Group; 1996.
40. Chao CH, Lu HY. Crystallization of Na2O-doped colloidal gel-derived silica. Mater Sci Eng A-Struct Mater Prop Microstruct Process. 2000;282(1–2):123–30.
41. Venezia AM, La Parola V, Longo A, Martorana A. Effect of alkali ions on the amorphous to crystalline phase transition of silica. J Solid State Chem. 2001;161(2):373–8.
42. Deer WA, Howie RA, Zussman J. An introduction to the rock-forming minerals. 3rd ed. London, UK: Mineralogical Society of Great Britain & Ireland; 2013. p. 498.
43. Damby DE, Llewellin EW, Horwell CJ, Williamson BJ, Najorka J, Cressey G, et al. The [alpha]-[beta] phase transition in volcanic cristobalite. J Appl Crystallogr. 2014;47(4):1025–215.
44. Horwell C, Williamson B, Donaldson K, Le Blond J, Damby D, Bowen L. The structure of volcanic cristobalite in relation to its toxicity; relevance for the variable crystalline silica hazard. Part Fibre Toxicol. 2012;9(1):44.
45. Rodriguez-Navarro C, Ruiz-Agudo E, Luque A, Rodriguez-Navarro AB, Ortega-Huertas M. Thermal decomposition of calcite: mechanisms of formation and textural evolution of CaO nanocrystals. Am Mineral. 2009;94(4):578–93.
46. Borm PJA, Tran L, Donaldson K. The carcinogenic action of crystalline silica: a review of the evidence supporting secondary inflammation-driven genotoxicity as a principal mechanism. Crit Rev Toxicol. 2011;41(9):756–70.
47. Steenland K, Mannetje A, Boffetta P, Stayner L, Attfield M, Chen J, et al. Pooled exposure–response analyses and risk assessment for lung cancer in 10 cohorts of silica-exposed workers: an IARC multicentre study. Cancer Causes Control. 2001;12(9):773–84.
48. Collins JF, Salmon AG, Brown JP, Marty MA, Alexeeff GV. Development of a chronic inhalation reference level for respirable crystalline silica. Regul Toxicol Pharmacol. 2005;43(3):292–300.
49. Donaldson K, Borm PJA. The quartz hazard: a variable entity. Ann Occup Hyg. 1998;42(5):287–94.
50. Meldrum M, Howden P. Crystalline silica: variability in fibrogenic potency. Ann Occup Hyg. 2002;46 suppl 1:27–30.
51. Tourmann JL, Kaufmann R. Biopersistence of the mineral matter of coal mine dusts in silicotic human lungs: is there a preferential release of iron? Environ Health Perspect. 1994;102 Suppl 5:265–8.
52. Cullen RT, Vallyathan V, Hagen S, Donaldson K. Protection by iron against the toxic effects of quartz. Ann Occup Hyg. 1997;41:420–5. inhaled particles VIII.
53. Duffin R, Gilmour PS, Schins RPF, Clouter A, Guy K, Brown DM, et al. Aluminium lactate treatment of DQ12 quartz inhibits its ability to cause inflammation, chemokine expression, and nuclear factor-κB activation. Toxicol Appl Pharmacol. 2001;176(1):10–7.
54. Nolan RP, Langer AM, Harington JS, Oster G, Selikoff IJ. Quartz hemolysis as related to its surface functionalities. Environ Res. 1981;26(2):503–20.
55. Stone V, Jones R, Rollo K, Duffin R, Donaldson K, Brown DM. Effect of coal mine dust and clay extracts on the biological activity of the quartz surface. Toxicol Lett. 2004;149(1–3):255–9.
56. Fubini B, Bolis V, Cavenago A, Volante M. Physicochemical properties of crystalline silica dusts and their possible implication in various biological responses. Scand J Work Environ Health. 1995;21 suppl 2:9–14.
57. Aladdin M, Jian J, Yang Q, Chen L-C, Finkelman RB, Huang X. Laboratory studies of the impact of calcite on *in vitro* and *in vivo* effects of coal dust: a potential preventive agent for coal workers' pneumoconiosis? Am J Ind Med. 2013;56(3):292–9.
58. Diler SB, Ergene S. Nuclear anomalies in the buccal cells of calcite factory workers. Genet Mol Biol. 2010;33(2):374–8.
59. Oscarson DW, Van Scoyoc GE, Ahlrichs JL. Lysis of erythrocytes by silicate minerals. Clay Clay Miner. 1986;34(1):74–80.
60. Vallyathan V, Schwegler D, Reasor M, Stettler L, Clere J, Green FHY. Comparative *In vitro* cytotoxicity and relative pathogenicity of mineral dusts. Ann Occup Hyg. 1988;32(VI):279–89.
61. Karlsson HL, Gustafsson J, Cronholm P, Moller L. Size-dependent toxicity of metal oxide particles–a comparison between nano- and micrometer size. Toxicol Lett. 2009;188(2):112–8.
62. Zhou YM, Zhong CY, Kennedy IM, Pinkerton KE. Pulmonary responses of acute exposure to ultrafine iron particles in healthy adult rats. Environ Toxicol. 2003;18(4):227–35.
63. Zhu MT, Feng WY, Wang B, Wang TC, Gu YQ, Wang M, et al. Comparative study of pulmonary responses to nano- and submicron-sized ferric oxide in rats. Toxicology. 2008;247(2–3):102–11.
64. Brunner TJ, Wick P, Manser P, Spohn P, Grass RN, Limbach LK, et al. *In vitro* cytotoxicity of oxide nanoparticles: comparison to asbestos, silica, and the effect of particle solubility†. Environ Sci Technol. 2006;40(14):4374–81.

65. Costantini LM, Gilberti RM, Knecht DA. The phagocytosis and toxicity of amorphous silica. PLoS One. 2011;6(2):e14647.
66. Pavan C, Tomatis M, Ghiazza M, Rabolli V, Bolis V, Lison D, et al. In search of the chemical basis of the hemolytic potential of silicas. Chem Res Toxicol. 2013;26(8):1188–98.
67. Duffin R, Tran CL, Clouter A, Brown DM, MacNee W, Stone V, et al. The importance of surface area and specific reactivity in the acute pulmonary inflammatory response to particles. Ann Occup Hyg. 2002;46 suppl 1:242–5.
68. Duffin R, Tran L, Brown D, Stone V, Donaldson K. Proinflammogenic effects of low-toxicity and metal nanoparticles *in vivo* and *in vitro*: highlighting the role of particle surface area and surface reactivity. Inhal Toxicol. 2007;19(10):849–56.
69. Schinwald A, Donaldson K. Use of back-scatter electron signals to visualise cell/nanowires interactions *in vitro* and *in vivo*; frustrated phagocytosis of long fibres in macrophages and compartmentalisation in mesothelial cells *in vivo*. Part Fibre Toxicol. 2012;9(1):34.
70. Chamberlain M, Davies R, Brown RC, Griffiths DM. *In vitro* tests for the pathogenicity of mineral dusts. Ann Occup Hyg. 1982;26(1–4):583–92.
71. Champion JA, Mitragotri S. Role of target geometry in phagocytosis. Proc Natl Acad Sci U S A. 2006;103(13):4930–4.
72. Ye J, Shi X, Jones W, Rojanasakul Y, Cheng N, Schwegler-Berry D, et al. Critical role of glass fiber length in TNF-α production and transcription factor activation in macrophages. Am J Physiol Lung Cell Mol Physiol. 1999;276(3):L426–34.
73. Schinwald A, Murphy FA, Jones A, MacNee W, Donaldson K. Graphene-based nanoplatelets: a new risk to the respiratory system as a consequence of their unusual aerodynamic properties. ACS Nano. 2012;6(1):736–46.

22

Health risks in international container and bulk cargo transport due to volatile toxic compounds

Xaver Baur[1,2*†], Lygia Therese Budnik[1,3†], Zhiwei Zhao[4], Magne Bratveit[1,5,6,7], Rune Djurhuus[8], Louis Verschoor[9], Federico Maria Rubino[10], Claudio Colosio[10] and Jorgen R Jepsen[1,11]

Abstract

To ensure the preservation and quality of the goods, physical (i.e. radiation) or chemical pest control is needed. The dark side of such consents may bear health risks in international transport and production sharing. In fact, between 10% and 20% of all containers arriving European harbors were shown to contain volatile toxic substances above the exposure limit values. Possible exposure to these toxic chemicals may occur not only for the applicators but also the receiver by off gassing from products, packing materials or transport units like containers. A number of intoxications, some with lethal outcome, occur not only during the fumigation, but also during freight transport (on bulk carriers and other transport vessels), as well as in the logistic lines during loading and unloading. Risk occupations include dock-workers, seafarers, inspectors, as well as the usually uninformed workers of importing enterprises that unload the products. Bystanders as well as vulnerable consumers may also be at risk. Ongoing studies focus on the release of these toxic volatile substances from various goods. It was shown that the half-lives of the off-gassing process range between minutes and months, depending on the toxic substance, its chemical reactivity, concentration, the temperature, the contaminated matrix (goods and packing materials), and the packing density in the transport units. Regulations on declaration and handling dangerous goods are mostly not followed. It is obvious that this hazardous situation in freight transport urgently requires preventive steps. In order to improve awareness and relevant knowledge there is a need for more comprehensive information on chemical hazards and a broader implementation of the already existing regulations and guidelines, such as those from ILO, IMO, and national authorities. It is also necessary to have regular controls by the authorities on a worldwide scale, which should be followed by sanctions in case of disregarding regulations. Further, fumigated containers must have a warning sign corresponding to international recommendations and national regulations, and freight documents have to indicate any potential hazard during stripping the goods.

Introduction

Transporting more than 70% of all international freight, container ships represent the majority of the c. 40,000 merchant ships that are larger than 1,000 gross register tonnes. A minor fraction of transported goods are carried by bulk carriers, tankers, reefers, roll-on/rill-off ships. All these ships may be categorized by their operations with liners running regularly and operating on a schedule and tramps without fixed runs that will go wherever a suitable cargo takes it.

* Correspondence: xaver.baur@charite.de
† Equal contributors
1 European Society for Environmental and Occupational Medicine (EOM), Berlin, Germany
2 Institute for Occupational Medicine, Charité University Medicine, Charité-Campus Benjamin Franklin, Berlin, Germany

Freight on board ships in containers as well as in other forms is frequently disinfected by use of toxic fumigants. All fumigants, which are used to protect the transported freight from alien species and to inhibit their spread to foreign countries comprise a potential health hazard which draws attention to, the role of exposure situation for risk assessment, especially for exposed dockers, other port staff and transport workers involved in unloading imported production parts and goods, but presumably also to vulnerable end consumers. They affect mainly the central and peripheral nervous system and the respiratory tract, but may also cause cancer. Further, recent studies identified a varying spectrum of toxic industrial chemicals released from the newly manufactured transported products (see chapter on Intoxication incidents).

Unfortunately, so far, there is limited communication on potential health risks from volatile toxic substances in globally transported freight between producing companies, logistic companies along the transport line, national controlling agencies, and the end-user. Further, common information and communication systems do not exist at all. Appropriate national and supra-national common databases comprising all relevant health information of transported freight are urgently needed. This would give full transparency, stimulate precautions and allow the reduction of time consuming, expensive and cumbersome controls and measurements. It would reduce the health risks and provide protection against intoxications.

This review aims to give an overview of the most prominent toxicants in transport containers, published intoxications, and show findings from examined cases (including case histories and exposure assessment). We suggest biomonitoring and medical examination scheme for exposed workers. The legislative framework and the practice of handling transport containers in different settings are reviewed and appropriate preventive measures are presented. Additionally a questionnaire based survey on practical handling of transport container in China (exporting country) and Denmark (importing country) were performed.

The objective of this overview was to give a state of the art presentation on endangering exposures to volatile substances in freight transport, on the associated possible adverse health effects, diagnostics, regulations and appropriate preventive measures.

Outline

The review is divided into several paragraphs, discussing various aspects of health issues associated with international container and bulk cargo transport. The separate sections deal with the following issues.

1. Health effects of toxic substances in container transport
   a. Health effects of individual fumigants
   b. Health effects of preservatives and ripening inhibitors
   c. Health effects of toxic substances released from cargo
2. Medical examination of subjects with suspected intoxications
   a. Case report: intoxications in a storage room from off gassing fumigants
3 Practice of handling transport containers in exporting and receiving countries. Pilot studies in China and Denmark
   a. Pilot study in China
   b. Pilot study in Denmark
   c. Discussion of the pilot studies in China and Denmark
4. Occurrences of intoxications with chemicals used for pest control in transport containers and on bulk cargo ships
   a. Fumigant intoxications – general
   b. Fumigated transport containers
   c. Fumigated bulk cargo ships
   d. Summary of incidents
   e. Concluding remarks
5. Regulations on fumigants
6. Preventive measures
   a. Applied preventive measures
   b. Labelling
   c. Knowledge and awareness
   d. Guidelines for safe procedures
   e. Measurements
   f. Ventilation
   g. Personal protective equipment

Health effects of toxic substances in container transport

Container transport over sea has expanded enormously in the last thirty years. The use of toxic substances for fumigation and preserving (i.e. ripening inhibition) goods has increased concordantly with a tendency to decay during transport [1]. Other sources of toxic substances in container transport are the encasement material and the transported cargo itself. During the whole process of loading, transporting and unloading, people are at risk for exposure to these toxic substances. Even consumers at the end of the chain may be at risk [2]. The occurrence and severity of the health effects depend on a number of factors (see below).

Factors determining occurrence and severity of health effects

- The concentration of the substance the subject is exposed to
- The duration of exposure
- Whether the exposure was acute and/or chronic
- The individual sensibility of the exposed subject

Additive or synergistic effects from co-exposure to the substances.

It is important to keep in mind that acute intoxications with these substances can lead to health effects that persist for months to years or even lifelong. The Expertise Centre Environmental Medicine (ECEMed) Rijnstate Teaching Hospital in Rijnstate, the Netherlands, and in the outpatient departments have primarily seen health complaints due to exposure during unloading containers or drivers, who had to open the container in order to drive their truck to the dock for unloading [2,3]. In this chapter we will briefly discuss the health effects of the most common toxic substances people are exposed to in container transport (see Table 1).

Health effects of individual fumigants

Phosphine

Phosphine is used especially in the transport of grain in containers as well as as bulk carrier transport in trains or ships. Tablets containing aluminium- or magnesium phosphide are combined in small sockets or long sleeves. The phosphide reacts with the moisture in the air of the container to produce phosphine. Mostly, the containers are holding silica gel for drying the container in order to prevent too much formation of phosphine during the transport. Thus a crucial moment is the opening of the container. The remaining phosphide starts forming phosphine when humidity enters the container from outside. The same reaction takes place for loads in the holds of ships at the presence of remaining phosphide. Especially this moment leads to acute intoxications. After this acute moment continuous exposure may take place due to the absorption of phosphine to the clothes of the person.

In the western world, intoxications were previously seen primarily in employees of phosphine producing plants and with agricultural use. In Asia phosphine is reported as a suicidal agent with death rates as high as sixty percent [4].

Phosphide reacts with moisture (i.e. water) to form gaseous phosphine [5]. Phosphine interferes with the electron transport chain in the mitochondria [6,7]. Already within one minute after exposure, effects on the respiratory and gastrointestinal tract are found. Respiratory symptoms are irritation of the (upper) airways leading to pain and cough, shortness of breath and eventually hypoxia and a feeling of severe pressure on the thorax. The gastrointestinal symptoms are nausea, abdominal discomfort, diarrhea and vomiting. Neurological and skeletal muscle effects occur rapidly thereafter. Involvement of the central as well as the peripheral nervous system lead to dizziness, disorientation, headache, neuropathic pain, mainly in arms and legs, and eventually decreased consciousness and coma. All skeletal muscles can be involved with severe pain and loss of tonus. Single acute exposure leads to muscular damage with a peak after 24 to 48 hours after the acute incident and lasting for weeks to months. In severe intoxication, the cardiovascular system is also involved. Cardiac arrhythmia, hypotension, hypoxia and renal failure ultimately lead to death [8]. The majority of patients that come to the attention of doctors are seen at the emergency room in general hospitals. Due to unfamiliarity with the clinical syndrome, the correct diagnosis is often not made and patients are discharged from the emergency room under the diagnosis of hyperventilation syndrome. Measurement of PaO2 and oxygen saturation can rapidly distinguish between hyperventilation and phosphine intoxication, the latter showing decreased values [9].

Table 1 Major toxic substances in container atmosphere

Fumigation	Preservation	Encasement	Cargo
Phosphine	Carbon monoxide	Formaldehyde	Benzene
Bromomethane (methyl bromide)	Carbon dioxide		Xylene
Sulfuryl difluoride			1,2-Dichloroethane
Formaldehyde			Ethylbenzene
Ethylene oxide			Toluene
1,2-Dichloroethane (ethylene dichloride)			Dichloromethane
Dichloromethane			Other organic solvents
Chloropicrin (trichloro(nitro) methane)			

Methyl bromide (bromomethane)

Since 1938 methyl bromide has been used widespread as an agricultural fumigant. During the last twenty years there has been a rapid rise in the use of methyl bromide for fumigation in transport containers [10].

The Montreal Protocol on Substances that Deplete the Ozone Layer (http://ozone.unep.org/new_site/en/montreal_protocol.php) has put an end to the broad use of methyl bromide in agriculture in order to prevent further reduction of the ozone layer caused by halogenated methyl/ethyl bromides and –chlorides (i.e. methyl bromide/bromomethane). Due to its toxicity, the use of methyl bromide in the European Union has been forbidden since 2010, but exceptions are made, especially with regard to the International Standards for Phytosanitary Measures 15, ISPM 15 (https://www.ippc.int/publications/regulation-wood-packaging-material-international-trade-0). Consequently, the use of methyl bromide for fumigation of stow wood in sea containers remains allowed until 2015 (and continues to be used, if no alternative product is available, as a part of CUEs, critical use examples). The increasing use as a fumigant in sea container (a part of the CUE) transport leads to exposure to methyl bromide of a new group of workers, handling import containers.

28 fatal cases of methyl bromide intoxication [10] have been described in the literature [11]. In 1983, this has risen above 950 fatal cases [11]. Acute intoxication is characterized by early symptoms like headache, vomiting, sore throat, vertigo and visual disturbances, followed by reduced consciousness, coma and convulsions [10,12]. Chronic effects can last for years and are confined mainly to the central (chronic toxic encephalopathy) and peripheral

nervous system (painful neuropathy) together with general complaints of fatigue [13]. See Table 2 for limit values.

1,2-Dichloroethane (ethylene dichloride)

Acute exposure to 1,2-dichloroethane (ethylene dichloride) leads to headache, dizziness and hypoxia. Chronic exposure elicits chronic toxic encephalopathy (see organic solvents) and is frequently accompanied by liver function tests [14]. See Table 2 for limit values.

Sulfuryl difluoride (sulfuryl fluoride)

Sulfuryl difluoride is considered as a less toxic substitute for methyl bromide. However, it does have ozone-depleting as well as toxic effects including acute and chronic encephalopathy, disturbances in the olfactory function, and neuropathy with reduced nerve conduction velocity [12]. See Table 2 for limit values.

Formaldehyde

Acute intoxication is characterized by dizziness, nausea and vomiting, fatigue, feeling of drunkenness, disturbance in coordination and concentration followed by headache, malaise, hypersensitivity for noise and light, and upper airway symptoms like cough, shortness of breath, a hoarse voice and sometimes skin eruptions. Symptoms and complaints last for days or weeks [15].

More than 90% of inhaled formaldehyde is taken up in the upper airway system and leads to local irritation and neuro-cognitive effects. Severe exposure may cause additional complaints from the lower respiratory tract like shortness of breath, increased sputum production and coughing.

Formaldehyde may also impose severe long-term effects since it is carcinogenic to humans [16].

Chloropicrin (trichloro(nitro)methane, nitrochloroform)

This previously used fumigant may be added as an indicator to (odourless) methyl bromide or other fumigants due its strong odour. See Table 2 for limit values.

Health effects of preservatives and ripening inhibitors

Carbon monoxide

Exposure to carbon monoxide leads to non-specific complaints like headache, dizziness, somnolence to unconsciousness, flu-like symptoms, and seizures. If such symptoms occur in the context of handling containers, especially with fruits, one should be alarmed. The primary measures to be taken are immediate removal of the victim from the site and dispense oxygen. Omitting these measures can eventually lead to death. Since carbon monoxide has a much higher affinity for hemoglobin than oxygen, severe hypoxia rapidly develops [17].

Carbon dioxide

Carbon dioxide, frequently combined with reduced oxygen levels, is added to sea containers with fruits as cargo in order to prevent ripening during transport. It acts as an asphyxiant and in addition has toxic effects at the cellular level.

Low concentrations (up to 5%) lead to headache, dizziness, sweating and shortness of breath. Concentrations up to ten percent cause hyperventilation, tachycardia and worsening of headache and dizziness with laboratory findings of metabolic acidosis. Severe intoxications occur at concentrations above 10% with additional symptoms of drowsiness, muscle twitching and loss of consciousness with severe hypoxia. Higher concentrations elicit convulsions, coma and death. Immediate removal of the person from the area of exposure should be done along with administration of oxygen and general life support [18].

Table 2 Health based occupational exposure limits values for major fumigants

Fumigant	Acute effects/workplace	Carcinogenic effects (potential)
Chemical	Occupational exposure limit, OEL [mg/m^3]	Carcinogen = + (Class)
Phosphine	0.14	-
Bromomethane (methyl bromide)	3.89	+ (3)
Sulfuryl difluoride	20.9	-
Formaldehyde	0.37	+ (4)
Ethylene oxide	1.80	+ (2)
1,2-Dichloroethane (ethylene dichloride)	4.05	+ (2)
Dichloromethane (chloromethane)	86.75	+ (3)
Chloropicrin (trichloro(nitro)methane)	0.672	-

Sources: NIOSH; National Institute for Occupational Safety and Health, Center for Disease Control and Prevention (www.cdc.gov/niosh/npg).
IRAC, International Agency for Research on Cancer (http://monographs.iarc.fr/ENG/Monographs/vol100F/mono100F.pdf).
(see [19] for further details on community exposure levels and thresholds).

Health effects of toxic substances released from cargo

Organic solvents (benzene, xylene, ethyl benzene and toluene, chloromethane)

All kinds of organic solvents and degreasing agents fall into this category. These solvents are emitted from goods such as furniture or shoes that have been manufactured with the use of paint, lacquer or glue. Given the long duration of transport over sea in a closed container (usually without ventilation), high concentrations may build up [19]. As soon as the doors are opened people entering the container may be exposed to high concentrations of solvents.

All organic solvents give rise to acute and chronic toxic encephalopathy (CTE) the severity of which depends on the amount and duration of the exposure and the presence and amount of peak exposures [20]. Acute neurotoxic effects resemble alcohol intoxication with comparable narcotic features like dizziness, disorientation, euphoria and a feeling of drunkenness [21]. Chronic effects are seen after exposure duration of up to 3 – 10 years and are categorized in stages I to III (WHO, see Table 3).

In the case pressed wood panels are used, formaldehyde is often emitted from the panels during transport. See for health effects of formaldehyde in the section on fumigants.

In addition to the neurotoxic effects benzene is also carcinogenic to humans (IARC Monographs, 100 F, 2012). Accumulating evidence indicates effects on several blood cell types at ever lower concentrations, suggesting risk of developing malignancies of the hematopoietic system [22-24].

Medical examination of subjects with suspected intoxications

As mentioned, acute or chronic intoxications by fumigants or toxic industrial chemicals are typically associated with non-specific symptoms and therefore frequently misdiagnosed. The consequence may be ongoing hazardous exposures in the workplace with serious and frequently non-reversible disorders. This requires that workers as well as physicians are aware of these potential dangerous exposures at the workplace.

The crucial initial step is the detailed occupational and clinical history, which should be taken by an experienced physician who is aware of potential risk exposures to volatile toxic substances in the workplace (see dignostic set-up below). A well-known detailed questionnaire is available from Safe Work Australia [25]. Based on the literature as well as on our own clinical experience we have developed a new comprehensive questionnaire (FumEx), which is now available in three languages [26]. It was shown in various applications to be very useful in field studies as well as for individual intoxication cases. It is not too time-consuming and it is easy to handle by the patient by adding information by the physician performing the crucial personal interview. FumEx allows to settle/fix the time, the duration and the type of workplace exposures [27], the applied protective devices, and to detect acute and chronic symptoms related to workplace exposures and to exposures outside the workplace. For the full diagnosis, the work history is followed by physical examination and functional tests that reflect the potentially affected organs such as lung function testing, blood analyses, and neurological and neuropsychological investigations [28,29]. Abnormal findings may require sophisticated examinations by other medical disciplines such as neurology or pneumology. Imaging such as MRT or cranial CT may also be indicated. Early starting of biomonitoring may help to identify the causative toxic substance. Unfortunately, there is no specific therapy and no available antidote; only symptomatic treatment is possible.

Immediate diagnostic set-up, which requires an experienced physician in case of assumed intoxication is outlined below (see also the questionnaire in Additional file 1)

- Diagnostic set-up in case of suspected intoxication
- *Case history, questionnaire*
  - headache, dizziness, forgetfulness, concentration disorders, feeling impatient or depressed, sleepiness, emotional problems, shortness of breath, diarrhea, change of sense or taste, loss of sexual interest etc.

Table 3 Classification of CTE according to the WHO

	Symptoms	Cognitive defects	Neurological abnormalities
Class I	Fatigue, diminished memory, concentration and initiative	No objective dysfunction	No objective abnormalities
Organic affective syndrome	Change in personality. Poor impulse control, lowered mood and motivation, irritability, anxiety, emotional lability		
Class II Mild chronic toxic encephalopathy	Difficulties in concentration and attention, impairment of memory, decrease in learning capacity	Objective evidence of cognitive impairment	Minor neurological signs
Class III Severe chronic toxic encephalopathy	Marked global deterioration in intellect and memory	Marked global deterioration in intellect and memory	Neurological signs and/or neuroradiological abnormal findings

  - Fum-Ex2 Questionnaire is accessible online at: www.EOMsociety.org
- *Physical and neurological examination*
- *Lung function testing*
  - spirometry, gas exchange measurement, methacholine challenge test, spiroergometry
- *Clinical chemistry/Blood tests:*
  - liver enzymes, muscle enzymes
  - intoxication markers
  - bromide and fluoride in serum and urine
- *Human Biomonitoring*
  - residual fumigants in blood and urine (methyl bromide, ethylene oxide, ethylene dichloride, chloropicrin, methylene chloride, co-exposure to solvents like benzene, toluene, xylene etc.; headspace tubes – Gas-Chromatography-Mass-spectrometry analyses
  - hemoglobin adducts in blood (methylvaline and hydroxyethyl valine)
- *Sniff sticks (olfactory test)*
- *Colour vision test*
- *Comprehensive neurological and neuropsychological tests, e.g.*
  - physical performance (grooved pegboard and finger tapping test)
  - test of crystallized and fluid intelligence
  - information processing speed
  - selective attention/concentration tests, divided attention
  - sustained attention/vigilance
  - learning/memory tests
  - decision making and pre-morbid verbal intelligence
  - logical thinking and abstraction
- *MRT, cranial CT*

Case report: intoxications in a storage room from off gassing fumigants

In a medium sized European company, which received electronic production parts from south east Asia and South America, several employees developed signs of intoxication on three occasions within two years [30]. Six storage room workers were exposed to fumigants off gassing from shipped products. They were unloading approximately two overseas shipments a week at the time of the incident. They all worked 8 hours per day day in a storage room. Patients 1,3,4,5 and 6 unloaded the delivered items on a regular basis, and unpacked wooden pellets with paper boxes covered with plastic. Patient 2 supervised the working place. The workers were responsible for unloading and distributing the delivered items into several separate areas on different floors. Following each incident, the workers (patients 1, 3, 4, 5 and 6) noticed itchy skin, very red eyes and suffered from recurrent epistaxis, headaches and intention tremor. After the second incident, four individuals (Pat. 1, 3, 4 and 5) additionally complained about paresthesia (pins and needles in the legs), dizziness, breathing difficulties and increasing irritability. After the third incident, patient 4 was on sick leave for several weeks; patients 1 and 3 developed immediate epistaxis with a severe headache [30]. Air samples taken in the space between the packed electronic parts with trapped gas residues (in the breathing zone of the workers) showed presence of ethylene oxide and methyl bromide. Patients ($n = 6$, aged from 32 to 54 yrs.) were compared with a healthy control group ($n = 30$, with median age of 40 yrs.). Patients underwent standardized medical examination for the symptoms of fumigant intoxication as described earlier [31,27,30]. No significantly elevated bromide levels in any of the analyzed serum samples were detected. However, we detected low methyl bromide levels (0.24 μg/L) in the blood of patient 5 collected five days after the second incident (BM2). No increased levels of ethylene dichloride, chloropicrin, methyl iodine or dichloromethane were detected in the blood samples (all were below the limit of detection). Patients 1, 3, 4, 5 and 6 showed slightly increased levels of ethylene oxide in blood and two patients displayed elevated methanol levels, Patient 5 showed presence of small amounts of methyl bromide in blood [30]. In-vivo dose monitoring by means of adducts to macromolecules after exposure to methylating agents showed elevated levels of hemoglobin adducts: methylvaline and hydroxyethylvaline. The monitoring of hemoglobin adducts additionally allows to monitor past exposures and to generate extrapolated data that might enhance the risk assessment strategy. We have calculated the theoretical exposures to methyl bromide and ethylene oxide at the time of the individual incidents. Based on these data, the intoxication could be confirmed for three patients out of six (patients, 3, 4 and 5); data for patients 1, 2 and 6 did not allow any extrapolation. The clinical examination data from these patients (data not shown here) support the evidence of intoxication. No intoxication could be confirmed for patients 1, 2 and 6. Patient 2 supervised the other workers and after the first incident patients 1 and 6 were mostly engaged in other areas of the storage room with less direct contact with (newly delivered) unloaded products. Notably, after the first accident the company reorganized the storage area with a separate zone for unpacking the incoming shipment. As reported, the patients showed serious intoxication symptoms with itchy skin, very red eyes, dizziness, breathing difficulties and increasing irritability. They suffered from headache, acrotaxia, (intention tremor) paresthesia, and/or developed immediate or recurrent epistaxis. Our case studies indicate a need for an early and comprehensive prevention system including dedicated rules for the occupational hygiene and biomonitoring procedures [30].

Practice of handling transport containers in exporting and receiving countries. Pilot studies in China and Denmark

This section addresses the local interpretation and implementation of international and national regulations for safe container handling in China (as exporting country) and Denmark (as importing country). This is found of relevance since the involved workers may not always sufficiently know the legal regulations and the required precautions that may consequently not be properly integrated in the daily occupational health practises.

Pilot study in China

With more than 30 years economic reform, the Chinese government is now paying more attention to the working conditions and health and safety of workers than before. However, little notice has been paid to these issues in the field of container fumigation in China [31].

Firstly, the operation of the fumigation of export containers in China is discussed in general, mainly considering the following two questions: who is operating the business and how work has been organized. It also looks at the working conditions and the health issues of workers. The research draws on a case study of a Chinese state-owned company, established in 2007, operating the fumigation of containers. It is a subsidiary company of the Provincial Administration of Inspection and Quarantine. Qualitative methods are utilised, with two first line managers being interviewed extensively and four workers being group-interviewed under the 'supervision' of their managers. The presence of the managers may prevent workers from expressing their concerns to some extent and hence weakens the analysis. However, available data still provide a meaningful explanation as to what is going on within that particular field.

In China, the business of fumigating export containers is under the administration of the General Administration of Inspection and Quarantine of the P.R. China. This government agency also formulates relevant policies and regulations, such as 'Measures for Supervision and Management of Fumigation and Disinfection' and 'Rules of Operating Container Fumigation'. In each province, there is Provincial Administration of Inspection and Quarantine responsible for implementing the regulations and policies. The provincial agency sets up local subsidiary companies that monopolize the business of fumigation. The interviewed managers introduced:

> *"Only the subsidies can operate the fumigation of exported containers. Other companies are not allowed" (interviewed manager No.2)*

The monopolization of the business of fumigation by the subsidiary companies is a result of special supports of the provincial agency to the subsidies. Firstly, the subsidies obtain credentials to provide training to the workers and issue them professional certificates. More importantly, the subsidies obtain credentials of operating fumigation and issues official certificates to the fumigated containers, which are highly recognized by foreign consignees. None of these credentials can be obtained by any other company. Last but not least important, these subsidies are supported financially by their parent agency. By monopolizing the business, the subsidies are faced with little competition in the market and do not have to concern much about lowering down the costs.

This may have some positive implications to the working condition of workers who seem very happy with their jobs. The workers in the case study received professional training and are issued nationally recognized certificates at the end of the course. They are very familiar with the operation of fumigation and operate fast. Two workers can finish the fumigation of one 20 feet container in less than 5 minutes. They work at the 'Specified Fumigation Area' and wear working suits, masks, and gloves during fumigation. They know the existence of health and safety regulations of fumigating and said they learnt them at the training course but could not remember them specifically. They know that they use methyl bromide for fumigation and that it is highly toxic. They are not sure whether the masks are dust masks or gas filter masks. However, they seem pretty sure that their masks can prevent them from any harm. They seem fearless. They do not report any symptoms that might be related to chemical exposure or any diseases that might be related to chemical exposure. They said they are very satisfied with their work:

> *"Although there are many detailed instructions about the operation, for instance the environmental factors such as wind direction that can influence the operation, in practice it is rather straightforward – nothing complicated at all"*

> *"No exposure to the chemicals". "No danger to health" "I am very happy with my job". "I think it is a good one". "Yes, I am happy with it"*

However, this may not be the whole story because according to the managers, the fumigation job is not a good at all. The managers said:

> *"I do not think it is a good job. At least, it is not decent and it does not pay much." (Manager No.1). "Honestly, it is the peasants (land man) who are doing the job. Even the peasant workers are not willing to do the job. It is a simple, but NOT a very good job!" (Manager No.2)*

Most of the workers in the company are peasant workers. They are temporarily employed, offered low wages, have little job security, are not provided with any social insurance and most of them received little education from school. The managers explained:

> *"When there is a need, the workers are called to work" (Manager No.1). "Peasant workers are not under the social insurance scheme. Before the economic reform, workers were provided with food subsidy and work protection subsidy. But now, there is nothing. If the peasant workers want to do the job, they do it. If not, they can just leave." (Manager No.1)*

These peasant workers are specifically trained for fumigating containers, without many other skills. They are in a very weak position and depend on their managers for job opportunities. Because of the presence of their managers, it is possible that workers did not thoroughly express their concerns about their working condition or occupational health issues, especially the problems. However, the limited alternatives of their jobs in the labour market can be another important explanation as to why the workers express their content with their current jobs.

In conclusion, the study suggests that peasant workers are in lack of job security and basic protection, especially concerning the social insurance aspect. Their weak position due to the lack of protection and support from the society is an important issue that needs addressing. It is also important to notice that fumigation of export containers is monopolized by subsidiary companies of the Provincial Administration of Inspection and Quarantine. Without much pressure for high profits, state-owned subsidies provide relatively satisfactory working condition to their workers.

It was also seen from the case study that since the European countries improved the inspecting standards of the levels of methyl bromide in the imported containers, fumigation using toxic chemicals has been gradually replaced by heat treatment in this state-owned company. This might imply that a stricter regulation may reduce the use of using toxic chemicals in this industry and improve workers' health and safety standard.

Pilot study in Denmark

The practice of container work was investigated in a series of semi-structured interviews with key informants including managers and safety representatives of two organizations the employees of which may be chemically exposed while handling containers [31].

Two major working populations are potentially exposed to hazardous chemicals when handling containers in Danish harbours: workers who unload freight and government officers in charge of inspecting transported goods. The practices and perceptions of workers was assessed by approaching the staff of the custom office and a container logistics company both located in Aarhus – the largest Danish container port. The selection of respondents was based on a purposeful snowball sampling method of individuals that were rich in information and experiences related to the topic. The interviews followed a template that included questions about work activities, potential chemical exposures, experienced health effects, health and safety regulations and applied preventive measures. A semi-structured face-to-face method was used to support the respondents to share their views and to gain in-depth information about the topic.

The approaches to prevention were quite different for the two populations. Group policies in the logistic company aimed to follow the vision for conducting business in a safe manner and to comply with applicable laws and regulations. The safety instructions were structured and easily available but had no stated relation to national and international regulations. In case of suspicion caused by the presence of a fumigation certificate, labeling as "dangerous goods" or closed container ventilation valves, ventilation, filter mask and gloves were prescribed. The custom office had safety instructions applying to control of containers, storage and warehousing that relate to the IMDG code, to European and Danish directives as well as to a chemical database established by the Danish occupational health service for seafarers (Seahealth).

In spite of limited knowledge about the potential health risks from exposure to fumigated containers, all the interviewees agreed on their existence. They expressed concern about frequent chemical exposure and estimated the proportion of polluted containers to be high, up to 50%. According to their experiences, 20% to 50% of the containers have a distinct perceivable odour. In contrast, they recalled that few containers were documented and labelled as previously fumigated or chemically treated. Methyl bromide was the only fumigant encountered in practice that all interviewed persons could quote. Some interviewees expressed their awareness about general industrial chemicals and noted experience with signs of exposure, such as a white powder in some containers, but could not specify the chemicals.

Most interviewees assumed that chemical exposures from transport containers may chronically damage workers' health. Inspectors were increasingly aware of the risk, but had very limited specific knowledge. Manual workers were also rather unknowledgeable about the problem and fear was not typical among them.

Headache as the most commonly reported acute health effect was more frequently experienced in the past and tends to be related to special types of freights. Eye irritation and unspecified discomfort are also experienced occasionally. However, no interviewees recalled chronic intoxications with medically established connection to previous chemical exposures.

The interviewed managers were aware of the existence of relevant international and national regulations although they were typically not able to specify them. On the other hand, the interviewees were more knowledgeable about the local instructions of their organisations. Besides the general provisions for workplace health and safety, e.g. risk assessment, education, use of safety equipment and personal protective equipment, the local instructions, however, give insufficient guidance for several practical challenges of preventing chemical exposures during work with containers.

In practice, the preventive measures are primarily based on the attempt to identify the containers that carry occupational health risks. Although the review of documentation was reported to be the main way to get information about previous chemical treatment it was rarely seen and likely to be absent in a major proportion of fumigated containers. Apart from the documents, strange odour, the type of goods and the country of origin may create suspicion. Containers arriving from developing countries with food, footwear, furniture and other wood products were most frequently regarded as carrying chemical hazards. Equipment for monitoring of container air is available in some of the organisations only, but even if available, it can detect only methyl bromide but no other potentially harmful chemicals. In some organisations a suspicion is sufficient for applying specific preventive measures while others would require positive results of air measurements to take action.

The decision and choice of preventive measures to be used in practice tend to be left to the directly involved employees and the actions taken show considerable variation. The main preventive measure to reduce chemical exposure is passive ventilation; active ventilation is not applied in practice. The conditions of aeration are not consistently prescribed. The applied ventilation times vary between 2 and 48 hours without knowledge of whether this amount of time is sufficient. The other major way of preventing adverse health effects of chemical exposures is the use of personal protective equipment. Dust masks are usually provided to the workers, but do not prevent passage to the airways of chemical vapours. Gloves are typically provided and the use of coveralls reported by some interviewees. In practice, however, the overall frequency of wearing personal protective equipment is low.

Discussion of the pilot studies in China and Denmark

Both presented experiences from China and Denmark are likely to represent "best cases". In China, the state monopoly of fumigation without competition permits a certain level of training and protection of workers. Even heat treatment was used when adequate. Still, the peasant workers are disfavoured by the absence of social security. The importing countries experience adequate labelling as being rare even when most containers arrive from China. In Denmark, the set standards aimed to provide full protection. Still, monitoring and ventilation practices and e.g. the use of respiratory protection were clearly inadequate. We have little information about fumigation practices elsewhere in exporting countries, but the level of protection might well be inferior compared to China. Denmark has relatively high standards relating to chemical exposure at work, and exposure levels may well be much higher in other importing countries with lower standards of protection. Some Incidents of intoxications with chemicals used for pest control in transport containers and on bulk cargo ships.

Occurrences of intoxications with chemicals used for pest control in transport containers and on bulk cargo ships

Fumigant intoxications – general

Incidents with fumigants used for pest control are reported frequently [32-35]. A lot of cases occur in the agricultural use of pesticides, and in some cases affecting both applicators and people living in the neighbourhood [36]. Some incidents occur in relation to fumigation of buildings, both public buildings and private homes [37,38]. A recent incident was reported in in January 2014 where a private home in Jerusalem, Israel, was fumigated with phosphine by a professional exterminator, and two children died. Two other children were seriously harmed but survived.(http://www.jpost.com/National-News/Family-of-6-believed-poisoned-by-pesticides-in-Jerusalem-home-toddler-dies-338999).

Fumigated transport containers

Although adverse health effects after occupational exposures to pesticides seem to occur frequently, the documentation of these incidents are often insufficient, lacking traceable description of exposure with respect to site and time, well documented exposure data, adverse health effects, clinical symptoms and not at least: publication of the incidents/cases in well-respected and traceable sources.

In particular, incidents related to opening of transport containers or fumigant intoxications on bulk cargo ships are seldom reported in scientific journals or described in public available reports. For those that are reported, the sources are variable, ranging from a few scientific papers, conference presentations to newspaper articles and short notes in organisations like Marine Accident Investigation Branch (MAIB).

To address container incidents a literature survey was conducted on PubMed in October 2014 with the following search string in the Title/Abstract field: "(toxic* OR poison* OR intoxic*) AND (fumiga* NOT fumigatus)

AND container*". The search returned 43 references. Nearly 30% of all papers regarding fumigants or hazardous volatile chemicals in transport containers were by Baur and various co-partner, who started to collect the cases (see Table in Additional file 2). The PubMed search revealed only one paper with sufficient documentation of an intoxication case related to opening of transport containers: Two dock workers who opened a container in the port of Rotterdam in 2006 were acutely intoxicated, and subsequent field analysis by the fire brigade confirmed the presence of methyl bromide as the likely causative agent, although the paper did not contain any data showing the methyl bromide levels [39].

Two papers reported exposure incidents in detail. Preisser et al. described 26 patients referred to a clinic in Germany with symptoms of pesticide intoxication after opening of transport containers [29]. The authors were able to confirm the diagnosis based on typical symptoms and extensive clinical examination. Additionally by laboratory analysis ethylene dichloride, methyl bromide, phosphine and methylene chloride were identified. The predominant symptoms were headaches, concentration and memory problems, dizziness and nausea, irritation of the skin and mucous membranes and a reduced ability to do exercise. In addition to the neurological and neuropsychological impairments the analyses verified the development of reactive airways dysfunction syndrome (RADS) in 14 of 26 patients with long lasting symptoms due to their contact with fumigants.

Later Budnik et al. has performed more comprehensive exposure assessment using biomonitoring data for 164 subjects exposed to halogenated hydrocarbon pesticides (methyl bromide and ethylene dichloride) [27]. Another paper described 33 cases of presumed intoxication by transport containers [40]. The cases indicated phosphine and ethylene dichloride as the fumigants. However, the paper lacked detailed documentation of exposure data and for two of the cases there were no information of where the incident took place. A recent case report documented phosphine intoxication on board of bulk carrier in France [41].

Similar search on Web of Science added a single reference; this was a meeting abstract presenting a case report with two dock-workers being poisoned by methyl bromide as they opened a transport container. The abstract did not contain any information of location and date, but the incident most probably occurred in the Netherlands since the authors were from the National Institute for Health and the Environment in the Netherlands. No exposure data were included [42]. A Google search reveals two short notes describing patients referred to the Expertise Centre Environmental Medicine in Arnhem, The Netherlands after intoxication by container fumigants [9,40].

Fumigated bulk cargo ships

Incidents related to transport of bulk cargo on ships seem to be slightly more frequently reported in relevant publications, e.g. as Safety Flyers/Accidents Flyers by MAIB internet site (www.maib.gov.uk). A similar, systematic literature survey as for container contamination was conducted for fumigation on bulk cargo ships. A search on PubMed in October 2014 with the following search string in the Title/Abstract field: "(toxic* OR poison* OR intoxic*) AND ship" returned 223 references. Replacing "ship" with "freighter" gave 3 additional results. Another search with the string "(fumiga* NOT fumigatus) AND (ship OR crew)" in the Title/Abstract field returned 21 references. The search results identified 3 scientific papers describing incidents on board bulk cargo ships: One on a Polish ship in Vietnam, 1967 [43], one on a grain freighter on the Canadian/American East Coast in 1978 [44], and a survey on Danish merchant ships 1988–1996 carried out by the Institute of Maritime Medicine and Danish Maritime Authority in Denmark [45,46]. The latter investigation [45] showed 6 intoxication incidents due to fumigation of cargo with pesticides, 4 of these were fatalities. The oldest publication was not assessed due to difficulties in retrieving the paper.

The PubMed search was then supplemented with searches for incident reports on the web sites of International Labour Organization (ILO), the International Maritime Organization (IMO, the International Maritime Health Association (IMHA), Marine Accident Investigation Branch (MAIB), and the international maritime insurance companies Gard, Skuld and Norwegian Hull Club. The two latter companies did not have any incident reports made public, but Gard described several incidents in Gard News 204 (November 2011/January 2012). Neither ILO (http://www.ilo.org), IMO (http://www.imo.org) nor International Maritime Health Association had any publications on incidents/case reports. MAIB showed two incidents in the period from 1999 to date: One fatality with phosphine on a bulk cargo ship loaded with grain in 2007 was released by MAIB as an Accident Flyer. Another hazardous incident happened by unloading a maize cargo in 2012 without any serious injuries was released by MAIB as a Marine incident report 21/2013 (MAIB, 2013; http://www.maib.gov.uk/publications/index.cfm).

The majority of reported cases are bulk transport of foodstuffs like grain, flour etc., and nearly all of these are treated with aluminium or magnesium phosphide in solid form. The phosphide then reacts with water (as moisture in the air or in the cargo) and releases phosphine (PH_3) gas as the active pesticide. A unique feature of this way of administrating the fumigant is that the moisture/water may be a limiting factor and cause the reaction to stop, leaving solid phosphide in the cargo. When it arrives at the destination and the holds are opened, replenishment with ambient, moist air may restart the reaction liberating phosphine gas.

Summary of incidents

A brief summary of the incidents with fumigated containers and bulk cargo ships that have implied health effects on humans are shown in Tables 4 and 5, respectively (see also Table in Additional file 2 for more detailed list of incidences). The majority of cases consist of dock workers and seafarers. However, the incidents with bulk cargo ships also include some stowaways. The Tables show the reported incidents with approximate location, date, number of affected subjects, the number of fatalities and the sources of information.

Concluding remarks

Both incidents with fumigated containers and bulk cargo ships are scarcely reported in the scientific literature. However, based on the literature survey and the reports referenced above it might seem as if there is a difference with regard to the severity of outcomes in the two cases: So far, there has been only limited reports of fatalities in relation to opening of transport containers (Table 4 and Additional file 2), while fumigation of bulk cargo ships has led to several fatalities, including several stowaways (Table 5). A possible explanation may be that the exposure on a bulk cargo ship may be of considerable longer duration, and that it is more difficult to escape. In addition, the fumigants may be present in the living compartments on the ship without recognised until the exposure has become fatal.

It is important to emphasise that the numbers of incidents reported in Tables 4 and 5 (and the Table in Additional file 2) may be highly underestimated since input from several representatives from both research institutions and national regulatory bodies suggest that a lot of near-accidents and intoxications with serious outcomes are never reported in public. This view was also supported by several presentations and participants at the Berlin workshop in May 22-23rd, 2014 (http://www.eomsociety.org/index.php/meetings).

The literature surveys add to this and illustrate one of the major challenges pursuing this field: providing adequate and sufficient documentation of incidents relating to fumigated transport containers including adverse health effects, clinical symptoms, and well documented exposure data, and to make these data public available in well-respected sources.

Regulations on fumigants

Contemporary trans-continental shipping of consumer goods largely uses tropical softwood to manufacture short-lived or disposable shipping boxes and pallets (wood packaging materials). These items can easily host and transport tropical parasites to other geographical areas, where these foreign organisms often thrive in the absence of their natural predators, and can exert considerable damage to endemic flora, wild animals, cultivated crops and reared animals in temperate areas. This phenomenon is at least as old as the mid-1800 trade of European wine in wooden casks to Northern America. The scarcity of European cask-quality oak forced to manufacture wine casks in the USA, by using local varieties of oak, which carried to Western continental Europe their parasites, mainly *Phyloxera* and *Peronospera.* These foreign parasites quickly expanded in the continent, essentially wiping out most local vine varieties and leading to the treatment of the surviving vineyards with early pesticides, such as the copper-based Bordeaux mixture and later lead and copper arsenates.

The concern that such events may repeat led to discuss at the 6th Conference of the Food and Agriculture Organization of the United Nations (FAO), and to establish in 1952 an international agreement, the International

Table 4 Examples of reported incidents/intoxications with fumigants in transport containers (see Table in attachment for more detailed case reports)

Date	Location	Fumigant	No. of subjects		Reference/source
			Affected	Fatalities	
Nov. 2008 2008 - 2006	-	PH_3	1	0	Case reports [28] (PubMed)
	-	PH_3?	1	0	
	Warehouse, Germany	1,2-dichloroethane	2	0	
2006	Rotterdam	CH_3Br	2	0	[39] (PubMed)
2008-2009	Rotterdam	1,2-dichloroethane	20	0	[40] (Google)
		PH_3	9	0	
		CO_2	2	0	
		CH_3Br	2	0	
2007-2008	The Netherlands	CH_3Br	2	0	[42] (Web of Science)

Table 5 Examples of reported incidents/intoxications with fumigants on bulk cargo ships

Date	Location	Fumigant	No. of subjects		Reference/source
			Affected	Fatalities	
September 1978	Bulk grain freighter, East coast Canada/USA	PH_3	31[1)]	2[1)]	[46] (PubMed)
1988-1996	Danish bulk carriers	PH_3	2	1[2)]	[45] (PubMed)
		Unknown pesticide	4	3[2)]	
October 2007	General cargo ship, Russia – UK	PH_3	1	1	MAIB Accident Flyer 1/2008
2010	General cargo ship, Latvia – Antwerp	PH_3	2	1	Gard News 204 Nov 2011/Jan 2012 http://www.gard.no/
2010	Bulk carrier US East coast	PH_3	16	0	
2009	General cargo ship, Lagos, Nigeria	PH_3	6[3)]	1[3)]	
2000	Bulk carrier US West coast	PH_3	12	0	
1997	Geared bulker Brazil – Ireland	PH_3	5	0	

[1)]2 children.
[2)]4 stowaways.
[3)]6 stowaways.
See Table in Additional file 2 for additional cases investigated in detail (Incidents with fumigants/or toxic industrial chemicals. Intoxication cases from 1993–2013).

Plant Protection Convention (IPPC), aiming to protect cultivated and wild plants by preventing the introduction and spread of pests. The number of signatory Countries is currently of 181, and the Food and Agriculture Organization of the UN provides the Secretariat of the IPPC. The International Standards for Phytosanitary Measures (ISPMs) are recognized by the World Trade Organization (WTO) for managing pest risks associated with trade, and cover the movement of pests and apply to vehicles, ships, aircraft, containers, storage places, soil, wood packaging and other objects that could harbour plant pests. More than 50 ISPMs, as of 2012, cover issues such as plant quarantine and international trade; pest risk analysis; pest free areas; wood packaging material in international trade; and inspection protocols. Among the technical interventions to counter the spread of pests is the preventive treatment of goods and materials by thermal, irradiation and chemical means. The treatment of materials and goods with volatile chemical agents is referred to as fumigation.

The major fumigant that is subject to regulations at national or to regulated agreements at the international level is methyl bromide. This low-boiling liquid has been used since the late 1930s to protect from spoilage grains shipped in the trans-oceanic routes, as well as in storage silos and in processing facilities, such as in wheat mills, and as a pesticide for greenhouses and for the tilled land. In the late 1980s, it was found that the far-UV absorbing layer of ozone in the upper stratosphere of Antarctica was rapidly vanishing, and therefore the narrowing of the ozone layer in the upper atmosphere above the planetary boundary layer would increase the intensity of carcinogenic far-UV radiation on the Earth and thus have significant deleterious effects on human health. Along with several other synthetic chemicals, such as chloro-fluoro-carbons (CFCs) that were widely used in several fields of technology and of everyday life in consumer products, methyl bromide was identified as an ozone layer-depleting substance. Anticipated by talks and negotiations that started in 1981, a convention was agreed within the UN as early as 1985 to gradually limit, substitute and ban such substances from industrial uses. The Vienna Convention for the Protection of the Ozone Layer is the first treaty ever to achieve universal participation by 1988, and is often called a framework convention, because it served as a framework for efforts to protect the globe's ozone layer. This Convention paved the way to the later Montreal Protocol on Substances that Deplete the Ozone Layer, which was agreed on September 16, 1987, and entered into force on January 1, 1989. The Montreal Protocol includes a unique mechanism that enables to respond quickly to new scientific information and to accelerate the reductions required on chemicals that are already covered by the Protocol, since these adjustments are then automatically applicable to all countries that ratified the Protocol. Central to the Montreal Protocol is the definition of lists of chemical substances that are recognized to have ozone-depleting characteristics and of programs to phase-out their production and use.

In particular, for methyl bromide there was a need to balance the consequences of two equally binding international treaties, each of which addresses a crucial issue of planet stewardship. Therefore, for methyl bromide a specific exemption was authorized for the amounts used for quarantine and pre-shipment applications (Article 2H: Methyl bromide; para. 6) and a specific identification of the substance in the treaty was provided (Annex E). In addition, the original agreement of the Montreal Protocol allowed a large group of 147 developing countries (Article 5(1) Parties) a slower path to reduction of production, of use and to final ban of several of the controlled substances. The phase-out agreement is articulated into three steps: the first one defining a base level of production, the second a freeze of production at the base level amounts, the third a stepwise gradual reduction in the amounts used, to finally reach 100 per cent reduction of use or its effective cease at a specified date. All uses of methyl bromide by all countries should cease by January 1, 2015. The phase-out schedules of the original agreement and of that following the Adjustments agreed in 1999 in Beijing at the Eleventh Meeting of the Parties are reported in the Tables below (see Tables 6 and 7), as taken from the official UNEP Ozone Secretariat website (http://ozone.unep.org/en/).

Other major authorized fumigants are phosphine and phosphine-generating chemicals (metal phosphides) and sulphuryl difluoride. To protect the health of workers at all steps of the maritime logistic chain, a number of bodies at the international and national levels have issued regulations that cover a number of different issues, including the use of hazardous chemicals, such as pesticides and fumigants.

The framework international agreement is the United Nations IMO Safety of Life at Sea (SOLAS) Convention that stems from the first, never enacted agreement of 1914. It was only as late as 1960 that the long sought for UN International Maritime Organization started to develop and maintain a comprehensive regulatory framework for shipping that includes maritime security, safety and environmental concerns, enacting obligation on all Governments to ensure all activities on ships showing their flag are carried out safely. The SOLAS Convention specifically deals with shipping of hazardous items in two of its Chapters, VII and IX. Chapter VII – Carriage of dangerous goods requires that transport of all kinds of dangerous goods comply with the International Maritime Dangerous Goods Code (IMDG Code). Chapter IX - Management for the Safe Operation of Ships, establishes as mandatory the International Safety Management (ISM) Code, which in turn requires the ship owner to establish a safety management system and to empower the ship's Master to maintain the security of the ship without constraints by the Company, the charterer or any other person.

The IMO further issued several Codes and Recommendations aimed at specific issues. The IMO IMDG Code is the international guideline for the safe transportation or shipment of dangerous goods or hazardous materials by water and is aimed at protecting crewmembers and at preventing marine pollution when hazardous materials are transported on water vessels. The IMO Recommendations on the Safe Use of Pesticides in Ships (revised 2002) is a guide to all those involved in the use of pesticides and fumigants on ships and to governments to comply with their legal obligations under the SOLAS Convention. The IMO last issued a Revised Recommendation On The Safe Use Of Pesticides In Ships Applicable To The Fumigation Of Cargo Transport Units (MSC.1/Circ.1361 27 May 2010) where a number of active substances, still including methyl bromide and its mixture with carbon dioxide, are listed.

The International Maritime Fumigation Organisation (IMFO) is a private non-profit organization to which companies, which provide maritime fumigation services freely adhere. It was constituted with the objective of enabling member companies to provide levels of treatment in accordance to the Code and the Recommendations. IMFO issued a Code of Practice (COP) as a guidance to fumigators and ships' masters in respect of bagged and bulk cargoes, packaged goods (at: http://www.imfo.com; www.imfo.com/IMFO_Code_of_Practice.pdf). The COP recognizes in its Introduction that phosphine is the only fumigant that can be used during shipping, and provides fumigators with specific instructions, labelling and checklists.

Own requirements of individual countries

Most countries directly require all vessels in their territorial waters to comply with the IMO recommendations. The US and the Canadian Coastguards issue their own regulations and specifications (*e.g.*, for Canada: https://www.tc.gc.ca/eng/marinesafety/bulletins-1997-06-eng.htm) and the European Union has issued regulations for the Fumigation of packaged goods only (freight container fumigation) under Regulation CE 1107/2009 and Directives 2008/40/EC, 2006/39/EC e 2003/68/EC.

Preventive measures

Lessons must be learned from the presented studies, especially since the fumigants are often colourless and odourless, and dangerous even at low concentrations. Since no reliable indication of the absence of toxic gases in closed import containers exist, each container has to be regarded as potentially hazardous. Therefore, such import containers should be entered only if hazardous airborne exposures are excluded, i.e. only after appropriate measurement of air samples or after appropriate aeration, where forced extraction ventilation was shown to be most effective (which necessitates some redesign of containers, e.g. by a hole in the back for applying the extraction pipe). Forced ventilation rapidly reduces toxic concentrations in the container atmosphere; however off gassing within the following hours or days from the goods, which may have absorbed toxic substances, have to be taken into consideration. Thus ventilation should be on-going in initially contaminated containers during stripping due to such off-gassing from goods.

Measuring gases has to be extended from fumigation to include volatile toxic industrial chemicals arising from the production processes. However, it is important to

Table 6 Summary of control measures under the Montreal Protocol - Annex E - Group I: Methyl bromide

Non-Article 5(1) Parties		*Article 5(1) Parties (developing countries)*	
Base level:	1991	Base level:	Average of 1995-98
Freeze:	January 1, 1995.	Freeze:	January 1, 2002.
25 per cent: reduction	January 1, 1999.	20 per cent: reduction	January 1, 2005.
50 per cent: reduction	January 1, 2001.	100 per cent: reduction	January 1, 2015 (with possible critical use exemptions).
70 per cent: reduction	January 1, 2003.		
100 per cent: reduction	January 1, 2005 (with possible critical use exemptions).		

Applicable to production and consumption, amounts used for quarantine and pre-shipment applications exempted.

measure not only directly behind the container door (where concentrations may be low due to leakages), but rather to assess the levels deep inside at the bottom, middle, and top of the container. A new flat lancet facilitates this procedure.

It is difficult to measure all possible toxic substances in the container atmosphere; especially formaldehyde and phosphine are not adequately analysed by many devices. So far, no ideal portable non-expensive device is on the market.

More effectively, alternatives for fumigation (such as heat treatment, use of oxygen-depleted air) should be promoted and introduced and toxic industrial chemicals replaced by harmless substances.

The many still existing knowledge gaps, e.g. potentially structural modifications of food by fumigants and health risks for consumers, have to be taken into consideration by future research projects.

The previously mentioned severe and broad health hazards demonstrate an urgent need of common databases, which comprise all health relevant data of each container from the production site, along the transport line, till the end-user. Due to the globalized economy this has to done on national as well as supra-national scales, providing authorities as well as recipients/audience full access to them.

The first comprehensive preventive measures system – which can be considered to be a "State of the art model" – has been implemented in the harbor of Hamburg. The existing risk assessment system is a part of the daily routine to protect the controlling bodies from incidents associated with all kinds of terrorist or criminal threats in the container air and freight. The concept was developed during 2006 till 2010 on the basis of on-site experiences in cooperation with the Institute of Occupational and Maritime Medicine (ZfAM) and the State labor inspection office (Health & Safety Executive Hamburg). It contains a catalog of the minimal requirements for inspections, analyses and an evaluation system. If a potentially toxic gas group (comprising structurally related compounds) is identified by a screening measuring device, additional mandatory analytical toxicological measurements in a specialized analytical laboratory are required [31].

Applied preventive measures

Appropriate preventive measures for safe handling and stripping of freight containers rely on several factors such as correct labeling, knowledge and awareness among managers and workers, guidelines for safe procedures, measurements, ventilation and personal protective devices.

Labelling

The first step for taking preventive action is based on the identification of containers with hazardous content. Although labeling is mandatory with warning signs accompanied with transportation documents specifying

Table 7 Allowance for production to meet the basic domestic needs of Article 5(1) Parties following the Beijing Adjustments

Non-Article 5(1) Parties		*Article 5(1) Parties*
Base level:	Production in 1991.	No additional production allowed for basic domestic needs.
January 1, 1995	10 per cent of base level until July 28, 2000.	
New base level for basic domestic needs (effective July 28, 2000)	Annual average production for basic domestic needs of Article 5(1) Parties for the period 1995 to 1998 inclusive.	
July 28, 2000	15 per cent of base level until January 1, 2002.	
January 1, 2002	100 per cent of base level.	
January 1, 2005	80 per cent of new base level.	
January 1, 2015	Zero.	

Annex E - Group I: Methyl bromide.

the fumigation procedures for fumigated containers, several articles and reports between the years 2002 to 2011 have described violations of these regulations. In a study from Rotterdam [46] only three of 303 randomly selected containers had some kind of warning sticker, although methyl bromide or phosphine were detected in 23% of the containers. In Hamburg in 2006 only 3.6% of the 2113 examined containers carried any form of fumigation hazard warning, but none of these corresponded to those required by the IMDG Code and they mostly consisted of fragments of old, presumably outdated, warning [1]. Residual fumigants were detected in a total of 541 (26%) the containers. None of the containers had valid Dangerous Goods Transport Documentation. Safe Work in Australia found that none of 76 surveyed containers displayed any external notice that they had been fumigated, although methyl bromide was identified in 68% of them [25]. In Gothenburg none of the 101 randomly selected containers were labeled [47] http://ki.se/sites/default/files/2011-1_0.pdf They argued that lack in compliance with the labeling regulations raises serious concerns as warning sign is the first, and perhaps only, message the worker receives that suggests the container atmosphere to be hazardous. A Danish study concluded that in practice, the measures applied to prevent harmful chemical exposures released from transport containers are primarily based on the attempt to identify the containers that carry occupational health risks [48]. Discussions with managers and workers in an Australian study suggested that no systematic assessment of containers took place prior to entry by workers [25]).

Knowledge and awareness

The employers are obliged to inform the workers on all hazards in their work environment and provide adequate training in health and safety at work. The practice of handling containers was recently investigated in a qualitative study in Denmark based on semi-structured interviews with nine key informants, including managers and health and safety representatives of organizations that handle containers [48]; (for details see chapter IV. Practice of handling transport containers in exporting and receiving countries. Pilot studies in China and Denmark). They concluded that there was limited knowledge among managers, workers and even among occupational health professions about the types of chemicals that can be released from containers.

In Australia informal discussions were held with five experienced managers and 15 workers [25]. Also in this study the numbers of workers who completed the surveys was low, and the authors argued that the results should not be used to make generalizations for broader industry or occupational groups. However, about 70% of the workers had completed specific work health and safety training on unpacking shipping containers. None of them knew much about the risks of fumes in containers but 67% knew a little. The most significant reason for not taking safety precautions was lack of training (33%), followed by lack of awareness that the container atmosphere may contain chemical fumes (29%). Thus, although most workers had received work health and safety training there was still a large degree of uncertainty regarding the risks associated with fumigated containers and their ability to identify such containers.

Guidelines for safe procedures

In addition to the international and national regulations related to container handling there are also local safety instructions from organizations and from employers (e.g. [48-52]).

In the Danish study the interviewed managers were aware of the existence of relevant international and national regulations but were typically not able to specify them [48]. The interviewees were more familiar with the local instructions but these were reported to give insufficient guidance for several practical challenges of preventing chemical exposures during work with containers.

Measurements

At present there is no single portable instrument available to detect all types of relevant hazardous substances at sufficient sensitivity. However, different approaches, including direct-reading devices and air sampling for later analysis have been used to detect selections of fumigants and toxic gases in various harbors.

The commercial company EWS in Belgium dealing with fumigation suggested that for ad hoc situations handhold technology could be used. Examples of those technologies are [50]:

- Photo ionization detector (PID) for volatile organic compounds (VOC)
- Infrared (spectra) only for sulfuryl difluoride
- Sensors (CO, CO_2, O_2, PH_3)
- Colorimetrical gas detector or indicator tubes, mainly for methyl bromide + 1,2-dichloroethane, benzene, toluene, chloropicrin, styrene, xylene.

Further, measurements for oxygen depletion are recommended.

Onsite measurements/samples from unopened containers should preferably be taken at the middle or top of the container and not only at the bottom of the door where concentrations are lowest [51]. The openings in the top corners of the containers and possible leaking rubber seals around the doors may explain the observation of uneven concentrations in the container. Recently a new flat lancet was developed to facilitate onsite measurements from unopened containers. The lancet was further connected to a direct-reading instrument with detectors for VOCs, formaldehyde, hydrogen cyanide, phosphine and carbon monoxide [51].

In Hamburg, measurements were performed onsite with a gas detector array instrument (GDA, Airsense) by sampling through the online probe inserted into the container. After the measurements with the hand held instrument, special 1 liter air bags were filled with the air of the containers. The air bags were transported to the laboratory for analysis with gas chromatography–mass spectrometry (GC-MS), which requires a well-equipped lab and a well-trained lab technician; in addition, it is time-consuming [5,19,52,53].

Svedberg & Johanson [47] described that on arrival to Sweden, the fumigated and labeled containers are normally handled as all other containers, except when the Swedish Food Agency has border control campaigns during which about 20 containers per year are controlled by measurements. They also reported that as far as they knew most of the central stores and end costumers in Sweden do not have systems to control and handle potentially fumigated/gassed containers, although good examples exist. One large storehouse had a Fourier Transform Infrared–instrument in the central unit. However, they claimed that it is not realistic to require every costumer handling containers, small-sized terminals in particular, to have expensive measurement instruments, but rather rely on sufficient ventilation before entry.

Based on interviews with nine key informants in the Danish study, equipment for monitoring of container air is available in some of the selected organizations only, and even when available, the measuring device can detect only methyl bromide but no other potentially harmful chemicals [48]. In some of these organizations a suspicion is sufficient for applying specific preventive measures while others would require positive results of air measurements to take action.

Ventilation

The container should be efficiently ventilated before opening when high concentrations of harmful substances have been detected or when measurements have not been done.

Containers normally have small openings in the top corners to provide limited natural ventilation. Svedberg & Johanson [47] evaluated different ventilation methods by tracer gas, and reported that natural ventilation (open doors) and blowing ventilation (open doors, fan blowing air towards goods) had virtually no impact on gas levels in deep container air 12 m from the doors. In contrast, forced extraction ventilation (fan sucking air via a tube inserted all the way into the container and fresh air entering via the doors) resulted in rapid washout of the gas. They concluded that unfortunately the current container design makes safe and speedy sampling and ventilation prior to opening the doors technically difficult. Ventilation must preferably be ongoing during stripping, and a ventilated container that is closed for stripping the following day must be re-ventilated.

In the Australian study [25] the containers were often left to ventilate naturally. The also concluded that for those containers with known high levels of fumigants, natural ventilation may require supplementation with forced ventilation to reduce the concentrations of residual chemicals to acceptable levels for unloading. Industry representatives expressed concern that ventilation systems for extracting fumigants from containers were not effective because the levels of fumigants within containers simply rose again after termination of ventilation and close up of the containers. Thus, it may be useful to set a time limit (e.g. 2 hours) after which unloading should be stopped and the container would have to be ventilated again.

The workers that performed stripping of containers in the Swedish study expressed that the containers frequently carried unpleasant odors that from time-to-time prevented stripping. Such containers were left for natural ventilation before re-entry [47].

The interviewed personnel in the Danish study reported that the main preventive measure to reduce chemical exposure is natural ventilation; active ventilation is not used in practice [48]. The conditions of aeration were not consistently applied; the reported ventilation times varied between 2 and 48 hours without any knowledge of whether this amount of time was sufficient or not.

Personal protective equipment

In published articles and reports the use of PPE during container stripping has only been briefly mentioned, and it has not been described which type of protective mask or other PPE that have been used. The types of required PPE differ from one toxicant to another and it is emphasized that the correct PPE should be used. In addition, rescue strategies should be available to individuals who need to enter unventilated containers with unknown hazards [47,31].

In the Australian study one-third reported use of PPE, but they did not specify which kind of PPE they used [54]. Knol-de Vos [46] noted that staff wore personal PPE when opening containers in Rotterdam. Pedersen et al. [48] reported that although masks are usually provided to the workers in Denmark, they are mainly dust masks that do not prevent exposure to gaseous chemicals. The also described that the decision and choice of preventive measures to be used in practice are often left to the directly involved employees and the actions taken show considerable variation. When the workers in Sweden experienced unpleasant odors, the containers were left for natural ventilation, or, alternatively, the workers were instructed to wear respiratory equipment [47].

WorkSafe [54] summarizes that consistent with the risk assessment for containers with methyl bromide mixtures, PPE considerations could include:

- Elbow length chemical gloves;
- Full coveralls;
- Full face mask equipped with:
  - multi-gas filters; or
  - an organic vapor cartridge filter, that is designed to cover methyl bromide and chloropicrin
  - mixed gas (filter type will depend upon the brand & type of full face mask that you purchase); or
- Self-Contained Breathing Apparatus (SCBA).

It is important to ensure regular training and instruction about the procedures and the maintenance and use of PPE to ensure that staffs are competent in its use. Records of this training should be maintained.

Competing interests
The authors declare that they have no competing interests.

Authors' contributions
Study design and literature review: XB, LTB, ZZ, MB, RD, LV, FMR, CC, JRJ); LV overview of Health effects of fumigants; XB, LTB diagnostic methods and analyses; ZZ, JRJ pilot studies in Denmark and China; MB, RD overview on accidents with fumigants; FMR, CC regulations on fumigants; XB, JRJ manuscript draft version; XB, LTB final version of the manuscript; all authors accepted the final manuscript version submitted.

Acknowledgments
Die authors would like to thank Dr. Preisser, Dr. Heblich and Dr. Kloth from the Institute for Occupational and Maritime Medicine (ZfAM), University Medical Center Hamburg-Eppendorf for the support with the data extraction of the intoxication case reports in the attachment.
This study is a part of a WHO CC collaborative global cross-sectional project between the Transport group (lead by Prof. Dr. Lygia T Budnik) and the Agricultural group (lead by Prof. Dr. Claudio Colosio).

Author details
[1]European Society for Environmental and Occupational Medicine (EOM), Berlin, Germany. [2]Institute for Occupational Medicine, Charité University Medicine, Charité-Campus Benjamin Franklin, Berlin, Germany. [3]Institute for Occupational and Maritime (ZfAM), University Medical Center Hamburg-Eppendorf, Division Occupational Toxicology and Immunology, University of Hamburg, Hamburg, Germany. [4]Dalian Maritime University (DMU), Dalian, Ganjingzi, China. [5]Department of Occupational Medicine, Haukeland University Hospital, Bergen, Norway. [6]Occupational and Environmental Medicine, University of Bergen, Bergen, Norway. [7]Department of Global Public Health and Primary Care, Occupational and Environmental Medicine, University of Bergen, Bergen, Norway. [8]Norwegian Center for Maritime Medicine, Department of Occupational Medicine, Haukeland University Hospital, Bergen, Norway. [9]Expertise Centre Environmental Medicine (ECEMed), Rijnstate Teaching Hospital, AA Velp, the Netherlands. [10]Department of Health Sciences of the University of Milano and International Centre of Rural Health, San Paolo University Hospital Milano, Milan, Italy. [11]Centre of Maritime Health and Society, Institute of Public Health, University of Southern Denmark, Odense, Denmark.

References

1. Baur X, Poschadel B, Budnik LT. High frequency of fumigants and other toxic gases in imported freight containers–an underestimated occupational and community health risk. Occup Environ Med. 2010;67(3):207–12. doi:10.1136/oem.2008.043893.
2. Verschoor AH, van Leeuwen HJ, Verschoor L. Gibt es Gefaehrdungen der Verbraucher durch Begasungsmittelrueckstaende? Zentralblatt Arbeitsmedizin. 2012;62:44–5.
3. Baur X, Budnik LT, Preisser AM. Health risks of residual fumigants in international transport containers. Dtsch Med Wochenschr. 2010;135(11):516–21. doi:10.1055/s-0030-1249198.
4. Shadnia S, Mehrpour O, Soltaninejad KA. A simplified acute physiology score in the prediction of acute aluminium phosphide poisoning outcome. Ind J Med Sci [serial online]. 2010;64:532–9. Available from: http://www.indianjmedsci.org/article.asp?issn=0019-5359;year=2010;volume=64;issue=12;spage=532;epage=539;aulast=Shadnia.
5. Fahrenholtz S, Huhnerfuss H, Baur X, Budnik LT. Determination of phosphine and other fumigants in air samples by thermal desorption and 2D heart-cutting gas chromatography with synchronous SIM/Scan mass spectrometry and flame photometric detection. J Chromatogr A. 2010;1217(52):8298–307. doi:10.1016/j.chroma.2010.10.085.
6. Proudfoot AT. Aluminium and zinc phosphide poisoning. Clin Toxicol. 2009;47(2):89–100. doi:10.1080/15563650802520675.
7. Anand R, Binukumar BK, Gill KD. Aluminum phosphide poisoning: an unsolved riddle. J Appl Toxicol. 2011;31(6):499–505. doi:10.1002/jat.1692.
8. Chugh SN, Aggarwal HK, Mahajan SK, Chugh SN, Aggarwal HK, Mahajan SK. Zincphosphide intoxication symptoms: analysis of 20 cases. Int J Clin Pharmacol Ther. 1998;36:406–7.
9. Verschoor AH, van Leeuwen HJ, Verschoor L. Hydrogen phosphide intoxication. Zentralblatt Arbeitsmedizin. 2011;61:424–5.
10. Budnik LT, Kloth S, Velasco-Garrido M, Baur X. Prostate cancer and toxicity from critical use exemptions of methyl bromide: environmental protection helps protect against human health risks. Environ Heal. 2012;11:5. doi:10.1186/1476-069X-11-5.
11. Alexeeff GV, Kilgore WW. Methyl bromide. Residue Rev. 1983;88:101–53. 1983;88:101–53.
12. Calvert GM, Mueller CA, Fajen JM, Chrislip DW, Russo J, Briggle T, et al. Health effects associated with sulfuryl fluoride and methyl bromide exposure among structural fumigation workers. Am J Public Health. 1998;88(12):1774–80.
13. Reidy TJ, Bolter JF, Cone JE. Neuropsychological sequelae of methyl bromide: a case study. Brain Inj. 1994;8(1):83–93.
14. Brautbar N, Williams 2nd J. Industrial solvents and liver toxicity: risk assessment, risk factors and mechanisms. Int J Hyg Environ Health. 2002;205(6):479–91. doi:10.1078/1438-4639-00175.
15. Cogliano VJ, Grosse Y, Baan RA, Straif K, Secretan MB, El Ghissassi F, et al. Meeting report: summary of IARC monographs on formaldehyde, 2-butoxyethanol, and 1-tert-butoxy-2-propanol. Environ Health Perspect. 2005;113(9):1205–8.
16. Humans IWGotEoCRt. Chemical agents and related occupations. IARC monographs on the evaluation of carcinogenic risks to humans/World Health Organization, International Agency for Research on Cancer. 2012;100(Pt F):9–562.
17. Balzan MV, Agius G, Galea DA. Carbon monoxide poisoning: easy to treat but difficult to recognise. Postgrad Med J. 1996;72(850):470–3.
18. Langford NJ. Carbon dioxide poisoning. Toxicol Rev. 2005;24(4):229–35.
19. Budnik LT, Fahrenholtz S, Kloth S, Baur X. Halogenated hydrocarbon pesticides and other volatile organic contaminants provide analytical challenges in global trading. J Environ Monit. 2010;12(4):936–42. doi:10.1039/b918428g.
20. van Valen E, van Thriel C, Akila R, Nilson LN, Bast-Pettersen R, Sainio M, et al. Chronic solvent-induced encephalopathy: European consensus of

neuropsychological characteristics, assessment, and guidelines for diagnostics. Neurotoxicology. 2012;33(4):710–26. doi:10.1016/j.neuro.2012.03.010.
21. Preller L, Burstyn I, De Pater N, Kromhout H. Characteristics of peaks of inhalation exposure to organic solvents. Ann Occup Hyg. 2004;48(7):643–52. doi:10.1093/annhyg/meh045.
22. Lan Q, Zhang L, Li G, Vermeulen R, Weinberg RS, Dosemeci M, et al. Hematotoxicity in workers exposed to low levels of benzene. Science. 2004;306(5702):1774–6. doi:10.1126/science.1102443.
23. Vlaanderen J, Portengen L, Rothman N, Lan Q, Kromhout H, Vermeulen R. Flexible meta-regression to assess the shape of the benzene-leukemia exposure-response curve. Environ Health Perspect. 2010;118(4):526–32. doi:10.1289/ehp.0901127.
24. Thomas R, Hubbard AE, McHale CM, Zhang L, Rappaport SM, Lan Q, et al. Characterization of changes in gene expression and biochemical pathways at low levels of benzene exposure. PLoS One. 2014;9(5):e91828. doi:10.1371/journal.pone.0091828.
25. Safe-work-Australia Questionnaire. http://www.safeworkaustralia.gov.au/sites/swa/about/publications/pages/hazard-surveillance-residual-chemicals-in-shipping-containers.pdf.
26. FumEx2 Questionnaire. http://eomsociety.org/attachments/FUM-EX%202_%20QUESTIONNAIRE_EOM%20ENGLISH%20VERSION.pdf F-EFEQ.
27. Budnik LT, Kloth S, Baur X, Preisser AM, Schwarzenbach H. Circulating mitochondrial DNA as biomarker linking environmental chemical exposure to early preclinical lesions elevation of mtDNA in human serum after exposure to carcinogenic halo-alkane-based pesticides. PLoS One. 2013;8(5):e64413. doi:10.1371/journal.pone.0064413.
28. Preisser AM, Budnik LT, Baur X. Health effects due to fumigated freight containers and goods: how to detect, how to act. Int Marit Health. 2012;63(3):133–9.
29. Preisser AM, Budnik LT, Hampel E, Baur X. Surprises perilous: toxic health hazards for employees unloading fumigated shipping containers. Sci Total Environ. 2011;409(17):3106–13. doi:10.1016/j.scitotenv.2011.04.053.
30. Kloth S, Baur X, Goen T, Budnik LT. Accidental exposure to gas emissions from transit goods treated for pest control. Environ Health. 2015;14:110. doi:10.1186/1476-069X-13-110.
31. Baur X, Horneland AM, Fischer A, Stahlmann R, Budnik LT. How to handle import containers safely. Int Marit Health. 2014;65(3):142–57. doi:10.5603/IMH.2014.0029.
32. Sudakin DL. Occupational exposure to aluminium phosphide and phosphine gas? A suspected case report and review of the literature. Hum Exp Toxicol. 2005;24(1):27–33.
33. Alavanja MC, Bonner MR. Occupational pesticide exposures and cancer risk: a review. J Toxicol Environ Health B Crit Rev. 2012;15(4):238–63. doi:10.1080/10937404.2012.632358.
34. Oriel M, Edmiston S, Beauvais S, Barry T, O'Malley M. Illnesses associated with chloropicrin use in California agriculture, 1992–2003. Rev Environ Contam Toxicol. 2009;200:1–31. doi:10.1007/978-1-4419-0028-9_1.
35. Burgess JL, Morrissey B, Keifer MC, Robertson WO. Fumigant-related illnesses: Washington State's five-year experience. Clin Toxicol. 2000;38(1):7–14.
36. Lee SJ, Mehler L, Beckman J, Diebolt-Brown B, Prado J, Lackovic M, et al. Acute pesticide illnesses associated with off-target pesticide drift from agricultural applications: 11 States, 1998–2006. Environ Health Perspect. 2011;119(8):1162–9. doi:10.1289/ehp.1002843.
37. Yamano Y, Nakadate T. Three occupationally exposed cases of severe methyl bromide poisoning: accident caused by a gas leak during the fumigation of a folklore museum. J Occup Health. 2006;48(2):129–33.
38. Lemoine TJ, Schoolman K, Jackman G, Vernon DD. Unintentional fatal phosphine gas poisoning of a family. Pediatr Emerg Care. 2011;27(9):869–71. doi:10.1097/PEC.0b013e3182348e40.
39. Breeman W. Methylbromide intoxication: a clinical case study. Adv Emerg Nurs J. 2009;31(2):153–60. doi:10.1097/TME.0b013e31819dca1b.
40. Verschoor AH, van Leeuwen HJ, Verschoor L. Health problems in handling gassed containers. Zbl Arbeitsmed. 2010;60:246–7.
41. Lodde B, Lucas D, Letort JM, Jegaden D, Pougnet R, Dewitte JD. Acute phosphine poisoning on board a bulk carrier: analysis of factors leading to a fatal case. J Occup Med Toxicol. 2015;10:10. doi:10.1186/s12995-015-0050-0.
42. Spijkerboer H, de Vries I, Meulenbelt J. Use of fumigants in sea containers can lead to serious human poisonings. Toxicol Lett. 2008;180S:S139–40.
43. Brodniewicz A. Poisoning of seamen with methyl bromide due to fumigation of a Polish cargo ship in Haiphong (Vietnam). Arh Hig Rada Toksikol. 1967;18:19–24. http://www.ncbi.nlm.nih.gov/pubmed/6043110.
44. Wilson R, Lovejoy FH, Jaeger RJ, Landrigan PL. Acute phosphine poisoning aboard a grain freighter: epidemiologic, clinical, and pathological findings. JAMA. 1980;244(2):148–50.
45. Hansen HL, Pedersen G. Poisoning at sea: injuries caused by chemicals aboard Danish merchant ships 1988–1996. Clin Toxicol. 2001;39(1):21–6.
46. Knol-de Vos T. Measuring the amount of gas in import containers. 2002 http://rivm.openrepository.com/rivm/bitstream/10029/9020/1/609021025.pdf.
47. Svedberg U, Johanson G. Work inside ocean freight containers - personal exposure to off-gassing chemicals. Ann Occup Hyg. 2013;57(9):1128–37.
48. Pedersen R, Jepsen JR, Adam B. Regualtion and practice of workers' protection from chemical exposures during container handling. JOMT. 2014;9(1):33.
49. Boels DK, Fahrenholtz S, Baur X, Budnik LT. Anforderungen an die Messung und Begutachtung der Schadstoffbelastung in der Luft von Importcontainern. Zbl Arbeitsmed. 2010;60:130–6.
50. Lyts L. Security of import containers: Practical experiences at Benelux terminals. 2010. http://www.ews-fumigation.com/fileadmin/user_upload/docs/TGAV_conference_231110_workshop_Ludo_Luyts_EWS.pdf.
51. Johanson G, Svedberg U. Occurance and levels of VOCs in containers arriving in Sweden, including aspects of personal exposure, ventilation and sampling position. 2014. (see abstracts in attchment to reference [31]).
52. Baur X, Yu F, Poschadel B, Veldman W, Vos TK. Health risks by bromomethane and other toxic gases in import cargo ship containers. Int Marit Health. 2006;57(1–4):46–55.
53. Walte A, Münchmeier W, Lund, H. Onsite measurements of fumigated containers: possibilities and problems 2014. see abstracts in attchment to reference [31].
54. WorkSafe NT. Ventilation of Fumigated Freight Containers with Methyl Bromide Mixtures. http://www.worksafe.nt.gov.au/Bulletins/HealthAndSafetyTopics/Workplace%20Hazards/Forms/AllItems.aspx.

Anicteric hepatoxicity: a potential health risk of occupational exposures in Nigerian petroleum oil refining and distribution industry

Tobias I Ndubuisi Ezejiofor[1*], Anthonet N Ezejiofor[3], Orish E Orisakwe[3], Hariet C Nwigwe[1], Ferdinand OU Osuala[2] and Moses OE Iwuala[2]

Abstract

Background: Literature abounds linking one's job to certain unpalatable health outcomes. Since exposures to hazardous conditions in industrial environments often results in sundry health effects among workers, we embarked on this study to investigate the hepatic health effects of occupational activities in the petroleum refining and distribution industry.

Method: Biochemical markers of liver functions were assayed in plasma, using Reflotron dry chemistry spectrophotometric system. The study was conducted on randomly selected workers of Port Harcourt Refining Company (PHRC) and Pipelines and Petroleum Product Marketing Company (PPMC) both in Alesa-Eleme near Port Harcourt, Nigeria, as well as non-oil work civil servants serving as control subjects.

Result and conclusion: Results showed that, bilirubin ranged 0.3-1.6 mg/dl with a mean of 0.66±0.20mg/dl among the oil workers as against 0.5-1.00mg/dl with a mean of 0.58±0.13mg/dl in non-oil workers, Alkaline phosphatase ranged 50.00-296.00u/l (mean: 126.21±39.49u/l) in oil workers as against 40.20-111u/l (mean: 66.83±18.54u/l) for non-oil workers, Aspartic transaminases (AST) ranged 5.80-140.20u/l (mean: 21.81±11.49u/l) in oil workers against 18.00-44.00u/l (mean: 26.89±6.99u/l) for non-oil workers, while Alanine transaminases (ALT) ranged 4.90-86.00u/l (mean: 22.14±11.28u/l) in oil workers as against 10.00-86.60u/l (mean: 22.30±10.22u/l) for the non-oil workers. A close study of the results revealed that although the mean values for all the studied parameters were still within the parametric reference ranges, however, relative to the referents, there were significant increases ($P<0.05$) in plasma bilirubin (though anicteric) and alkaline phosphatase that was not matched with a corresponding increase in the plasma transaminases, suggesting a possibility that toxic anicteric hepatoxicity is part of the potential health effects of sundry exposures in the Nigeria petroleum oil refining and distribution industry. Gender differentiation data showed that though the mean values for the parameters were higher in males than females, the increases were not significant in most cases ($P>0.05$), whereas data for age and exposure period classifications revealed that irrespective of the age of the worker, the effects are likely to start after the first five years, manifesting fully after the first decade of occupational exposures. Thus, an update of industrial/occupational health measures is necessary for a safer and healthier work environment.

Keywords: Anicteric hepatoxicity, Occupational exposures, Petroleum refining and distribution industry, Nigeria

* Correspondence: tinezejiofor@gmail.com
[1]Department of Biotechnology, School of Science, Federal University of Technology, Owerri, Nigeria
Full list of author information is available at the end of the article

Background

Petroleum- components, ecological distribution and toxicological impacts

Petroleum consists of crude oils and a variety of refined oil products, and is also a significant source of polycyclic aromatic hydrocarbons (PAH) [1]. Pollution by petroleum hydrocarbons being widespread and frequent, can arise accidentally wherever oil is produced, transported, stored, processed, or used at sea or land. On land, petroleum products can account for a large proportion of the chemicals at contaminated sites [2]. Wilson and LeBlanc). Contamination of groundwater and soil by specific hydrocarbon compounds (e.g. benzene leaking from underground fuel storage tanks) has led many countries to enact regulatory requirements for action and cleanup of these compounds [3]. An estimated 2 to 3 million tons of petroleum hydrocarbons reach the world's seas and oceans each year [4]. Municipal and industrial wastes, urban and river runoff account for a significant proportion of petroleum products in fresh water systems and in the marine environments. Oil refineries discharge waste water containing some petroleum hydrocarbons. The receiving waters are therefore subject to low level chronic pollution [2]. Due to its complicated composition, petroleum has the potential to elicit multiple types of toxic effects. It can cause acute lethal toxicity, sub-lethal chronic toxicity, or both depending on the exposure, dosage, and organism exposed. Some PAH components of petroleum have the potential to bioaccumulate within susceptible aquatic organisms and be passed by trophic transfer to other levels of the food chain [5,6]. Petroleum can also affect living organisms by other means such as through physical oiling and through alterations in their habitat. When an oil spill occurs, toxicities are not limited to acute effects restricted to the immediate vicinity of the discharge. Due to dispersion, dilution and deposition of oil into the water column and onto shores and into sediments via weathering and other mechanisms, all organisms within the area may be exposed to petroleum hydrocarbon components for an extended period of time. Crude oil and many of its individual components have been reported to cause a variety of some lethal effects in a wide array of living organisms. Some of the most frequently observed long-term petroleum pollution on individual organisms include impaired reproduction [7], reduced growth [5], tumours and lesions [8]), blood disorders [9], and morphological abnormalities [10]. Female rats exposed to petroleum hydrocarbons showed evidence of nephrotoxic effects [11].

Petroleum refining and distribution industry: exposures and health implication

Petroleum refining and distribution are among the occupational activities perceived to be hazardous. Petroleum refining has evolved continuously in response to changing consumer demands for better and different products. Once extracted, crude oil is transported to an oil refinery where complex hydrocarbon compounds are separated and converted through various refining operations (fractional distillation, cracking, solvent extractions, then other treatments including formulating and blending) to become useable fuel sources. Finally, impurities are removed through chemical treatment of each product. The process of refining oil manufactures nearly 2,500 useful products [12]. The major end product of oil is gasoline, followed by diesel fuel, jet fuel, fuel oil, kerosene, lubricating oil and asphalt used for road paving. Apart from the products, oil refineries also contribute various forms of pollution including thermal and noise pollution. Thermal pollution involves the discharge of effluents that are significantly warmer than surrounding water, while noise level in refineries can exceed 90 decibels, posing a significant threat to the health and safety of oil refinery employees and even the surrounding community because leakage of noise pollution can have significant psychological effects on local residents, decreases aesthetics of the area and can interfere with wildlife [13].

Oil refinery workers are continuously exposed to numerous hazardous materials and working conditions that place them at continuous risk of injury and death. Such chronic hazards include exposure to noise, heat, polluted air, wide varieties of numerous hazardous chemical substances used either as process chemicals and/or present in resultant effluents/wastes, as well as in the usually invisible emissions, which include petroleum itself and other aromatic hydrocarbons (benzene, toluene, phenol, etc.), hydrogen sulphide and other natural gases (methane, propane, butane, etc.), carbon monoxide, asphalt, toxic heavy metals (arsenic, chromium, cadmium, nickel, zinc, etc.), coke dust, lead alkyls, silica, asbestos etc. [14,15]. Asphalt for example, can cause severe burns and eye irritation, and its fumes may contain unacceptable levels of benzene and hydrogen sulphide, which may lead to dermatitis, bronchitis and chemically induced pneumonia [16]. Continuous exposure to carbon monoxide can lead to headaches and mental disturbances, and at high concentrations may bring about death from asphyxiation. Long-term exposure to coke dust, silica and hydrogen sulphide can lead to chronic lung disease, while Lead alkyls used as gasoline additives can lead to psychosis and peripheral neuropathies. Asbestos, often used in oil refineries for the thermal insulation of boilers and pipes, has long been associated with pulmonary fibrosis, lung cancer and malignant mesothelioma among maintenance, repair and removal workers [16]. Even though the use of asbestos is banned in some countries, it is still widely used in many parts of the world. The use of asbestos in developing countries is a major problem as these nations often lack legislation regarding the use of asbestos, and the long-term health and safety of workers is often a low priority [12].

Oil refineries are inherently complex in their equipment and structural design that combined with the multitude of chemicals used, workers are at a continuous risk of accidents involving fires, explosions, chemical spills and burns as well as numerous health effects, many of which may remain latent even onto or post-retirement from active service. Accidental oil spills and leaks harm both workers and surrounding ecosystems because of exposure to petroleum and petroleum derivatives. Explosions and fire potentials stem from natural gases such as methane, propane, and butane produced at the refineries. Microscopic flaws in metal pipes fittings or fixtures in "hydro crackers" that operate at pressures ranging from 500 to 3200 pounds per square inch and temperatures ranging from 500 to 1800°f [14] can also lead to dangerous explosions. Accidental oil spills and leaks harm both workers and surrounding ecosystems because of exposure to petroleum and petroleum derivatives. Although oil spills most commonly occur during transport, leaking oil storage tanks and barrels contribute significantly to chemical and oil spills at refineries. Oil refineries and transport efforts account for approximately 46% of the estimated 3.2 million tons of oil entering the ocean each year [16]. The oil and oil waste products eventually find their way into the atmosphere, water column, bottom sediments and beaches. The resulting build-up of petroleum waste matter in an area has impact on surrounding biota and ecosystems [17].

Operational area facilities, activities and products: potential sources of hazards

Alesa-Eleme near Port Harcourt, Nigeria, West Africa, is the location of the main operational facilities of both PHRC and PPMC, and lies within latitude 4.7706° and longitude 7.1056°. Petroleum refining and distribution industry in Nigeria, as elsewhere, constitute a giant industry with many complicated systems. It consists of two refineries in one: the old Port Harcourt refinery (Area 5), and the New Port Harcourt Refinery (Areas 1- 4). Both refineries have combined installed capacity of 210,000bpsd [18]. The PHRC has five process areas, areas1-5 each of which houses several operational units such as the following: crude distillation unit (CDU), saturated gas concentration unit (SGCU), vacuum distillation unit (VDU)- area1; Naphtha hydrotreating unit (NHU), catalytic reforming unit (CRU) with continuous catalyst regeneration (CCR) section, kerosene hydrotreating unit (KHU)-area2; fluid catalytic cracking unit (FCCU), gas concentration unit (GCU), gas treating unit (GTU), merox unit- area3; dimersol units, HF alkylation unit, butamer unit- area4; crude distillation unit (CDU) crude reforming unit (CRU) and liquefied petroleum gas (LPG) plant- area5. Beside these, the refinery also has a power plant and utility (PPU) section equipped with boilers and other facilities that generates its power and other utilities, as well as a waste water treatment (WWT) section, which treats refinery waste water before being discharged to the neighbouring creek. These units or sections are named according to the nature of activities or work performed in them, and accordingly, they also constitute potential sources of exposures to the workers performing those activities, and particularly so when the facilities or parts thereof become defective and consequent outlets to misty and gaseous fumes of various process materials, products or wastes/effluents. The process of production and the actual products are both sophisticated. The major end product of oil is gasoline, followed by diesel fuel, jet fuel, fuel oil, kerosene, lubricating oil and asphalt used for road paving. PHRC processes crude oil (Bonny Light) into liquefied petroleum gas (LPG), Premium Motor Spirit (PMS), Dual purpose Kerosene (DPK) (Aviation and Domestic), Automotive Gas Oil (AGO– Diesel), Low Pour Fuel Oil (LPFO), and High Pour Fuel Oil (HPFO) as well as many other intermediate products that are industrially and domestically very useful. Through complex network of pipelines and storage tanks, these products of the refineries are passed over to the Pipelines and Petroleum Marketing Company (PPMC) for subsequent distribution. Behind all these facilities and their operations are workers, who are therefore, considered liable to certain health effects and/or impacts on account of several hazards from sundry job exposures in the various work units. Unraveling the actual nature and extent of these health effects/impacts is the main thrust of this study.

The knowledge that most human diseases and sufferings are sometimes related to the hazards of their workplace meant that appropriate remedies to the situation would come only when these hazards are properly assessed, their very nature, extent and impacts firmly established. Consequently, the need for toxicological data regarding industrial exposures and their health effects has been variously expressed by industrial stakeholders and researchers. However, for most of the industrial establishments in Nigeria particularly the numerous small and medium scale industries that form the bedrock of her industrial activities, and even some of the large scale industrial concerns (inclusive of the petroleum and petrochemical industry that is the mainstream of her economy), such occupational studies for proper assessment/establishment of the hazards are yet to be carried out. Thus, there is need for concerted effort towards providing some of the industrial exposures-health effects data called for by Loewenson [19], and particularly Scala [20] who had emphasized a three-fold need for toxicological data on the part of petroleum or petrochemical industry. In the Nigerian setting, available data regarding petroleum industry are based on studies using animal models, but non on humans, who for occupational reasons are subjected to long term, low-level continuous exposures to petroleum fractions, intermediates and finished products, as well as other hazardous conditions in their work environments, as is the case with petroleum refining and distribution industry workers. To the best of our knowledge, it is most uncertain that these workers have been directly investigated for any health effects or toxicological impacts of their occupational activities in the industry. Consequently, there is dearth of data regarding the nature and extent of health effects of sundry job exposures in this industry in Nigeria. Studies done elsewhere with regard to workers in the oil and gas industry had documented some organs/systems health effects, producing various morbidities and mortalities [21-32]. Although previous Nigerian studies have reported the effects of petroleum exposures in animal models that could possibly be extrapolated for humans [33-39], there is need for a direct human assessment of the situation using human biological samples. Results to be obtained from such direct human studies is expected to give a more assured situation with regards to human toxicology of petroleum products than an extrapolated result, which might be affected by species differences.

Meanwhile, risk assessment of petroleum refining and distribution industrial work environment revealed that the workers are furnished with sundry hazardous exposures [40], just as a study of some anthropometrical and biochemical markers also showed cardiovascular diseases and toxic nephropathy as part of diverse health hazards of this work cohorts [41,42]. Presently, the impacts of these exposures, particularly as it concerns the hepatic systemic effects remain uncertain in Nigeria, and thus forms the major focus of this study aimed at exploring the implications of workplace conditions and exposures to a wide range of potentially hepatotoxic substances present in emissions in the environment of petroleum refining and distribution industry. These include petroleum itself, benzene, dioxins, furans, other aromatic hydrocarbons (toluene, phenol, etc.), hydrogen sulphide and other natural gases (methane, propane, butane, etc.), carbon monoxide, asphalt, toxic heavy metals (arsenic, hexavalent chromium, cadmium, nickel, zinc, etc.) [14,15], all of which have deleterious effects on human body, and have also been recognized as carcinogens by the International Agency for Research on Cancer (IARC) [8]. In relation to their metabolic functions, the liver in humans, animal models or naturally exposed fauna, are target organs for several substances and metals (at least Cd or As), and accumulations of these beyond its metabolic detoxification capacity portend serious dangers to the hepatic health, and by extension, the overall health of the individual. Meanwhile, data from the plant clinic jointly used by the two establishments being studied revealed liver diseases as making reckonable contribution to the morbidities and mortalities recorded in this industry [43,44], suggesting that these diseases might be prevalent among the workers, and thus warranting further studies. Here lies the justification for the present evaluation of hepatic health risk among workers of this sector, using relevant biomarkers.

Objective of the study

This study hopes to contribute towards providing some of the necessary data called for by Loewenson [19] and in particular, Scala [20] who had emphasized a three-fold need for toxicological data on the part of petroleum or petrochemical industry. In the Nigerian setting, available data are based on studies using non-human animal species as can be gleaned from the studies cited above, but definitely non-existent for the humans who for occupational reasons are subjected to long term, low-level continuous exposures to petroleum fractions, intermediates and finished products, as well as other hazardous conditions in their work environments, as may be the case with petroleum refining and distribution industry workers. Although most toxicological studies conducted with respect to petroleum industry in the Nigerian environment had reported some biological effects of petroleum products on the animal models used, it is most uncertain that workers of this industrial sector have been directly investigated for any health effects or toxicological impacts of their occupational activities in the petroleum refining and distribution industry. Consequently, there is dearth of data regarding the nature and extent of health effects of occupational exposures in this industry in the Nigerian setting. This forms the scope of what this study seeks to address. Thus, the objective of the study is to evaluate these workers for possible health effects of occupational exposures in this industry, though with particular focus on the hepatic system, and to determine the role of gender, age and exposure period in defining any observed effect. Since our present attention is on the hepatic system, liver function markers would be assayed in the biological samples to be provided by the study participants. The outcome of this research would among other things:

1. clear the uncertainties about the dangers of occupational exposures in the petroleum refining and distribution industrial sector,
2. provide a firmer ground to sue (or not to sue) for health compensation for the retired/disengaged or estranged workers who may have already fallen victims of various organic ailments, particularly hepatic disease conditions, following several years of service in this sector, and
3. provide data-based evidence for update of industrial/occupational health measures aimed at improving health of workers and eventually their productivity

Materials and methods

Subjects

The participants of this study consisted of three hundred and thirty three (333) human subjects aged between 28 and 60 years old. Of this number, three hundred and three (303) study participants (273 males and 30 females) were randomly drawn from the staff of the two industrial establishments studied: Port Harcourt Refining Company Ltd (PHRC) (Petroleum refiners) and Pipelines and Petroleum Products Marketing Company (PPMC) (Petroleum distributors); the remaining 30 were non-oil sector civil servants considered healthy (20 males and 10 females) also randomly recruited to serve as referents or comparison group, and these were mainly classroom teachers in institutions of higher learning. The nature and purpose of the study was explained to the participants, following which they willingly consented to participation in the study.

Ethical clearance

Ethical Clearance was obtained from the Institutional Review Committee of the Department of Petroleum Resources (DPR), Federal Ministry of Petroleum Resources (the supervisory ministry). The nature and purpose of the study was explained to the management and staff of the establishments studied, following which approval for study and consent for voluntary participation respectively were obtained.

Inclusion and exclusion criteria

For the study participants from the industry, only those on the job for a period not less than 3 years (service period of 3 years or more) were included, while those with less service period were excluded. For the referents, exclusion criteria were involvement(s) in petroleum refining and distribution activities or any other activity that warrants prolonged and close contact/exposure to petroleum and gas products. Based on these criteria, 27 oil workers and 3 Non oil workers were excluded.

Sample

Using syringes and needles, blood (5 ml) was collected from each of the participants and dripped into a Lithium heparin anticoagulant specimen container. The sample was gently but thoroughly mixed to ensure the blood did not clot. The heparinized tube sample was subsequently centrifuged and the resultant plasma separated from the cells and then stored in the refrigerator for subsequent hepatic biochemical profile assays.

Methodology/data analysis

The biochemical markers of liver function determined include plasma bilirubin, Alkaline phosphatase, Aspartic and Alanine transaminases. The resultant data were analyzed using statistical programme for social sciences (SPSS) Version11. Descriptive statistics, student's T-test, ANOVA, multiple comparisons analyses using least significant difference (LSD) (Post Hoc tests), regression and correlation analyses were some of the statistical tools adopted for analyses.

Determination of plasma total Bilirubin

Plasma total bilirubin assay was performed based on the reaction principle of Freitag et al. [45]. After application of the sample (Plasma) to the Bilirubin test strip (made by Roache Diagnostic GmbH (Germany), the sample flows into the reaction zone. Before the beginning of reaction however, the protein-bound indirect bilirubin is released by means of dyphylline [7-(2, 3-dihydroxypropyl) – theophyline], so that both the direct and indirect bilirubin react with the diazonium salt, 2-methoxy-4-nitrophenyl-diazonium-tetrafluoroborate Bilirubin + 2-methoxy-4-nitrophenyldiazonium tetrafluoroborate Azobilirubin.

At a temperature of 37°C, the dye formed is displayed after about 135 seconds in mg/dl.

Determination of plasma aspartic transaminase (AST), formerly glutamate oxaloacetate transaminase (GOT) activity

The assay of this enzyme activity was done based on the reaction principle of Deneke et al. [46] using the Reflotron dry chemistry spectrophotometric system. After application to the AST Test Strip (made by Roache Diagnostic GmbH (Germany), the sample flows into the reaction zone. In the presence of GOT, ∝ – ketoglutarate and Alanine sulfinate are converted to pyruvate and glutamate. In a second reaction step catalyzed by pyruvate Oxidase (PyOD), the resulting pyruvate is cleaved into acetyl phosphate, carbon dioxide and hydrogen peroxide. In the presence of peroxidase (POD) the hydrogen peroxide converts an indicator into its oxidized blue form:

$$\propto\!-Ketoglutarata + alanine\,sulfinate(Aspartate)^{GOT}\; glutamata + SO_3^{2-}$$

$$Pyruvate + PO4^{3-} + O^{2-} + H_2O^{PyOD}\; acetylphosphate + H_2O_2 + CO_2$$

$$H_2O_2 + Indicator(red)^{POD}\; indicator(ox) + H_2O$$

Endogenous Pyruvate is eliminated in a preliminary reaction. At a temperature of 37°C, the formation of the dye is measured kinetically at 567 nm as a measure of the enzyme activity of GOT and the result displayed after 124 seconds in U/L.

Determination of plasma Alanine transaminase (ALT), formerly glutamate pyruvate transaminase (GPT) activity

The assay of this enzyme activity was done based on the principle of Deneke and Rittersdorf [47], using the Reflotron dry chemistry spectrophotometric system. After application to the ALT Test Strip (made by Roache Diagnostic GmbH (Germany), the sample flows into the reaction zone. In the presence of ALT (GPT), ∝ – ketoglutarate and Alanine are converted to glutamate and pyruvate. In a second reaction step catalyzed by pyruvate oxidase, the resulting pyruvate is cleaved into acetyl phosphate, carbon dioxide and hydrogen peroxide. In the presence of POD, the hydrogen peroxide converts an indicator into its oxidized blue form:

$$\propto\text{-}Ketoglutarate + alanine^{GPT}\ glutamate + pyruvate$$

$$Pyruvate + PO_4^{2-} + O^{2-} + H_2O^{PYOD}\ acetylphosphate + H_2O_2 + CO_2$$

$$H_2O_2 + Indicator(red)^{POD}\ indicator(ox) + H_2O$$

Endogenous Pyruvate is eliminated in a preliminary reaction. At a temperature of 37°C, the formation of the dye is measured kinetically at 567 nm as a measure of the enzyme activity of GPT and the result displayed after 140 seconds in U/L.

Determination of plasma alkaline phosphatase (ALP) activity

The assay of this enzyme activity was done based on the reaction principle of Heins et al. [48] using the Reflotron dry chemistry spectrophotometric system. After application to the ALP Test Strip (made by Roache Diagnostic GmbH (Germany), the sample flows into the reaction zone. ALP hydrolyzes O-cresolphthalein phosphate to O-cresolphthalein and transfers the phosphate group to the acceptor molecule methylglucamine. The coloured hydrolysis product, O-cresolphthalein that is produced per unit of time under alkaline conditions is directly proportional to alkaline phosphatase activity:

$$O\text{-}cresolphthalein\ phosphate + methylglucamine^{ALP}\ O\text{-}cresolphthalein + methylglucamine\ phosphate.$$

At a temperature of 37°C, the formation of the coloured reaction product is measured kinetically at 567 nm as a measure of the enzyme activity of ALP and the result displayed after 135 seconds in U/L.

Results

The results of the hepatic function markers studied in the oil workers and referents are summarized in the following tables:

Table 1 reported on the ranges and mean values of hepatic function markers studied in the oil workers (PPMC and PHRC put together) as compared with those of the non-oil workers (referents). A close look at these values showed that despite a significantly lower mean age of oil workers relative to that of their non-oil work counterpart (43.3±7.03 yrs vs. 47.37±6.74 yrs, $P < 0.01$) and a significantly lower mean value for service (exposure) period in the oil workers than non-oil workers (16.18 ±6.42 yrs vs. 20.03±8.77 yrs, $P < 0.01$), the mean values of the studied health markers were significantly higher in oil workers for plasma Total bilirubin (0.66±0.20 mg/dl vs. 0.58±0.13 mg/dl, $P < 0.01$) and ALP (126.21±39.49u/l vs. 66.83±18.54u/l) but lower in oil workers than the referents for AST (21.81±11.49u/l vs. 26.89±6.99u/l, $P < 0.05$) and ALT (22.14±11.28u/l vs. 22.30±10.22u/l, $P > 0.05$), with the difference in AST being significant while that of ALT was not. Also, the oil workers and their control counterparts were separated according to gender and age groupings, and the mean values of studied parameters for these groupings were as presented in Tables 2 (Males), Table 3 (Females), and Table 4 (Age groups). For these groupings, the presentation pattern was as earlier observed, however, though the mean values for the parameters were higher in males than females, the increases were not significant in most cases ($P > 0.05$).

In all age groups, while bilirubin was non-significantly higher ($P > 0.05$) in oil workers, alkaline phosphatase remained very significantly higher ($P < 0.01$) in oil workers than in non-oil workers. AST and ALT remained consistently insignificantly lower ($P > 0.05$) in oil workers for all age groups except in age groups 40-49 years where the decrease in AST was significant ($P < 0.05$) among oil workers.

Finally, the oil workers were also grouped according to their service years or exposure periods (i.e. number of years the worker had been engaged in the work, amounting to his/her cumulative years of exposure to the hazards of his/her workplace) and the studied parameters compared between the various exposure groups of oil workers with those of the non-oil workers, and the results were as presented in Table 5. The results here revealed that, in all exposure groups, alkaline phosphatase was significantly higher ($P < 0.05$) in oil workers than non-oil workers; bilirubin, though also increased in oil workers for all exposure groups, the increase was significant ($P < 0.05$) only for exposure periods 6–10, 21–25 and 26–35 years respectively. AST was decreased in all exposure periods of oil work with the decrease being significant ($P < 0.05$) only for exposure periods 11–15, 16–20 and 26–35 years respectively. On the other hand, ALT was insignificantly lower ($P > 0.05$) in oil workers for all exposure periods except exposure periods 6–10 and 11–15 years.

Discussion

As the data were subjected to statistical analyses using Student's T-test, the mean values for Total bilirubin and Alkaline phosphatase (ALP) were significantly higher ($P < 0.05$) in oil than non-oil workers, while Aspartic transaminases (AST) and Alanine transaminases (ALT) were lower, with the decrease in AST being significantly different ($P < 0.05$) in oil workers than non-oil workers (Table 1). This remained the pattern of presentation even as the study participants were separated according to gender and equivalent sexes also compared using Student's T-test. The increase observed in the mean values of bilirubin for oil workers over the non-oil workers did not differ

Table 1 Value ranges and means of liver function parameters studied in the oil workers (PPMC and PHRC put together) compared with the NON-OIL WORKERS

Parameter	Non-oilworkers (N = 30) Range	Mean ± SD	Oil workers (N = 303) Range	Mean ± SD	P-value (2-tailed)	Normal range & unit of parameter
Age	35.00-59.00	47.37 ± 6.74*	28.00-60.00	43.30 ± 7.03	0.003	
Service period**	3.00-34.00	20.03 ± 8.77*	3.00-34.00	16.18 ± 6.42	0.003	Up to 35 yrs
Total bilirubin	0.50-1.00	0.58 ± 0.13	0.30-1.60	0.66 ± 0.20*	0.000	0- 1.00 mg/dl
ALK. PHOS	40.00-111.00	66.83 ±18.54	50.00-296.00	126.21 ± 39.49*	0.000	50-250 U/L
AST	18.00-44.00	26.89 ± 6.99*	5.80-140.20	21.81 ± 11.49	0.018	0-45 U/L (M), 0-35 U/L (F)
ALT	10.00-55.00	22.30 ± 10.22	4.90-86.60	22.14 ± 11.28	0.941	0-45 U/L (M), 0-35 U/L (F)

T-test was the statistical tool applied. * indicates statistically significant difference [**Service Period = number of years the worker had been engaged in the work, amounting to his/her cumulative years of exposure to the hazards of his/her workplace (i.e. exposure period). Presently, 35 yrs is the maximum service period that qualifies an average civil servant for retirement in Nigeria, and is therefore considered as the upper limit of normal for service period in this report].

significantly (P > 0.05) (Tables 2 and 3). Though the mean values for the parameters were higher in males than females, the increases were not significant in most cases.

When the population was separated into age groups, and their data subjected to Multiple Comparisons using Least Significant Difference (LSD) (Table 4), the findings showed that in all age groups, while bilirubin was non-significantly higher (P > 0.05) in oil workers, alkaline phosphatase remained very significantly higher (P < 0.01) in oil workers than in non-oil workers. AST and ALT remained consistently insignificantly lower (P > 0.05) in oil workers for all age groups except in age groups 40-49 years where the decrease in AST was significant (P < 0.05) among oil workers. As the oil work population was separated on the basis of exposure period and then compared with non-oil work population by the method of Multiple Comparisons using Least Significant Difference (LSD) (Table 5), it was observed that, in all exposure groups alkaline phosphatase was significantly higher (P < 0.05) in oil workers than non-oil workers; bilirubin, though also increased in oil workers for all exposure groups, the increase was significant (P < 0.05) only for exposure periods 6–10, 21–25 and 26–35 years respectively. AST was decreased in all exposure periods of oil work with the decrease being significant (P < 0.05) only for exposure periods 11–15, 16–20 and 26–35 years respectively. On the other hand, ALT was insignificantly lower (P > 0.05) in oil workers for all exposure periods except exposure periods 6–10 and 11–15 years. Thus, from all considerations we have a pattern of consistently significant increase in alkaline phosphatase among oil workers than the control group; consistent increase in bilirubin among oil workers that was significant in some instances and insignificant in other instances; and consistent decrease in AST and ALT among oil workers. Thus, Age and exposure group separations revealed that irrespective of the age of the worker, whatever the effects indicated by these parameters start showing up after the first five years (i.e. exposure period 6-10 years) with a possibility of becoming fully established after the first decade of occupational exposures in this industrial sector (i.e. exposure period 11-15 yrs and above).

To verify the relationships between the parameters under study, data of the entire study participants were jointly subjected to the Pearson's (2-tailed) correlation analyses, and the results showed that no correlation existed between age and the various parameters except with ALP where there was significant negative correlation (= -0.131, P < 0.017). Similarly, exposure period correlated with no other parameter except ALP, still with negative correlation (=-0.154, P < 0.005). However, there were significant

Table 2 Mean values of liver function parameters studied in male oil workers & non-oil male workers

Parameter	Non-oilworkers (N = 20) Mean ± SD	Oil workers (N = 273) Mean ± SD	P-value (2-tailed)	Normal range & unit of parameter
Age	49.75 ± 5.15*	43.63 ± 6.98	0.000	
Service period	23.20 ± 7.81*	16.32 ± 6.47	0.000	Up to 35 yrs
Total bilirubin	0.60 ± 0.14	0.67 ± 0.20	0.124	0- 1.00 mg/dl
ALK. PHOS	65.90 ± 19.56	126.69 ± 39.57*	0.000	50-250 U/L
AST	28.02 ± 6.71*	22.25 ± 11.88	0.033	0-45 U/L (M), 0-35 U/L (F)
ALT	22.80 ±9.00	22.55 ± 11.51	0.925	0-45 U/L (M), 0-35 U/L (F)

T-test was the statistical tool applied. *indicates statistically significant difference.

Table 3 Mean values of liver function parameters studied in female oil workers & non-oil female workers

Parameter	Non-oilworkers (N = 10) Mean ± SD	Oil workers (N = 30) Mean ± SD	P-value (2-tailed)	Normal range & unit of parameter
Age	42.6 ± 7.25	40.33 ± 6.9	0.379	
Service period	13.7 ± 7.21	14.97 ± 5.84	0.579	Up to 35 yrs
Total bilirublin	0.54 ± 0.07	0.61 ± 0.17*	0.228	0- 1.00 mg/dl
ALK. PHOS	68.7 ± 17.13	121.87 ± 39.16	0.000	50-250 U/L
AST	24.63 ± 7.34*	17.73 ± 5.67	0.004	0-45 U/L (M), 0-35 U/L (F)
ALT	21.3 ± 12.79	18.41 ± 8.15	0.408	0-45 U/L (M), 0-35 U/L (F)

T-test was the statistical tool applied. *indicates statistically significant difference.

positive correlations between bilirubin and ALP (=0.224, P < 0.000), bilirubin and AST (=160, P < 0.003), bilirubin and ALT (=0.203, P < 0.000). In all instances, there were strong positive correlation among the enzymes: ALP and AST (=0.163, P < 0.003), ALP and ALT (=0.279, P < 0.000), AST and ALT(= 0.545, p < 0.000).

Liver function profiles: implications for the oil workers

The plasma enzymes including ALP, AST and ALT together with the bilirubins form part of the major functional markers of the liver [49-52]. However, because the liver performs several roles including synthetic, storage, metabolic, excretory and detoxification functions [50-52], it stands out clearly as one organ whose true functional assessment involves the assemblage of a battery of general body functional markers including blood glucose, plasma proteins, plasma lipids and some haematological markers. However, within the confines of the four parameters assayed in this study and presently under consideration- ALP, AST, ALT and bilirubin, though none of these exceeded their individual parametric reference values, the fact that both AST and ALT were consistently lower in the face of a consistently elevated alkaline phosphatase and total bilirubin values in the oil workers in comparison with the referents clearly points to the existence of certain conditions among the oil workers that does not obtain among the non-oil workers.

AST is present in high concentration in cells of cardiac and skeletal muscles, liver, kidney and erythrocytes. Thus, damage to any of these tissues may increase plasma AST levels. In like manner, ALT is present in high concentrations in liver and to a lesser extent in skeletal muscle, kidney and heart [51]. Marked increase of the enzymes

Table 4 Mean values of liver function parameters studied for the various age groups of the oil workers & control subjects

Age group	Parameter	Non-oilworkers Mean ± SD	Oil workers Mean ± SD	P-value
30-39 (Non-oil workers, n = 5), (Oil workers, n = 97)	Age	36.60 ± 1.52	35.55 ± 2.69	0.651
	Service period	10.00 ± 4.18	11.46 ± 4.34*	0.000
	Total bilirubin	0.52 ± 0.04	0.66 ± 0.18*	0.035
	ALK. PHOS	62.60 ± 19.83	133.41 ± 40.17*	0.000
	AST	23.00 ± 2.09	22.59 ± 9.17	0.066
	ALT	16.78 ± 6.30	24.02 ± 12.99	0.462
40-49 (Non-oil workers, n = 13), (Oil workers, n = 142)	Age	45.46 ± 2.60	44.27 ± 2.71	
	Service period	19.62 ± 7.30	16.82 ± 5.34*	0.005
	Total bikirubin	0.56 ± 0.09	0.66 ± 0.20*	0.041
	ALK. PHOS	66.23 ± 12.40	121.62 ± 39.18*	0.000
	AST	27.35 ± 8.85	20.38 ± 8.79*	0.004
	ALT	24.35 ± 13.80	21.30 ± 10.68	0.657
50-59 (Non-oil workers, n = 13), (Oil workers, n = 64)	AGE	53.92 ± 2.78	53.23 ± 2.61	
	Service period	24.67 ± 8.29	21.97 ± 5.64	0.106
	Total bilirubin	0.62 ± 0.17	0.66 ± 0.23*	0.052
	ALK. PHOS	69.25 ± 24.09	125.68 ± 39.08*	0.000
	AST	28.02 ± 5.77	23.76 ± 18.03	0.236
	ALT	22.37 ± 5.87	21.43 ± 9.68	0.768

Multiple Comparisons using Least Significant Difference (LSD) was the statistical method of analysis applied. * indicates statistically significant difference.

Table 5 Value ranges and means of liver function parameters studied for the various exposure periods (service years) of the oil workers & control subjects

Exposure period	N	Parameter	Range	Mean	P-value	Normal range & unit of parameter
1-5	23	Total bilirubin	0.5 -1.00	0.66 ± 0.14	0.134	0- 1.00 mg/dl
6-10	14		0.5 -1.20	0.71 ± 0.20	0.027	
11-15	128		0.4 -1.30	0.64 ± 0.18	0.123	
16-20	56		0.4 -1.00	0.64 ± 0.15	0.161	
21-25	61		0.4 -1.30	0.69 ± 0.23	0.011*	
26-35	21		0.3 -1.60	0.75 ± 0.31	0.001*	
Control	30		0.5-1.00	0.58 ± 0.13		
Total	333		0.3-1.60	0.65 ± 0.19		
1-5	23	ALK. PHOS	82.00 -193.00	127.00 ± 32.09	0.000*	50-250 U/L
6-10	14		84.00 - 220.00	137.50 ± 36.63	0.000*	
11-15	128		58.00 - 270.00	129.68 ± 40.17	0.000*	
16-20	56		50.00 - 286.00	125.59 ± 43.81	0.000*	
21-25	61		51.00 - 296.00	120.51 ± 40.14	0.000*	
26-35	21		61.00 - 163.00	114.90 ± 28.14	0.000*	
Control	30		40.00-111.00	66.83 ± 18.54		
Total	333		40.00 - 296.00	120.86 ± 41.70		
1-5	23	AST	8.2 - 40.20	21.78 ± 6.88	0.101	0-45 U/L (M), 0-35 U/L (F)
6-10	14		11.1 - 38.30	22.94 ± 8.31	0.278	
11-15	128		6.7 - 50.20	22.05 ± 8.98	0.034*	
16-20	56		5.8 - 65.00	21.79 ± 10.86	0.045*	
21-25	61		6.6 - 140.20	22.08 ± 17.94	0.055	
26-35	21		8.1 - 39.30	18.87 ± 9.12	0.013*	
Control	30		18 - 44.00	26.89 ± 6.99		
Total	333		5.8 - 140.20	22.26 ± 11.25		
1-5	23	ALT	9.1 - 49.70	20.93 ± 10.65	0.657	0-45 U/L (M), 0-35 U/L (F)
6-10	14		10.7 - 42.40	23.76 ± 9.66	0.685	
11-15	128		7.0 - 86.60	24.11 ± 13.36	0.422	
16-20	56		6.7 - 52.20	21.21 ± 9.36	0.665	
21-25	61		4.9 - 48.60	19.34 ± 9.03	0.235	
26-35	21		6.7 - 37.30	20.97 ± 7.75	0.674	
Control	30		10.0 - 55.00	22.30 ± 10.22		
Total	333		4.9 - 86.60	22.15 ± 11.17		

Multiple Comparisons using Least Significant Difference (LSD) was the statistical method of analysis applied. * indicates statistically significant difference.
Key for letters in Normal Range.
M = Males.
F = Females.

(10 to 100 times the upper limit of adult reference range) may be caused by circulatory failure with 'shock' and hypoxia, myocardial infarction (particularly for AST) and acute viral or toxic hepatitis, while moderate increase may be caused by [51]:

- Cirrhosis (enzyme levels may be normal or up to twice the upper adult reference limit); infectious mononucleosis (due to liver involvement); cholestatic jaundice (levels may be up to 10 times the upper reference limit); liver congestion secondary to congestive cardiac failure (particularly ALT)
- Malignant infiltration of the liver (particularly for AST and this may be normal or rise to twice the upper reference limit); surgery or extensive trauma and skeletal muscle disease (ALT is much less affected than AST)

- Alkaline phosphatase – a group of enzymes that hydrolyze organic phosphates at high pH, are present in most tissues but are in particularly high concentration in the osteoblasts of bone and the cells of the hepatobiliary tract, intestinal wall, renal tubules and placenta [50,51]. According to these authors, possible causes of raised plasma Alp apart from physiological are:
- Bone disease: rickets and osteomalacia, Paget's disease of bone (Alp may be very high); secondary malignant deposits in bone; osteogenic sarcoma, only if extensive; primary hyperparathyroidism with extensive bone disease (Alp is usually normal but may be slightly elevated); Secondary hyperparathyroidism.
- Liver diseases: Intra or extra hepatic cholestasis; space-occupying lesions, tumours, granulomas, and other causes of hepatic infiltration.
- Malignancy with bone or liver involvement or direct tumour production. A placental-like (so-called 'Regan' Isoenzymes of Alp may occasionally be identified in plasma in patients with malignant disease, especially carcinoma of the bronchus [48,51].
- Leukaemia cells may also leak Alp. A raised plasma (and urinary) level is found in acute monocytic and myeloid leukaemia.

Given the multiple locations of these enzymes, i.e. their presence in many tissues, changes in their plasma activities may reflect damage to any of those tissues, thus allowing room for a needful differential diagnosis. Hence, a careful evaluation of the variously highlighted conditions above is relevant alongside consideration of the plasma bilirubin concentrations. Bilirubin, as a bile pigment, is a product of red blood cells (erythrocytes) broken down by the reticulo-endothelial system (RES) found mainly in the spleen. About 80% of bilirubin is derived from haem within the RES, other sources being the breaking down of immature red cells in the bone marrow and of compounds chemically related to haemoglobin such as myoglobin and the cytochromes. Bilirubin is bound to albumin and transported to the liver where it is conjugated, and after conjugation, excreted by active processes into the bile canaculi- a process that is largely dependent on active secretion of bile acids from hepatocytes. Thus, when bile secretion from the hepatocytes into the canaculi is impaired, intrahepatic cholestasis ensues as against extrahepatic cholestasis, which occurs when there is obstruction to the flow of preformed bile through the biliary tract. In these conditions plasma bilirubin levels and alkaline phosphatase activities are increased [51].

In the present study, the increases observed in both ALP and bilirubins were only in relative terms vis-a-vis oil workers and their control counterpart. The mean values of both parameters were still within their normal ranges and for bilirubin in particular, a state of jaundice is not yet reached- a condition of 'Anicteric' elevation of Alp without a corresponding increase in AST and ALT. This definitely rules out infective conditions such as viral hepatitis (as AST and/or ALT ought to have increased correspondingly) [51] but certainly not toxic hepatitis, which according to Davis [53], is possible as a result of enzyme induction in the face of certain environmental agents such as aromatic hydrocarbons (and these are superabundantly present in petroleum products), some food additives and some pesticides, which according to Conney [54] have enzyme-inducing properties. Again, chronic exposure to enzyme-inducing agents, according to Stamp et al. [55], may lead to osteomalacia (one of the possible causes of increases in plasma Alp concentration) as a result of diversion of vitamin D metabolism to biologically inactive metabolites. Also, many carcinogens and some hepatotoxins exert their toxic effects via metabolites, and enzyme induction potentiates the activation of these compounds and therefore their toxicity [56,57]. So, the question is: What does Anicteric elevation of AlP indicates for the oil work population?

The total alkaline phosphatase assayed consisted of several isoenzymes that can only be distinguished electrophoretically (not done in this study). These include isoenzymes from cells of bone, liver, biliary tract, intestine and placenta [49-51]. It is excessively rare to find all five fractions together in the same sample of serum. Placental AlP is present only in pregnant women (this is not applicable in this study). The presence of intestinal AlP seems related to liver cirrhosis and also the ABO secretor status, higher levels being found in individuals of blood groups O and B [58,59] though the concentration in the intestinal tissue is not related to blood groups [60]. The presence of both liver and bile isoenzymes in anicteric patients point to an impairment of the bile flow termed 'focal block'. The macromolecular bile components are refluxed back into the blood, which they cannot leave again. The low molecular weight components such as bilirubin are however, again extracted from the blood and secreted in zones where the bile flow is not blocked [61]. The most frequent cause of this type of obstruction is the presence of malignant primary or secondary tumour in the liver [49].

Another interesting change in serum alkaline phosphatase in malignancy is the appearance in the serum of an isoenzyme that cannot be distinguished from placental AlP (i.e. placental-like Alp) called 'Regan isoenzyme' after the patient in whom it was first demonstrated. Apart from this patient with bronchial carcinoma (the isoenzyme was found in both the serum and tumour), it was found in the serum of 27 out of 500 patients with various malignant diseases [59]. Warnock and Reisman [62] found a similar enzyme in extracts of eight out of 10 hepatomas and also in the serum of some of these patients. In all these instances as in this study, total serum alkaline phosphatase was increased.

Although serum electrophoresis was not done in this study to distinguish the isoenzyme fractions of the total AlP (elevated in the oil workers over their control peers) and possibly establish or rule out other conditions including presence of tumours or carcinomas, it is believed that a reasonable pointer has been shown as to the possible conditions indicated by Anicteric significant rise in alkaline phosphatase among oil workers. Based on these submissions, it could be said that part of the health risks associated with occupational exposures in the Oil and Gas industry are among others, the possible development of bone diseases with increased osteoblastic activity, liver diseases with involvement of the biliary tracts, toxic hepatitis, liver cirrhosis, malignancies of various body sites including bronchial carcinoma, hepatoma and leukaemia, etc. In fact, apart from the various degrees of accidents and injuries previously reported among these same petroleum refining and distribution workers [63], results also indicated that some of the above highlighted conditions including liver diseases, made reckonable contributions to the morbidities and mortalities recorded in this industry [64], thus suggesting the presence of organs/systems toxic agents in this work environment. Serum alkaline phosphatase electrophoreses study is therefore highly warranted in a further study of these oil refining and distribution workers to establish the actual isoenzyme fraction of alkaline phosphatase responsible for the increasing pattern observed for this enzyme among this segment of workers, and thus establish on a firmer basis some or all of these possible health risks among the oil workers.

Just like in our own study, previous works relating to occupational exposures had recorded variable levels of these same liver markers. Contrary to the findings in the present study, elevated levels of AST and ALT were reported for those occupationally exposed to toxic substances, indicating susceptibility to Anicteric hepatitis [63,64]. The study of Dioka et al. [65] revealed that while ALT and AST activities were elevated in occupationally exposed artisans than in controls, ALP activity was significantly lower in the exposed subjects than in controls. Waldman and Borman [66] had earlier reported similar findings of increased serum ALT and AST activities. Studies by Kapaki et al. [67] showed an ALT elevation in taxi drivers, while activities of both ALT and AST were elevated in gas station workers.

Similarly, other animal studies produced variable results in enzyme levels following exposure to petroleum products. In fish, serum levels of AST, ALT and ALP were increased following hepatocellular damage resulting from exposure to 2, 3, 4-triaminoazo benzene [68]. Other studies also indicated increase in the activities of the liver enzymes following liver damage in fish and albino mouse exposed to toxic substances [69-71]. Chu et al. [72] noted an increase in levels of serum aspartate aminotransferase (AST) in male rats and alkaline phosphatase (ALP) in female rats exposed to petroleum hydrocarbon, whereas administration of 200, 400, and 800 mg/kg of Bonny light crude oil in the study of Orisakwe et al. [34] caused a significant dose-dependent increase in AST and ALT, but a significant decrease in the alkaline phosphatase (ALP) level compared to the control. Thus, administration of the bonny light crude oil produced a dose-dependent damage of the liver cells.

A three months study of biochemical changes in the serum and liver of albino rats chronically administered with $5.0gkg^{-1}$, $7.5gkg^{-1}$ and $15.0gkg^{-1}$ of gasoline, kerosene, and crude petroleum (bonny light) respectively showed that the petroleum samples caused biochemical changes in the serum and liver parameters [38]. Thus, AST, ALT and ALP showed dose-dependent increase in levels from first month to the 3rd month for all the petroleum samples, with substantial to marginal increases that are significantly different from the control ($p < 0.05$) following administration of various combinations of the samples. Elevations of these enzymes reflect presence of some inflammatory disease or injury to the liver, while the maximum ALP activity (more than two fold) obtained for gasoline and kerosene for the third month showed the possibility of hepatocellular damage.

Histopathological study of Liver of rats administered with diesel fuel showed that this substance induced a dose-dependent effects ranging from narrowing of sinuses (LD_{50}) to severe hepatocellular necrosis (LD_{100}), thus qualifying to be included as a hepatotoxin [36]. Hepatotoxins are defined as agents that cause liver injury after a relatively short period, and which may cause liver cell necrosis alone or with altered enzyme activity and biliary tract dysfunction [73]. However, another study involving exposure of male and female mice to various doses (up to 2056 ppm) of PS-6 blend gasoline vapour 6 hr/day, 5days/week up to 13 weeks, showed that though the leaded gasoline increases hepatocellular proliferation in mice, it did not significantly affect serum ALT and AST activity or cause any histological changes in the liver [74]. Mechanism of gasoline toxicity or indeed other toxic substances may include inactivation of antioxidants such as Glutathione (GST), and this may explain the low activity of GST in gasoline-injected rats in the study of Ayalogu et al. [38]. Chiapotto et al. [75] had also reported inactivation of GST by different concentrations of acetaldehyde. Although GST assay was not done in the present study, these reports have shown that enzyme pattern in the serum or plasma reflects the physiological state of the organ.

Conclusion

The study revealed that though the levels of the assayed hepatic biochemical markers were still within the parametric reference ranges as at the time of this study, however, relative to the non-oil work referents that served as the control group, changes observed in the biochemical markers among the oil workers suggested that petroleum refining and distribution work environment is furnished with some hepatoxic substances and that anicteric hepatoxicity is a potential health effect of long term occupational exposures in the petroleum refining and distribution industry in Nigeria, hence, long-serving staff might be victims of anicteric toxic hepatitis.

Our inability to obtain and adjust data for the smoking habit of the study participants was a major deficiency of the study, which needs to be taken care of in any future study of these industrial workers. However, despite this shortcoming, the findings offer far reaching contributions in the area of occupational and environmental toxicology, given that most of what was known of petroleum toxicology in Nigeria were based on studies using animal models. To the best of our knowledge, this is the first study on this thematic area conducted directly on humans in Nigeria. While earlier studies have reported the effects of petroleum exposures in animal models for extrapolation to humans, our study was carried out using direct human biological samples. Thus, the results give a more assured situation than an extrapolated result, which might be affected by species differences

These study findings have important applications, since it provided the management of the establishments within this industrial sector with data-based evidence for upgrading the industrial/occupational health measures aimed at improving the health of their workers and eventually their productivity. In this regard, the study results indicated a need for frequent environmental and biological monitoring to ensure a safer and healthier workplace and workforce respectively in this very critical sector of the Nigerian economy. Again, in the realms of forensic toxicology, the study findings also offer immense benefit, since it provided scientific evidence for resolution of health compensation litigations, particularly those involving occupationally-facilitated hepatic diseases conditions. Finally, through this study, hepatic health data on petroleum refining and distribution industry workers have been provided, and this marks an important response to the calls for data by Loewenson (19) regarding industrially furnished exposures and their health effects, and also by Scala (20) for toxicological data on the petroleum/petrochemical industry. The situation as it affects other organs/systems still needs to be addressed, and remains the focus of our on-going studies.

Competing interests

The authors declare that they have no competing interests.

Authors' contributions

TINE conceived and designed the study, collected, analyzed and interpreted the data, and also drafted the manuscript. ANE and OEO assisted in drafting the manuscript, MOEI supervised the study while FOUO and HCN co-supervised the study. The authors have read and approved the final manuscript.

Acknowledgements

The authors are grateful to the Department of Petroleum Resources (DPR), Federal Ministry of Petroleum Resources for authorizing not only this study but also the release of relevant data by the studied establishments under her supervision. The management and staff of PHRC and PPMC are hereby appreciated for permitting and participating in this study. Credit for the success of this study goes to the entire staff of the plant clinic (used by both establishments) that were at the time of this study conducting periodic medical examination for the entire staff, an exercise that greatly smoothened our study. Special interest shown in this study and the various assistance rendered by Dr.Shaibu M, an occupational physician and then head (Pant Clinic), Dr.Idris F (who latter succeeded him) and their office secretaries, particularly miss Evangel Njoku were all very highly appreciated.

Author details

[1]Department of Biotechnology, School of Science, Federal University of Technology, Owerri, Nigeria. [2]Department of Biological Science, School of Science, Federal University of Technology, Owerri, Nigeria. [3]Department of Clinical Pharmacy, Toxicology Unit, University of Port Harcourt, Port Harcourt, Nigeria.

References

1. Neff JM: **Polycyclic aromatic hydrocarbons.** In *Fundamentals of Aquatic Toxicology.* Edited by Rand GM, Petrocelli SR. Bristol, PA: Taylor and Francis; 1985:416–454.
2. Wilson VS, LeBlanc GA: **Petroleum pollution.** *Review of Toxicology* 2000, **3**:77.
3. Oliver T, Kostecki PT, Kalabres EJ: *State summary of soil and ground water cleanup standards.* Massachusetts: Department of Environmental protection; 1993:48.
4. Clark RB: *Marine pollution.* Oxford: Clarendon press; 1992.
5. Eisler R: *Polycyclic aromatic hydrocarbon hazards to fish, wildlife, and invertebrates: A synoptic review. Fish and Wildlife Service.* Washington, DC: U.S: Department of Interior; 1987:85–111.
6. Gardner GR, Yevich PP, Harshbarger JC, Malcolm AR: **Carcinogenicity of Black Rock Harbor sediment to the eastern oyster and trophic transfer of Black Rock Harbor carcinogens from the blue mussel to the winter flounder.** *Enviro Health Perspective* 1991, **90**:53–66.
7. Feuston MH, Hamilton CE, Schreiner CA, Mackerer CR: **Developmental toxicity of dermally applied crude oils in rats.** *J Toxicol Environ Health* 1997, **52**:79–93.
8. Malins DC, Ostrander GK: *Aquatic toxicology: molecular, biochemical and cellular perspectives.* Chelsea, MI: Lewis Publishers; 1994.
9. Yamato O, Goto I, Maede YJ: **Hemolytic anemia in wild sea duck caused by marine oil pollution.** *J Wildl Dis* 1996, **32**:381–384.
10. Kennish MJ: *Practical Handbook of Estuarine and Marine Pollution.* Bocca Raton FL: CRC press; 1997:83.
11. Vyskocil A, Cizkova M: **Nephrotoxic effects of unleaded petrol in female rats.** *J Appl Toxicol* 1996, **16**(1):55–56.
12. Gennaro V, Finkelstein MM, Ceppi M, Fontana V, Montanaro F, Perrotta A, Puntoni R, Silvano S: **Mesothelioma and lung tumours attributable to asbestos among petroleum workers.** *Am J Ind Med* 2000, **37**(3):275–282.
13. Runion HE: **Occupational exposures to potentially hazardous agents in the petroleum industry.** *Occup Med* 1988, **3**(3):431–444.
14. Engler R: *Oil refinery health and safety hazards: their causes and the struggle to end them.* Philadelphia, U.S.A: Philadelphia Area Project on Occupational Safety and Health; 1975.
15. Gennaro V, Ceppi M, Boffeta P, Fontana V, Perrotta A: **Pleural mesothelioma and asbestos exposure among Italian oil workers.** *Scand J Work Environ Health* 1994, **20**(3):213–215.

16. Epstein PR, Selber J: *Oil- a life cycle analysis of its health and environmental impacts.* Harvard Medical School Boston and Massachusetts: Report of center for Health and the global Environment; 2002:73.
17. Whittle KJ, Hardy R, Mackie PR: **A quantitative assessment of the sources and fate of petroleum compounds in the marine environment.** *Philos Trans R Soc Lond B Biol Sci* 1982, **297**:193–218.
18. PHRC Brochure: *PHRC.* Nigeria: Premier Petroleum Refining Company; 2008:20.
19. Loewenson R: **Occupational health in small-scale industries in Africa.** *Afri Newsl on Occup Health and Saf* 1995, **13**:44–45.
20. Scala RA: **Motor Gasoline Toxicity.** *Toxicol Sci* 1988, **10**:(4):553–562.
21. International Agency for research on cancer (IARC): ***Occupational exposure in petroleum refining, crude oil and major petroleum fuels.*** **Lyons, France: IARC working group on the evaluation of carcinogenic risk to humans.** *Monogr on the Eval of Carcinog Risk to Humans* 1989, **45**.
22. Hayes RB, Yin SN, Dosemeci M, Li GL, Wacholder S, Chow WH: **Mortality among benzene-exposed workers in China.** *Environ Health Perspect* 1996, **104**(suppl 6):1349–1352.
23. Health Effects Institute (HEI): *Particulate air pollution and daily mortality: replication and validation of selected studies.* Boston, M A: The phase I report of the particle epidemiology evaluation Project; 1995.
24. Pukkala E, Auvinen A, Wahlberg G: **Incidence of cancer among finish airline cabin attendants, 1967–92.** *BMJ* 1995, **311**:649–652.
25. Dement JM, Hensley L, Kieding S, Lipscomb H: **Proportionate mortality among union members employed at three Texas refineries.** *Am J Ind Med* 1998, **33**(4):327–340.
26. Clap RW, Coogan PF: **Leukemia in petroleum refinery workers: a review of recent studies.** *New Solut* 1999, **9**:375–387.
27. National Institute of Environmental Health Science (NIEHS): *9th Annual report of suspected human carcinogens.* WashingtonDC: NIEHS; 2000.
28. Sebastian San M, Armstrong B, Cordoba JA, Stephens C: **Exposures and cancer incidence near oil fields in Amazon basin of Ecuador.** *Occup Environ Med* 2001, **58**:517–522.
29. Satin KP, Bailey WJ, Newton KL, Ross AY, Wong O: **Updated epidemiological study of workers at two California petroleum refineries, 1950–95.** *Occup Environ Med* 2002, **59**:248–256.
30. Tsai SP, Wendt JK, Cardarelli KM, Fraser AE: **A mortality and morbidity study of refinery and petrochemical employees in Louisiana.** *Occup Environ Med* 2003, **60**:627–633.
31. Parodi S, Vercelli M, Stella A, Stagnaro E, Valerio F: **Lymphohaematopoietic system cancer incidence in an urban area near a coke oven plant: an ecological investigation.** *Occup Environ Med* 2003, **60**:187–194.
32. Parodi S, Montanaro F, Ceppi M, Gennaro V: **Mortality of petroleum refinery workers (Letters).** *Occup Environ Med* 2003, **60**:304–307.
33. Orisakwe OE, Njan AA, Afonne OJ, Akumka DD, Orish VN, Udemezue OO: **Investigation into the nephrotoxicity of Nigeria bonny light crude Oil in albino rats.** *Int J Environ Res Public Health* 2004, **1**(2):106–110.
34. Orisakwe OE, Akumka DD, Njan AA, Afonne OJ, Okechi OO: **Hepatotoxic and haematological effects of Nigrian bonny light crude oil in male albino rats.** *Toxicol & Environ Chem* 2005, **87**(2):215–221.
35. Igbo NM, Dede EB, Ayalogu OE: **Acute toxicity effects of crude petroleum (bonny light), kerosene, and gasoline in albino rats.** *J Appl Sci Environ Mgt* 2001, **5**(2):73–75.
36. Dede EB, Kagbo HD: **Investigation of acute toxicological effects of diesels fuel in rats (Rattus Rattus).** *J Appl Sci Environ Mgt* 2001, **5**(1):83–84.
37. Gabriel UU, Allison ME, Alagoa KJ: **Effects of crude oil water dispersion on the haemoglobin and haematocrit of the afican catfish clarias gariepinus.** *J Appl Sci Environ Mgt* 2001, **5**(2):9–11.
38. Ayalogu OE, Igbo NM, Dede EB: **Biochemical changes in the plasma and liver of albino rats exposed to petroleum samples (gasoline, kerosene, and crude petroleum).** *J Appl Sci Environ Mgt* 2001, **5**(1):97–100.
39. Uba EC, Onyekonwu MO, Mbeledogu IU: **Modeling environmental contamination: case study of a potentially polluted area in the Niger delta.** *J Appl Sci Environ Mgt* 2001, **5**(2):77–84.
40. Ezejiofor TIN, Iwuala MOE, Osuala FOU, Nwigwe HC: **Risk assessment: Prevalent occupational hazards in Nigerian petroleum oil refining and distribution industry.** *J Med Invest Pract* 2012, **8**:24.
41. Ezejiofor TIN, Ezejiofor AN, Iwuala MOE: **Anthropometrical and biochemical markers of cardiovascular health risks among petroleum Oil refining and distribution industry workers, Nigeria.** *J Med Lab Sci* 2013, **22**:2. In Press.
42. Ezejiofor TIN, Ezejiofor AN, Iwuala MOE: **Toxic nephropathy: a potential health effect of occupational exposures in petroleum Oil refining and distribution industry workers in Nigeria.** *The J of Toxicol and Health. Photon* 2013, **103**:330–344.
43. Ezejiofor TIN: **Patterns of accidents and injuries in Nigerian petroleum Oil refining and distribution industry.** *Mary Slessor J of Med* 2010, **10**(1):23–28.
44. Ezejiofor TIN: **Morbidity and mortality patterns in Nigerian petroleum Oil refining and distribution industry.** *Mary Slessor J of Med* 2010, **10**(1):8–22.
45. Freitag H, *et al*: **Test for the quantitative determination of bilirubin in blood, serum or plasma with Reflotron.** *Clin Chem* 1987, **33**:1011.
46. Deneke U, *et al*: **Test for the quantitative determination of GOT (AST; ASAT; EC 2.6.1.1) in blood, serum or plasma with Reflotron.** *ClinChem* 1985, **31**:921.
47. Deneke U, Rittersdorf W: **Test for the quantitative determination of GPT (ALT; ALAT; EC 2.6.1.2) in blood, serum or plasma with Reflotron.** *ClinChem* 1984, **30**:1009.
48. Heins W, *et al*: **Test for the quantitative determination of the total activity of alkaline phosphatase (EC 3.1.3.1) in blood serum or plasma using Reflotron.** *Eur J ClinChem Biochem* 1995, **33**:231.
49. Wieme RJ, Demeulenaere L: **Enzyme assays in liver diseases.** *J Clin Path 24 Suppl (Ass Clin Path)* 1970, **4**:51–59.
50. Baron DN: *The Liver. A short textbook of chemical pathology.* 4th edition. Great Britain: ELBS/Hodder& Stoughton; 1982:188–206.
51. Mayne PD: *The Liver and Gall Stones, Plasma Enzymes in Diagnosis. Clinical chemistry in diagnosis and treatment ELST.* 6th edition. London: International Book Development Ltd; 1998:279–290. 299–312.
52. Balisteri WF, Shaw LM: **Liver function.** In *Fundamentals of clinical chemistry.* 5th edition. Edited by Tietz NW. USA: WB Saunders; 1999:1373–1433.
53. Davis M: **Enzyme induction by environmental agents.** *Proc Roy Soc Med* 1974, **67**:642.
54. Conney AH: **Pharmacological implications of microsomal enzyme induction.** *Pharmacol Rev* 1967, **19**:317.
55. Stamp TC, Round JM, Rowe DJ, Haddad JG: **Plasma levels and therapeutic effect of 25-hydroxycholecalciferol in epileptic patients taking anticonvulsant drugs.** *Br Med J* 1972, **4**(5831):9–12.
56. Udenfriend S: **Exertion of toxic effects by carcinogens and some hepatotoxins is via metabolites activation.** *Annals of the New York Acad Sci* 1971, **179**:295.
57. Seawright AA, Mclean AEM, Forrest BTM: **Enzyme induction potentiates activation and toxicity of compounds.** *Vet Rec* 1968, **82**:200.
58. Beckman L, Bjorling G, Heiken A: **Human alkaline phosphatase and the factors controlling their appearance in serum. In: wieme RJ, demeulenaere L. Enzyme assays in liver diseases.** *J Clin Path 24 Suppl (Ass Clin Path)* 1970, **4**:51–59.
59. Stolbach LL, Krant MJ, Fishman WH: **Ectopic production of alkaline phosphatase isoenzymes in patients with cancer.** *New Engl J Med* 1969, **281**:757–762.
60. Schreffler DC: **Relationship of alkaline phosphatase levels in intestinal mucosa to ABO and secretor blood group. In: wieme RJ, demeulenaere L. Enzyme assays in liver diseases.** *J Clin Path 24 Suppl (Ass Clin Path)* 1970, **4**:51–59.
61. Hill PG, Sammons HG: **An interpretation of the elevation of serum alkaline phosphatase in disease.** *J Clin Path* 1967, **20**:654–659.
62. Warnock ML, Reisman R: **Variant alkaline phosphatase in human hepatocellular cancers.** *ClinChimActa* 1969, **24**:5–11.
63. Ezeonu FC, Ezejiofor TIN: **Biochemical indicators of occupational health hazards in Nkalagu cement industry workers, Nigeria.** *Sci Total Environ* 1999, **228**:275–278.
64. Ezejiofor TIN: **Anicteric hepatitis: an occupational health hazard in cement industry workers.** *J of Med Investig and Pract* 2001, **3**:51–57.
65. Dioka CE, Orisakwe OE, Adeniyi FAA, Meludu SC: **Liver and renal function tests in artisans occupationally exposed to lead in mechanic village in Nnewi, Nigeria.** *Int J Environ Res Public Health* 2004, **1**:21–25.
66. Rk W, Borman EK: **A note on serum transaminase activity after lead absorption.** *Arch Indust Health* 1959, **7**:108–114.
67. Kapaki EN, Verlas PN, Spanaki MV, Andreadou E, Kakami AE, Papagiou C: **Blood lead levels of traffic and gasoline-exposed professional in the city of Athens.** *Arch Environ Health* 1998, **53**(4):287–291.
68. Krishan AG, Veena G: **2, 3,4-Triaminoazobenzene-inducedhaematobiochemical anomalies in fish (Chennapuntatus).** *Bull Environ Contam Toxicol* 1980, **25**:136–141.

69. Dheer JM, Dheer TR, Mahajan CL: **Haematological and haematopoietic response to acid stress in air breathing fresh water fish (channalpuntatus).** *Biochem J Fish Bio* 1987, **30:**577–588.
70. Mohssen M: **Inhalation toxicity studies of thimet (Phorate) in male Swiss albino mouse (Musmusculus).** *Environ Pollut* 1997, **96**(3):383–388.
71. Sharp L, Black RJ, Harkness EF: **Incidence of childhood leukaemia and Non-Hodgkin's lymphoma in the vicinity of nuclear sites in Scotland, 1968–93.** *Occup Environ Med* 1996, **53:**823–831.
72. Chu I, Villeneuve DC, Secours V, Otson R, Valli VE: **Short-term dermal toxicity and Mutagenicity of coal processing products in rat.** *J Toxicol Environ Health* 1991, **33:**317–326.
73. Jeffries GH: **Toxic and drug-induced liver disease.** In *Cecil textbook of medicine.* 15th edition. Edited by Beeson PB, McDermott W, Wyngaarden JB. Philadelphia: W.B Saunders; 1979:1657–1659.
74. Tiburyl L, Butterworth BE, Moss O, Goldsworthy TL: **Hepatocytes cell proliferation in mice after inhalation exposures to unleaded gasoline vapour.** *J Toxicol and Environ Health* 1993, **38**(3):293–307.
75. Chiapotto C, Biasi F, Scavazza A, Camandola S, Aragno M, Tamagno EO, Dianzan MU, Poli G: **Acetaldehyde involvement in ethanol induced potentiation of rats hepatocytes damage due to the carcinogen 1, 2- dibromoethanol.** *Alcohol* 1995, **30**(6):72–81.

24

Hospital physicians' work stressors in different medical specialities: a statistical group comparison

Grit Tanner[1*], Eva Bamberg[1], Agnessa Kozak[2], Maren Kersten[3] and Albert Nienhaus[2,3]

Abstract

Background: Some studies on the occupational health of hospital physicians have found that working conditions have different effects on physician's well-being and health in different medical specialities. There has been no comparative study of the effects of various work stressors in different specialities. This study aims to close this gap.

Methods: German hospital physicians were asked about their working conditions and aspects of health. The short version of the Instrument for Stress-Related Job Analysis for Hospital Physicians was used to measure working conditions. Irritation and emotional exhaustion were used to assess health. Physicians were also asked for socio-demographic aspects, including their medical speciality.

Results: Data from 763 hospital physicians were included in the analyses. Significant differences between medical specialities were demonstrated for time pressure, uncertainty, frustration about how work needs to be done and social stressors with patients. Physicians in internal medicine showed consistently high levels of stressors. Time pressure, frustration about how work needs to be done, and emotional dissonance were found to be significantly related to both aspects of health.

Conclusions: The results showed that some medical specialities are more affected by specific stressors. It is therefore discussed how improvements can be implemented. Furthermore, it is illustrated which stressors are especially relevant for health. These relationships to health should be investigated in further research and in longitudinal designs to allow hints of causal relationships.

Keywords: Work stressors, Physicians' everyday work, Comparison of medical specialities, Emotional exhaustion, Irritation

Background

There have been several scientific studies on the working conditions of hospital physicians [1-7]. The considered aspects include job satisfaction [1], work-life balance [2], multitasking and work interruptions [4,5]. Thereby, relationships to health have often been examined.

How specific working conditions can affect employees' health is described in the extension of the transactional stress model in work and organisational psychology [8]. Stress is seen as a process that arises by assessing and then mastering the situation (either problem- or emotion-focused). The starting points for this process are situation-related stressors (e.g., time pressure), person-related risk factors (e.g., illness), as well as situation-related resources (e.g., social support) and person-related resources (e.g., self-efficacy). Stressors are characteristics that increase the probability of stress-outcomes. Resources are characteristics that can be used to master demands [8]. Situation-related stressors and resources represent the work environment. Both influence the assessment and mastery of situations and – in unfavourable proportions – lead to stress-outcomes. Aside from the work environment, person-related factors influence this process and cause or prevent the stress-outcomes as well. On the other hand, stress-outcomes interact directly with the above mentioned starting points.

* Correspondence: grit.tanner@uni-hamburg.de
[1]University of Hamburg, Work and Organisational Psychology, Von-Melle-Park 11, 20146 Hamburg, Germany

In accordance with the transactional stress model of work and organisational psychology, studies have investigated specific situation-related stressors and resources within hospital physicians' work, as well as relationships to other health aspects. Longitudinal studies have found long-term effects on health aspects – particularly for resources. Especially, autonomy was shown to be related to depressive symptoms in long-term [9,10]. Several cross-sectional studies have investigated whether situation-related stressors, health aspects and their relationships differ with respect to other factors such as medical speciality. For example, one study has examined differences between emergency physicians and other physicians [11]. The results show that, for emergency physicians, poor collaboration with colleagues is more closely related to intention to quit and burnout than for other physicians. On the other hand, the relationship between worry about making errors and burnout was about the same in the two samples [11]. For work engagement and burnout in assistant physicians, one study showed that there were differences between the medical specialities [12]. A further study has also shown that there are differences between the different medical specialities with respect to the working time of hospital physicians in Germany [13].

These results illustrate that stressors may have different effects in different medical specialities. But there has not been any comparison of different specialities across various stressors that cover almost the whole physicians' working day. The current study aimed to bridge this gap by examining various situation-related stressors during the daily work of hospital physicians. These are compared for different specialities, so that any improvements could be developed specifically for the specialities. Moreover, relationships between stressors and stress-outcomes are examined. The current study primarily focuses only on stressors, as including other factors would increase the complexity to an excessive degree.

Methods

This project was entitled *Stress-Related Job Analysis for Hospital Physicians* (StArK) and was carried out by the Institute for Statutory Accident Insurance and Prevention in the Health and Welfare Services, University of Hamburg and University Medical Center Hamburg-Eppendorf, in order to examine hospital physicians' working conditions and their relationships to health.

Sample

Within the StArK project, hospital physicians throughout Germany were requested to evaluate their working conditions via questionnaire from February 2012 to December 2012. In addition, a link to the online survey was published in the newsletter of the official journal for German physicians (*Deutsches Ärzteblatt*). Thus, hospital physicians could take part in the survey independently of their hospitals. To ensure that the results were reliable, only medical specialities with more than ten participants were included.

Measures

The short version of the "Instrument for Stress-Related Job Analysis for Hospital Physicians" (ISAK-K) [14] was used to measure specific stressors of hospital physicians' work. This instrument includes seven different stressors. On the one hand, task-related stressors, such as time pressure and uncertainty (e.g., from insufficient information) as well as frustration about how work needs to be done were investigated. On the other hand, interaction-related stressors were considered, including problems in workflow due to physicians (supervisors and colleagues) and other professional groups (e.g., keeping to agreements, transmission of information), social stressors with patients and their families, and emotional dissonance (control of personal emotions). The stressors contain two to three items, which were rated on a 5-point Likert-scale.

Two aspects were selected to assess psychological health: Irritation [15] and emotional exhaustion [16]. Irritation describes work-related rumination after work. This includes additional effects on the state of mind (feeling of tension and irritability) [15]. Irritation represents a precursor to more serious psychological impairments. The eight items were answered on a 7-point Likert-scale, from 1 (*does not apply at all*) to 7 (*applies nearly completely*). Emotional exhaustion results in long-term from excessive efforts, both emotional and physical [17]. It is characterised by avolition and a feeling of weakness. One cause of emotional exhaustion may be that professional

Table 1 Sample characteristics

	Total sample (N = 817)	Study sample (n = 763)
Mean age	**41.0 (SD 9.8)**	**40.7 (SD 9.8)**
Gender		
Female	44.2%	43.0%
Male	55.8%	57.0%
Main medical specialities		
Internal medicine	21.8%	23.3%
Surgery	18.2%	19.5%
Anaesthesia	15.8%	16.9%
Professional position		
Assistant physician	39.7%	40.8%
Consulting physician	18.9%	18.3%
Senior physician	32.7%	32.5%
Chief physician	8.7%	8.4%

Table 2 One-way analyses of variance for the stressors by medical speciality

	Anaesthesia	Surgery	Obstetrics and gynaecology	Internal medicine	Paediatrics	Neurosurgery	Neurology	Orthopaedics	Psychiatry and psychotherapy	Radiology	Urology	F
	(n = 129)	(n = 149)	(n = 60)	(n = 178)	(n = 52)	(n = 20)	(n = 44)	(n = 46)	(n = 50)	(n = 23)	(n = 12)	
Time pressure	3.59	3.49	3.13[a]	3.76[a,b,c]	3.15[b]	3.85	3.74	3.45	3.14[c]	3.74	3.92	3.93***
Uncertainty[1]	3.32[d,e]	2.94[f]	2.53[d,g,h]	3.27[g]	2.68[e,i]	3.33	3.53[f,h,i]	3.00	2.83	3.09	3.04	4.71***
Frustration about how work needs to be done	2.78[j]	2.93[k]	2.80[l]	3.33[j,k,l]	2.78	2.93	3.35	3.05	2.96	2.58	3.28	3.85***
Problems in workflow due to supervisors and colleagues	2.45	2.29	2.43	2.47	2.09	2.38	2.19	2.47	2.28	2.52	2.58	1.47
Problems in workflow due to other professional groups	2.45	2.45	2.65	2.71	2.30	2.55	2.65	2.67	2.44	2.72	2.63	1.84
Social stressors with patients/ families	2.11[m, n, o, p, q]	2.54[m]	2.19[r,s,t]	2.85[n,r,u]	2.45	2.45	3.01[o,s,v]	2.75[p,w]	2.88[q,t,x]	1.89[u,v,w,x]	2.67	9.33***
Emotional dissonance[1]	2.52	2.41	2.33	2.54	2.15	2.43	2.48	2.75	2.97	2.28	2.71	1.96

N = 763. Post-hoc test: Bonferroni. [1]Because of the heterogeneous variance, tested with the Welch-test and Post-hoc test: Dunnett-T3.
Significant group differences are marked with the same high-ranking letters: [a]Internal medicine - Gynaecology ** ; [b]Internal medicine - Paediatrics * ; [c]Internal medicine - Psychiatry/Psychotherapy * ; [d]Anaesthesia - Gynaecology *** ; [e]Anaesthesia - Paediatrics * ; [f]Surgery - Neurology* ; [g]Gynaecology - Internal medicine*** ; [h]Gynaecology - Neurology *** ; [i]Paediatrics - Neurology ** ; [j]Internal medicine - Anaesthesia *** ; [k]Internal medicine - Surgery * ; [l]Internal medicine - Gynaecology * ; [m]Anaesthesia - Surgery** ; [n]Anaesthesia - Internal medicine*** ; [o]Anaesthesia - Neurology *** ; [p]Anaesthesia - Orthopaedics ** ; [q]Anaesthesia - Psychiatry/ Psychotherapy *** ; [r]Gynaecology - Internal medicine *** ; [s]Gynaecology - Neurology *** ; [t]Gynaecology - Psychiatry/Psychotherapy ** ; [u]Radiology - Internal medicine *** ; [v]Radiology - Neurology *** ; [w]Radiology - Orthopaedics * ; [x]Radiology - Psychiatry/Psychotherapy ***.
*$p < .05$; **$p < .01$; ***$p < .001$.

effort is not adequately rewarded (e.g., by appreciation) [18]. Emotional exhaustion was measured with six items [16], which were answered on a 7-point Likert-scale, from 1 (*never*) to 7 (*daily*). Furthermore, on the basis of other studies control variables were selected. These studies demonstrated effects related to the medical speciality [12,13], the professional position or age [10,19] and gender [10].

Statistical analyses

The comparison of medical specialities was conducted with one-way analyses of variance (ANOVA). The Bonferroni procedure (post-hoc test) was used to identify the groups with significant differences. If variance heterogeneity was confirmed, the Welch test was applied to examine the differences, followed by the Dunnett-T3 procedure for the post-hoc tests. The Bonferroni correction was used to counteract the accumulation of α-error [20]. Thus the significant ANOVA results presented here correspond to the corrected p-value.

Multiple hierarchical regression analyses were used to investigate the relationships between all stressors examined and each health aspect. In the first step, control variables were included, to ascertain whether, independently of these, there still is a relationship between the stressors and the health aspect. In the second step, all task-related stressors were included, followed by interaction-related stressors in the third step.

Results

In sum, data were collected from 817 German hospital physicians. The response rate of the acquisition via hospitals was 30.6% (705 hospital physicians). Additionally, with a response rate of 40.4% and a completion rate of 20.3%, 112 hospital physicians participated in the open online-survey. After excluding groups smaller than ten participants (e.g., ENT physicians, occupational physicians, ophthalmologists, and pathologists), 763 physicians were included in the analyses – split into eleven different medical specialities. Socio-demographic characteristics of the samples are presented in Table 1. Both samples are comparable with German physician statistics [21,22].

Comparison of specialities

Various differences were found between the medical specialities with respect to the examined stressors (see Table 2; for a schematic overview see Figures 1, 2, 3, and 4). *Time pressure* and the *frustration about how work needs to be done* were rated higher by physicians in internal medicine than by those in obstetrics and gynaecology or in paediatrics (see Figures 1 and 2). Surgeons reported lower levels of *frustration* than physicians in internal medicine. Psychiatrists and psychotherapists reported lower levels of *time pressure* than physicians in internal medicine. *Uncertainty* was rated lower by physicians in obstetrics and gynaecology than by physicians in internal medicine, anaesthesia and neurology (see Figure 3). Moreover, physicians in paediatrics rated *uncertainty* lower than physicians in anaesthesia and neurology. Neurologists rated *uncertainty* higher than did surgeons. Several significant differences were found with respect to *social stressors with patients and their families* (see Figure 4). Physicians in radiology, anaesthesia, and in obstetrics and gynaecology rated *social stressors* significantly lower than did physicians in internal medicine, neurology, and in psychiatry and psychotherapy. Physicians in orthopaedics and rehabilitation rated *social stressors* higher than did physicians in radiology and anaesthesia. Surgeons gave also higher rates for *social stressors* than did physicians in anaesthesia. On the other hand, for the stressors *problems in workflow due to physicians and other professional*

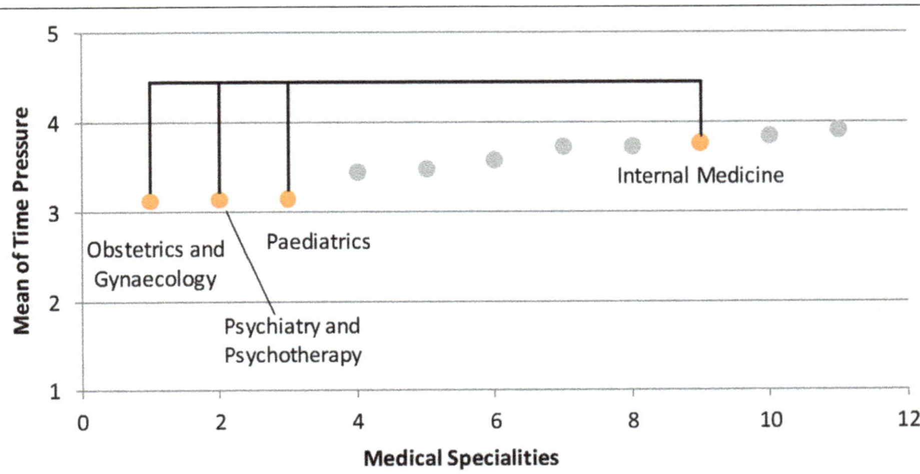

Figure 1 Differences between internal medicine and other specialities in time pressure. This is only a schematic figure of the differences found in time pressure. For detailed results use Table 2.

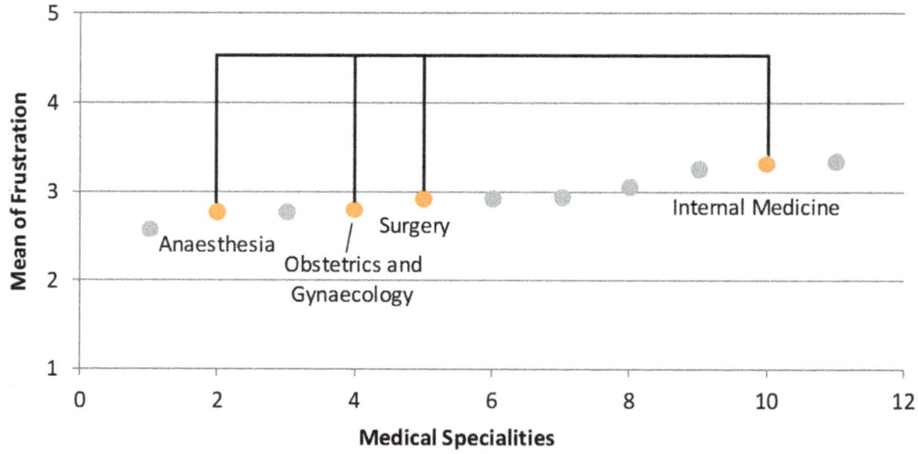

Figure 2 Differences between internal medicine and other specialities in frustration. This is only a schematic figure of the differences found in frustration about how work needs to be done. For detailed results use Table 2.

groups and *emotional dissonance*, there were no significant differences between the ratings in the medical specialities.

Relationships between Stressors and Health

As can be seen in Table 3, all stressors – as well as the control variables age, gender, and professional position – showed significant correlations with the health aspects irritation and emotional exhaustion. There was no significant correlation between the medical speciality and the two health aspects. In the multiple regression analyses with control for age, gender, professional position and medical speciality, results were different. Of the task-related stressors, *time pressure* and *frustration about how work needs to be done* showed significant relationships to both irritation and emotional exhaustion. Of the interaction-related stressors, only *emotional dissonance* showed a significant relationship to both stress-outcomes. In addition, *problems in workflow due to other professional groups* were significantly related to emotional exhaustion. Moreover, beyond task-related stressors, interaction-related stressors explained 5 to 7% of additional variance in the stress-outcomes.

Discussion

Especially physicians in internal medicine rated stressors more highly than do physicians in other specialities. Assuming that specific stressors (e.g., stressors with patients, lack of information) are negatively related to work engagement [23,24], these results support the findings of a study with Dutch assistant physicians [12]. In this study, physicians in internal medicine showed less work engagement than colleagues in other specialities, combined with high emotional exhaustion [12]. However, the latter finding was not confirmed in the current study, as no relationship between medical speciality and emotional exhaustion was found. The differences with respect to the social stressors

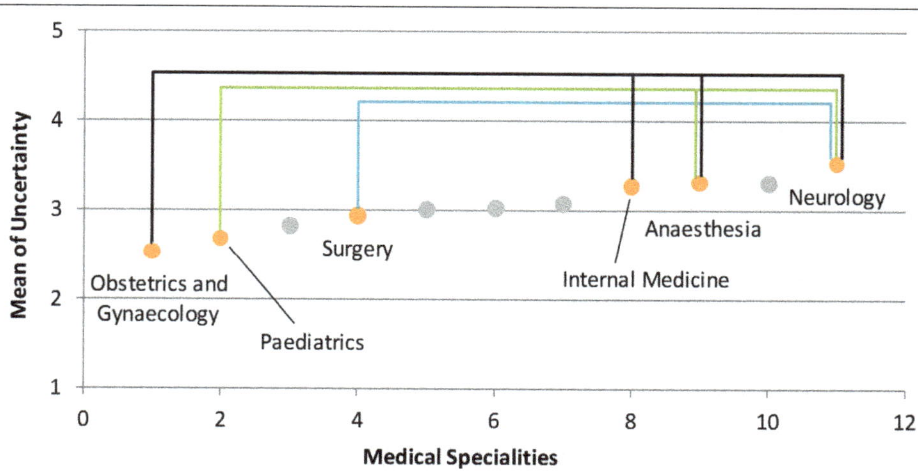

Figure 3 Differences between gynaecology, paediatrics, or surgery and other specialities in uncertainty. This is only a schematic figure of the differences found in uncertainty. For detailed results use Table 2.

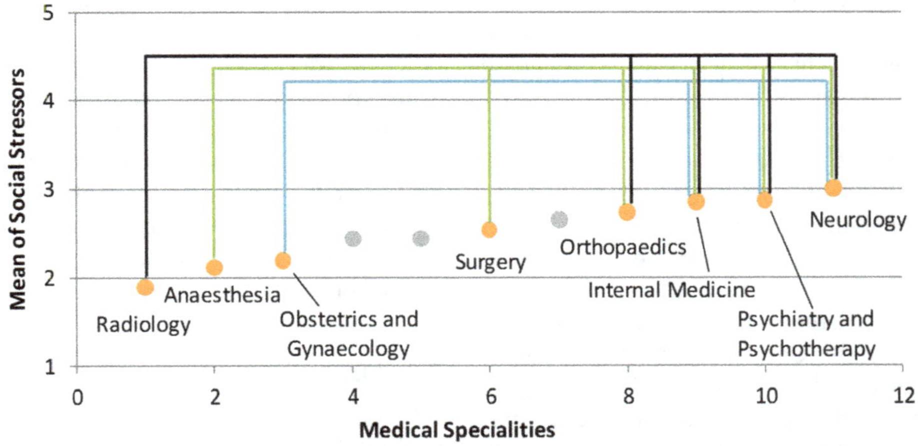

Figure 4 Differences between radiology, anaesthesia, or gynaecology and other specialities in social stressors with patients/families. This is only a schematic figure of the differences found in social stressors with patients/families. For detailed results use Table 2.

with patients and their families were predictable, if the differences in patient contact were considered for the different specialities. Specialities such as neurology, psychiatry and psychotherapy, and internal medicine inherently involve more communication with patients (e.g., for diagnosis) than in radiology or anaesthesia. Regarding uncertainty (e.g., consequences that are difficult to predict) and social stressors with patients, neurologists not only showed significant differences, but gave the highest ratings compared to the other specialities. As these stressors are presumably related to the medical problems in this speciality, it would be useful to investigate the role of resources (both, situation- and person-related) on stress-outcomes.

The results of the multiple regression analyses show that time pressure, frustration about how work needs to be done and emotional dissonance are related to different stress-outcomes. A prior study has already shown that time pressure is associated with a high feeling of stress in physicians [1]. The current results support this feeling perceived by physicians. The frustration about how work needs to be done means restrictions due to documentation and administration work. At least for surgeons and internal physicians, these tasks take up about

Table 3 Hierarchical multiple regression analyses explaining irritation and emotional exhaustion

	DV: irritation			DV: emotional exhaustion		
	r	β	ΔR^2	r	β	ΔR^2
Step 1: Control variables			.02**			.05***
Medical speciality	-.03	-.07*		.05	.00	
Professional position	-.12**	-.02		-.02***	-.15***	
Age	-.13***	-.04		-.18***	.01	
Gender	.11**	.12***		.10**	.07*	
Step 2: Task-related stressors			.21***			.32***
Time pressure	.37***	.16***		.48***	.28***	
Uncertainty	.36***	.05		41***	.02	
Frustration about how work needs to be done	.40***	.12***		.52***	.19***	
Step 3: Interaction-related stressors			.07***			.05***
Problems in workflow due to supervisors and colleagues	.27***	.08		.28***	.02	
Problems in workflow due to other professional groups	.28***	.03		.35***	.11**	
Social stressors with patients/families	.31***	.04		.36***	.03	
Emotional dissonance	.44***	.26***		.45***	.19***	

DV = dependent variable; r = Pearson correlation coefficient; β = standardised regression coefficient; ΔR^2 = changes in coefficient of determination R^2 to estimate source of variance. Numerical coding for control variables: medical speciality: 1 = Anaesthesia (sorted alphabetically) to 11 = Urology; Professional position: 1 = assistant physician (sorted in rising order), up to 4 = chief physician; gender: 1 = male, 2 = female.
*p < .05; **p < .01; ***p < .001.

one third of daily working hours [5]. This illustrates once again how important the relationship between frustration and stress-outcomes is. Thus, it seems to be useful to reduce high levels of frustration.

Strengths and limitations

As the sample was relatively large, it was possible to compare eleven different specialities. However, a selection bias cannot be excluded. For example, it is possible that unusually stressed physicians took part in this survey. Despite that, the current sample corresponds to the physician statistics of the German Medical Association [21] and the German Federal Bureau of Statistics [22], with respect to age, gender and medical specialities. Another advantage of this study is that it considers two potential stress-outcomes. Nevertheless, the relationships between stressors and health aspects should be interpreted with caution. Because of the cross-sectional design, no causal interpretations are possible. Hints for causal conclusions can only be drawn from longitudinal studies or studies with experimental designs [25]. Moreover, it should be emphasised that several situation-related stressors were considered in the current study, which represent a large part of the hospital physician's everyday work. Although the current analyses focused only on stressors, a further emphasis on resources should be considered because work-related resources are found to be relevant to health as well [26], as mentioned in the transactional stress model of work and organizational psychology.

Practical implications

Various approaches will be discussed to reduce the stressors of hospital physicians during their daily work. One way to handle social stressors with patients and their families can be found in reflecting these situations. Corresponding to Wilson [27], this could be realised by journaling, critical incident analysis, mentoring, and/or supervision. To reduce the frustration about how work needs to be done, it may be advantageous to introduce personalised training of key qualifications for handling administrative work. At the organisational level, it would be useful to improve staff planning and to reduce documentation and administrative work. One alternative could be to examine ways to facilitate the documentation and administrative tasks (e.g., easily manageable technical tools or more autonomy) and then to implement these. By reducing frustration about how work needs to be done, one could also reduce time pressure, as these two characteristics are closely correlated ($r = .51$, $p < .001$). The positive relationship between emotional dissonance (the suppression or control of the emotions) and emotional exhaustion has already been demonstrated for other professions, and high autonomy was shown to compensate the effects of high emotional dissonance [28]. For emotional exhaustion, problems in workflow due to other professional groups seem to be a relevant predictor. In order to reduce these problems, it seems to be useful to clarify the causes. There might be organisational reasons that agreements cannot be kept. But difficulties might also be caused by social conflicts, which have been found to be a frequent problem for assistant physicians [1]. In order to identify causes, interdisciplinary and cross-hierarchical working groups could be an adequate method [29] (e.g., focused on workflows and communication issues).

Conclusions

The results of the current study demonstrated that hospital physicians experience certain work stressors differently with respect to their medical speciality. Therefore, stress prevention programs should consider these differences. Additionally, the meaning of time pressure, frustration about how work needs to be done, and emotional dissonance for aspects of health was illustrated. Aside longitudinal studies are needed in order to verify these cross-sectional findings; these results suggest some approaches for health promoting improvements.

Competing interests

The authors declare that they have no competing interests.

Authors' contributions

GT made substantial contributions to conception and design of the study, to the acquisition of data, and to the analysis and interpretation of data; she was involved in drafting the manuscript as well as revising it critically. EB made substantial contributions to conception and design of the study; she was involved in drafting the manuscript as well as revising it critically. AK was involved in the acquisition of data, in the interpretation of the data, and in drafting the manuscript as well as revising it critically. MK was involved in conception and design of the study, in the acquisition of data, and in drafting the manuscript as well as revising it critically. AN was involved in conception and design of the study, and in drafting the manuscript as well as revising it critically. All authors read and approved the final manuscript.

Acknowledgements

This study was financed by the Institution for Statutory Accident Insurance and Prevention in the Health and Welfare Services.

Author details

University of Hamburg, Work and Organisational Psychology, Von-Melle-Park 11, 20146 Hamburg, Germany. [2]University Medical Center Hamburg-Eppendorf, Institute for Health Services Research in Dermatology and Nursing (IVDP), Martinistraße 52, 20246 Hamburg, Germany. [3]Institute for Statutory Accident Insurance and Prevention in the Health and Welfare Services (BGW), Principles of Prevention and Rehabilitation Department (GPR), Pappelallee 33/35/37, 22089 Hamburg, Germany.

References

1. Cohen JS, Patten S. Well-being in residency training: a survey examining resident physician satisfaction both within and outside of residency training and mental health in Alberta. BMC Med Educ. 2005;5:21–31.
2. Fuß I, Nübling M, Hasselhorn H-M, Schwappach D, Rieger MA. Working conditions and work-family conflict in German hospital physicians: psychosocial and organisational predictors and consequences. BMC Public Health. 2008;8:353–69.

3. Glaser J, Höge T. Spezifische Anforderungen und Belastungen personenbezogener Krankenhausarbeit. In: Badura B, Schellschmidt H, Vetter C, editors. Fehlzeitenreport 2004 Gesundheitsmanagement Krankenhäusern und Pflegeeinrichtungen. Berlin: Springer; 2004. p. 51–64.
4. Weigl M, Müller A, Vincent C, Angerer P, Sevdalis N. The association of workflow interruptions and hospital doctors' workload: a prospective observational study. BMJ Qual Saf. 2012;21:399–407.
5. Weigl M, Müller A, Zupanc A, Angerer P. Participant observation of time allocation, direct patient contact and simultaneous activities in hospital physicians. BMC Health Serv Res. 2009;9:110–21.
6. Buddeberg-Fischer B, Klaghofer R, Stamm M, Siegrist J, Buddeberg C. Work stress and reduced health in young physicians: prospective evidence from Swiss residents. Int Arch Occup Environ Health. 2008;82:31–8.
7. Unrath M, Zeeb H, Letzel S, Claus M, Escobar Pinzón LC. The mental health of primary care physicians in Rhineland-Palatinate, Germany: the prevalence of problems and identification of possible risk factors. Dtsch Arztebl Int. 2012;109:201–7.
8. Bamberg E, Keller M, Wohlert C, Zeh A. BGW-Stresskonzept. Hamburg: Berufsgenossenschaft für Gesundheitsdienst und Wohlfahrtspflege (BGW); 2006. p. 1–28.
9. Weigl M, Hornung S, Petru R, Glaser J, Angerer P. Depressive symptoms in junior doctors: a follow-up study on work-related determinants. Int Arch Occup Environ Health. 2012;85:559–70.
10. Buddeberg-Fischer B, Klaghofer R, Buddeberg C. Arbeitsstress und gesundheitliches Wohlbefinden junger Ärztinnen und Ärzte. Z Psychosom Med Psychother. 2005;51:163–78.
11. Estryn-Behar M, Doppia M-A, Guetarni K, Fry C, Machet G, Pelloux P, et al. Emergency physicians accumulate more stress factors than other physicians - Results from the French SESMAT study. Emerg Med J. 2011;28:397–410.
12. Prins JT, Hoekstra-Weebers JEHM, Gazendam-Donofrio SM, Dillingh GS, Bakker AB, Huisman M, et al. Burnout and engagement among resident doctors in the Netherlands: a national study. Med Educ. 2010;44:236–47.
13. Rosta J. Arbeitszeit der Krankenhausärzte in Deutschland. Dtsch Arztebl. 2007;104:2417–24.
14. Keller M, Bamberg E, Kersten M, Nienhaus A. Instrument for stress-related job analysis for hospital physicians: validation of a short version. J Occup Med Toxicol. 2013;8:10–20.
15. Mohr G, Rigotti T, Müller A. Irritation - ein Instrument zur Erfassung psychischer Beanspruchung im Arbeitskontext. Skalen- und Itemparameter aus 15 Studien. Zeitschrift für Arbeits- und Organ. 2005;49:44–8.
16. Enzmann D, Kleiber D. Helfer-Leiden: Streß Und Burnout in Psychosozialen Berufen. Heidelberg: Asanger; 1989.
17. Maslach C, Schaufeli WB, Leiter MP. Job burnout. Annu Rev Psychol. 2001;52:397–422.
18. Siegrist J. Adverse health effects of high-effort/low-reward conditions. J Occup Health Psychol. 1996;1:27–41.
19. Heinke W, Dunkel P, Brähler E, Nübling M, Riedel-Heller S, Kaisers UX. Burn-out in der Anästhesie und Intensivmedizin. Der Anästhesist. 2011;12:1109–18.
20. Victor A, Elsäßer A, Hommel G, Blettner M. Judging a plethora of p-values. Dtsch Arztebl Int. 2010;107:50–6.
21. Ärztestatistik 2012. [http://www.bundesaerztekammer.de/page.asp?his=0.3.11372].
22. Statistisches Bundesamt - Tabellen: Beschäftigte im Gesundheitswesen (Code 23621) [https://www-genesis.destatis.de/genesis/online/data].
23. Jenaro C, Flores N, Orgaz MB, Cruz M. Vigour and dedication in nursing professionals: towards a better understanding of work engagement. J Adv Nurs. 2011;67:865–75.
24. Sonnentag S, Mojza EJ, Demerouti E, Bakker AB. Reciprocal relations between recovery and work engagement: the moderating role of job stressors. J Appl Psychol. 2012;97:842–53.
25. Angerer P, Petru R, Nowak D, Weigl M. Arbeitsbedingungen und Depression bei Ärzten. Dtsch Medizinische Wochenschrift. 2008;133:26–9.
26. Richter A, Kostova P, Harth V, Wegner R. Children, care, career - a cross-sectional study on the risk of burnout among German hospital physicians at different career stages. J Occup Med Toxicol. 2014;9:1–9.
27. Wilson H. Reflecting on the "difficult" patient. N Z Med J. 2005;118:1–6.
28. Grandey AA, Fisk GM, Steiner DD. Must "service with a smile" be stressful? The moderating role of personal control for American and French employees. J Appl Psychol. 2005;90:893–904.
29. Münch E. Health promotion in hospitals - evaluation of health circles as a means of health promotion in workplaces and organization. J Public Health. 1996;4:318–34.

Permissions

All chapters in this book were first published in JOMT, by BioMed Central; hereby published with permission under the Creative Commons Attribution License or equivalent. Every chapter published in this book has been scrutinized by our experts. Their significance has been extensively debated. The topics covered herein carry significant findings which will fuel the growth of the discipline. They may even be implemented as practical applications or may be referred to as a beginning point for another development.

The contributors of this book come from diverse backgrounds, making this book a truly international effort. This book will bring forth new frontiers with its revolutionizing research information and detailed analysis of the nascent developments around the world.

We would like to thank all the contributing authors for lending their expertise to make the book truly unique. They have played a crucial role in the development of this book. Without their invaluable contributions this book wouldn't have been possible. They have made vital efforts to compile up to date information on the varied aspects of this subject to make this book a valuable addition to the collection of many professionals and students.

This book was conceptualized with the vision of imparting up-to-date information and advanced data in this field. To ensure the same, a matchless editorial board was set up. Every individual on the board went through rigorous rounds of assessment to prove their worth. After which they invested a large part of their time researching and compiling the most relevant data for our readers.

The editorial board has been involved in producing this book since its inception. They have spent rigorous hours researching and exploring the diverse topics which have resulted in the successful publishing of this book. They have passed on their knowledge of decades through this book. To expedite this challenging task, the publisher supported the team at every step. A small team of assistant editors was also appointed to further simplify the editing procedure and attain best results for the readers.

Apart from the editorial board, the designing team has also invested a significant amount of their time in understanding the subject and creating the most relevant covers. They scrutinized every image to scout for the most suitable representation of the subject and create an appropriate cover for the book.

The publishing team has been an ardent support to the editorial, designing and production team. Their endless efforts to recruit the best for this project, has resulted in the accomplishment of this book. They are a veteran in the field of academics and their pool of knowledge is as vast as their experience in printing. Their expertise and guidance has proved useful at every step. Their uncompromising quality standards have made this book an exceptional effort. Their encouragement from time to time has been an inspiration for everyone.

The publisher and the editorial board hope that this book will prove to be a valuable piece of knowledge for researchers, students, practitioners and scholars across the globe.

List of Contributors

Daniel Haile Chercos and Demeke Berhanu
Department of Environmental and Occupational Health and Safety, Institute of Public Health, University of Gondar, Gondar, Ethiopia

Tim Friede
Department of Medical Statistics, University Medical Center Göttingen, Humboldtallee 32, 37073 Göttingen, Germany

Tobias I Ndubuisi Ezejiofor, Hariet C Nwigwe, Ferdinand OU Osuala and Moses OE Iwuala
Department of Biological Science, School of Science, Federal University of Technology, Owerri, Nigeria

Anthonet N Ezejiofor and Orish E Orisakwe
Department of Clinical Pharmacy, Toxicology Unit, University of Port Harcourt, Port Harcourt, Nigeria

Ernst Hallier and Sebastian Straube
Institute of Occupational, Social and Environmental Medicine, University Medical Center Göttingen, Waldweg 37 B, 37073 Göttingen, Germany

Tolesa Bekele, Muhammedawel Kaso and Kemal Ahmed
Department of Public Health, College of Medicine and Health Sciences, Madda Walabu University, Oromia, Ethiopia

Alem Gebremariam
Department of Public Health, College of Medicine and Health Sciences, Adigrat University, Adigrat, Tigray, Ethiopia

Alexander Gerber, Alexander V Hofen-Hohloch, Johannes Schulze and David A Groneberg
Institute of Occupational, Social and Environmental Medicine, Goethe-University, Theodor-Stern-Kai 7, Haus 9b, 60590 Frankfurt am Main, Germany

Xaver Baur
European Society for Environmental and Occupational Medicine (EOM), Berlin, Germany
Institute for Occupational Medicine, Charité University Medicine, Charité-Campus Benjamin Franklin, Berlin, Germany

Lygia Therese Budnik
European Society for Environmental and Occupational Medicine (EOM), Berlin, Germany
Institute for Occupational and Maritime (ZfAM), University Medical Center Hamburg-Eppendorf, Division Occupational Toxicology and Immunology, University of Hamburg, Hamburg, Germany

Jorgen R Jepsen
European Society for Environmental and Occupational Medicine (EOM), Berlin, Germany
Centre of Maritime Health and Society, Institute of Public Health, University of Southern Denmark, Odense, Denmark

Magne Bratveit
European Society for Environmental and Occupational Medicine (EOM), Berlin, Germany
Department of Occupational Medicine, Haukeland University Hospital, Bergen, Norway
Occupational and Environmental Medicine, University of Bergen, Bergen, Norway
Department of Global Public Health and Primary Care, Occupational and Environmental Medicine, University of Bergen, Bergen, Norway

Zhiwei Zhao
Dalian Maritime University (DMU), Dalian, Ganjingzi, China

Rune Djurhuus
Norwegian Center for Maritime Medicine, Department of Occupational Medicine, Haukeland University Hospital, Bergen, Norway

Louis Verschoor
Expertise Centre Environmental Medicine (ECEMed), Rijnstate Teaching Hospital, AA Velp, the Netherlands

Federico Maria Rubino and Claudio Colosio
Department of Health Sciences of the University of Milano and International Centre of Rural Health, San Paolo University Hospital Milano, Milan, Italy

Rasa Šidagytė and Dovilė Šorytė
Occupational Health Centre, Institute of Hygiene, Didžioji str. 22, Vilnius, Lithuana

Sigita Vičaitė
Occupational Health Centre, Institute of Hygiene, Didžioji str. 22, Vilnius, Lithuana
Positive Health Team, Šviesos str. 4B-7, Vilnius, Lithuania

Maija Eglīte
Department of Occupational and Environmental Medicine, Riga Stradins University, Dzirciema str. 16, Riga, Latvia

Anne Salmi
Finnish Institute of Occupational Health, Aapistie 1, Oulu, Finland

Ivars Vanadziņš, Lāsma Kozlova and Svetlana Lakiša
Institute of Occupational Safety and Environmental Health of Riga Stradins University, Dzirciema str. 16, Riga, Latvia

Leila Hopsu and Jaana Lerssi-Uskelin
Finnish Institute of Occupational Health, Topeliuksenkatu 41 a A, Helsinki, Finland

Laima Bulotaitė
Department of General Psychology, Faculty of Philosophy, Vilnius University, Universiteto str. 9/1, Vilnius, Lithuania

C. Nattrass and C. J. Horwell
Institute of Hazard, Risk & Resilience, Department of Earth Sciences, Durham University, Durham DH1 3LE, UK

D. E. Damby
Department of Earth and Environmental Sciences, Ludwig-Maximilians-Universität München, Munich 80333, Germany

D. M. Brown and V. Stone
School of Life Sciences, Heriot-Watt University, Edinburgh EH14 4AS, UK

A. Kermanizadeh
School of Life Sciences, Heriot-Watt University, Edinburgh EH14 4AS, UK
Department of Public Health, Section of Occupational and Environmental Health, University of Copenhagen, Copenhagen DK-1014, Denmark

Sanja Terzic
Occupational Health Department, General Health Center "Savski Venac", Pasterova 1, Belgrade, Serbia

Boban Rakic
Institute of Occupational Medicine and Radiological Protection, Deligradska 29, Belgrade, Serbia

Aleksandar Milovanovic
Institute of Occupational Medicine and Radiological Protection, Deligradska 29, Belgrade, Serbia
School of Medicine, University of Belgrade, Dr Subotica 8, Belgrade, Serbia

Jelena Dotlic and Milan Terzic
School of Medicine, University of Belgrade, Dr Subotica 8, Belgrade, Serbia
Clinic of Obstetrics and Gynecology, Clinical Center of Serbia, Dr Koste Todorovica 26, Belgrade, Serbia

Stefanie Mache
Institute for Occupational Medicine and Maritime Medicine (ZfAM), University Medical Center Hamburg-Eppendorf, Seewartenstrasse 10, 20459 Hamburg, Germany

Stefan Linnig and Geraldine Preuß
Institute of Occupational Medicine, Charité – Universitätsmedizin Berlin, Free University and Humboldt University, Thielallee 69-73, 14195 Berlin, Germany

Sarah Jensen
Bremen International Graduate School of Social Sciences, Wiener Straße/Ecke Celsiusstraße, 28359 Bremen, Germany

Reimo Jahn
Institute of Technology & Innovation Management, Helmut Schmidt University, Hamburg, Holstenhofweg 85, 22043 Hamburg, Germany

Mirco Steudtner and Elke Ochsmann
Institute of Health Care Management, University of Applied Sciences Zwickau, Dr.-Friedrichs-Ring 2a, 08056 Zwickau, Germany

Mitrakrishnan R. Navinan, A C A Pathirana, H R I S Herath, Jevon Yudhishdran, Nilesh Fernandopulle and Aruna Kulatunga
National Hospital of Sri Lanka, Colombo 10, Sri Lanka

Isurujith K. Liyanage
National Hospital of Sri Lanka, Colombo 10, Sri Lanka
Department of Pharmacology, Faculty of Medical Sciences, University of Sri Jayewardenepura, Nugegoda, Sri Lanka

Henry Aidoo and Phyllis Aidoo
125 Row House, Michener Park, Edmonton, AB T6H, 4M4, Canada

Akye Essuman
Family Medicine Unit, Department of Community Health, School of Public Health, College of Health Sciences, University of Ghana, Korle-Bu, Accra, Ghana

Anita O. Yawson
Department of Anaesthesia, Korle-Bu Teaching Hospital, Korle-Bu, Accra, Ghana

Alfred E. Yawson
Department of Community Health, School of Public Health, College of Health Sciences, University of Ghana, Room 46, Korle-Bu, Accra, Ghana

Madeleine Dulon and Björn Kähler
Department of Occupational Health Research, German Social Accident Insurance Institution for the Health and Welfare Services, Pappelallee 33/35/ 37, 22089 Hamburg, Germany

Sandra Kirvel and Günter Schlanstedt
Society for Research and Consulting in the Health and Welfare Sector, Prälat-Otto-Müller-Platz 2, 50670 Cologne, Germany

Arno Villringer
Max-Planck-Institute for Human Cognitive and Brain Sciences, Leipzig, and Clinic for Cognitive Neurology, University Hospital Leipzig, Leipzig, Germany

Susel Rosário
Faculty of Engineering of the University of Porto, Porto, Portugal

João A. Fonseca
Faculty of Engineering of the University of Porto, Porto, Portugal
CINTESIS - Centre for Research in Health Technologies and Information Systems and Information and Decision Sciences Department, Faculty of Medicine, University of Porto, Porto, Portugal
Allergy Unit, CUF Porto Institute & Hospital, Porto, Portugal

Albert Nienhaus
Faculty of Engineering of the University of Porto, Porto, Portugal
Institute for Health Service Research in Dermatology and Nursing (IVDP), Center of Excellence for Epidemiology and Health Service Research for Healthcare Professionals (CVcare), University Medical Center Hamburg-Eppendorf, Martinistraße 52, Hamburg 20246, Germany
Principles of Prevention and Rehabilitation Department (GPR), Institute for Statutory Accident Insurance and Prevention in the Health and Welfare Services (BGW), Hamburg, Germany

José Torres da Costa
Faculty of Engineering of the University of Porto, Porto, Portugal
Faculty of Medicine of the University of Porto, Porto, Portugal

Stéphane Du Mortier, Silas Mukangu, Charles Sagna, Laurent Nyffenegger and Sigiriya Aebischer Perone
International Committee of the Red Cross, Geneva, Switzerland

Claudia Westermann
University Medical Center Hamburg-Eppendorf (UKE), Center of Excellence for Health Services Research in Nursing (CVcare), Hamburg, Germany

Ingmar Wolf
Department of Medical Statistics, University Medical Center Göttingen, Humboldtallee 32, 37073 Göttingen, Germany
Institute of Occupational, Social and Environmental Medicine, University Medical Center Göttingen, Waldweg 37 B, 37073 Göttingen, Germany

Madeleine Dulon and Dana Wendeler
Institution for Statutory Accident Insurance and Prevention in the Health and Welfare Services (BGW), Department of Prevention and Rehabilitation Principles (GPR), Hamburg, Germany

J. Knierer, E. N. Gallegos Morales, A. Schablon and J. F. Kersten
University Medical Center Hamburg-Eppendorf (UKE), Center of Excellence for Health Services Research in Nursing (CVcare), Hamburg, Germany

A. Nienhaus
University Medical Center Hamburg-Eppendorf (UKE), Center of Excellence for Health Services Research in Nursing (CVcare), Hamburg, Germany
Institute for Statutory Accident Insurance and Prevention in the Health and Welfare Services (BGW), Principles of Prevention and Rehabilitation Department (GPR), Hamburg, Germany

B. Loddé, R. Pougnet and JD. Dewitte
Université Européenne de Bretagne, Rennes, France
Université de Brest, EA 4686 - CS 93837 - 29238, Brest Cedex 3, France
Service de Santé au Travail et Maladies liées à l'environnement, CHRU Morvan, 2 avenue FOCH, Brest Cedex 29609, France
Société Française de Médecine Maritime, 22, Avenue Camille Desmoulins, Brest 29200, France

P. Cros and A. M. Roguedas-Contios
Service de dermato-vénéréologie CHRU Morvan, 2 avenue FOCH, Brest Cedex 29609, France

L. Misery
Service de dermato-vénéréologie CHRU Morvan, 2 avenue FOCH, Brest Cedex 29609, France
Société Française de Médecine Maritime, 22, Avenue Camille Desmoulins, Brest 29200, France

D. Lucas
Société Française de Médecine Maritime, 22, Avenue Camille Desmoulins, Brest 29200, France

Joachim Thiery
Institute of Laboratory Medicine, Clinical Chemistry and Molecular Diagnostics (ILM), University of Leipzig, Leipzig, Germany

Nathan Hutting, Josephine A. Engels and Yvonne F. Heerkens
Faculty of Health and Social Studies, Research Group Occupation & Health, HAN University of Applied Sciences, 6503 GL Nijmegen, Netherlands

Wiebke Oswald
Faculty of Health and Social Studies, Research Group Occupation & Health, HAN University of Applied Sciences, Therapy, HAN
University of Applied Sciences, Nijmegen, Netherlands

J. Bart Staal
Faculty of Health and Social Studies, Research Group Musculoskeletal Rehabilitation, HAN University of Applied Sciences, Nijmegen, Netherlands
Radboud Institute for Health Sciences, IQ Healthcare, Radboud University Medical Center, Nijmegen, Netherlands

Maria W. G. Nijhuis-van der Sanden
Radboud Institute for Health Sciences, IQ Healthcare, Radboud University Medical Center, Nijmegen, Netherlands

Hamideh Ghorbani and Arya Hedjazi
Legal Medicine Research Center, Legal Medicine Organization, Tehran, Iran

Mahnaz Ahmadimanesh
Legal Medicine Research Center, Legal Medicine Organization, Tehran, Iran
Department of Pharmacodynamics & Toxicology, Mashhad University of Medical Science, School of Pharmacy, Mashhad, Iran

Alireza Nezami
Department of Pharmacodynamics & Toxicology, Mashhad University of Medical Science, School of Pharmacy, Mashhad, Iran

Behjat Sheikholeslami
Faculty of Pharmacy, Lorestan University of Medical Sciences, Khorramabad, Iran

Daniel Sowah, Flora Balat and Sebastian Straube
Division of Preventive Medicine, Department of Medicine, University of Alberta, 5-30 University Terrace, 8303-112 Street, Edmonton, AB T6G 2T4, Canada

Daniela Ohlendorf, Jennifer Marx, Eileen M. Wanke, David A. Groneberg and Stefanie Uibel
Institute of Occupational Medicine, Social Medicine and Environmental Medicine, Goethe-University Frankfurt/Main, Theodor-Stern-Kai 7, Building 9A, 60590 Frankfurt/Main, Germany

Kathrin Clasen and Stefan Kopp
School of Dentistry, Department of Orthodontics, Goethe University Frankfurt/Main, Theodor-Stern-Kai 7, Building 9A, 60590 Frankfurt am Main, Germany

Melanie Luppa and Steffi G Riedel-Heller
Institute of Social Medicine, Occupational Health and Public Health (ISAP), Medical Faculty, University of Leipzig, Philipp-Rosenthal-Str. 55, 04103 Leipzig, Germany

Francisca S Then and Tobias Luck
Institute of Social Medicine, Occupational Health and Public Health (ISAP), Medical Faculty, University of Leipzig, Philipp-Rosenthal-Str. 55, 04103 Leipzig, Germany
LIFE - Leipzig Research Center for Civilization Diseases, University of Leipzig, Leipzig, Germany

Katrin Arélin and Matthias L Schroeter
LIFE - Leipzig Research Center for Civilization Diseases, University of Leipzig, Leipzig, Germany
Max-Planck-Institute for Human Cognitive and Brain Sciences, Leipzig, and Clinic for Cognitive Neurology, University Hospital Leipzig, Leipzig, Germany

Christoph Engel and Markus Löffler
LIFE - Leipzig Research Center for Civilization Diseases, University of Leipzig, Leipzig, Germany
Institute for Medical Informatics, Statistics and Epidemiology (IMISE), University of Leipzig, Leipzig, Germany

Grit Tanner and Eva Bamberg
University of Hamburg, Work and Organisational Psychology, Von-Melle-Park 11, 20146 Hamburg, Germany

Agnessa Kozak
University Medical Center Hamburg-Eppendorf, Institute for Health Services Research in Dermatology and Nursing (IVDP), Martinistraße 52, 20246 Hamburg, Germany

Albert Nienhaus
University Medical Center Hamburg-Eppendorf, Institute for Health Services Research in Dermatology and Nursing (IVDP), Martinistraße 52, 20246 Hamburg, Germany
Institute for Statutory Accident Insurance and Prevention in the Health and Welfare Services (BGW), Principles of Prevention and Rehabilitation Department (GPR), Pappelallee 33/35/37, 22089 Hamburg, Germany

Maren Kersten
Institute for Statutory Accident Insurance and Prevention in the Health and Welfare Services (BGW), Principles of Prevention and Rehabilitation Department (GPR), Pappelallee 33/35/37, 22089 Hamburg, Germany

Index

www.ingramcontent.com/pod-product-compliance
Lightning Source LLC
LaVergne TN
LVHW080738210926
848485LV00003B/576
* 9 7 8 1 6 3 9 2 7 4 4 7 5 *